SYMPTOMS OF PARKINSON'S DISEASE

Edited by **Abdul Qayyum Rana**

Symptoms of Parkinson's Disease
Edited by Abdul Qayyum Rana

Published by InTech
Janeza Trdine 9, 51000 Rijeka, Croatia

Publishing Process Manager Silvia Vlase

Technical Editor Teodora Smiljanic

Cover Designer InTech Design Team

Additional hard copies can be obtained from orders@intechopen.com

Symptoms of Parkinson's Disease, Edited by Abdul Qayyum Rana
p. cm.
978-953-307-464-1

For EU product safety concerns:
IN TECH d.o.o., Prolaz Marije Krucifikse Kozulić 3, 51000 Rijeka, Croatia,
info@intechopen.com or visit our website at intechopen.com.

Meet the editor

Dr. Abdul Qayyum Rana is a Canadian neurologist who specializes in the field of Parkinson's disease and Movement Disorders. He is a fellow of the Royal College of Physicians and Surgeons of Canada. After completing his neurology residency training, Dr. Rana undertook a clinical fellowship in Parkinson's disease and Movement Disorders at the University of Ottawa, Canada. He is currently the director of the Parkinson's Clinic of Eastern Toronto and Movement Disorders Centre located in Toronto, Canada. He is also founder of World Parkinson's Education Program. He is the author of "Frequently Asked Questions About Parkinson's Disease", which is a series of thirteen brochures about Parkinson's disease, translated in many languages and used in several countries around the world. Dr. Rana has also written the following books: "A Synopsis of Neurological Emergencies", "An Aid to Neuro-ophthalmology", "An introduction to Essential Tremor", "50 Ways Parkinson's Could Affect You", and "What is Parkinson's disease in Arabic?".

Contents

Preface

Parkinson's disease affects many different systems of human body and has both motor as well as non-motor symptoms. As the disease advances, both motor and non-motor symptoms progress and result in significant disability. Indeed with progression of time non-motor symptoms may become major cause of disease caregiver's burden and morbidity. This book discusses in detail the various symptoms of Parkinson's disease. Postural and gait problems have been discussed at length as they are the main cause of balance problems. Among the non-motor symptoms cognitive dysfunction which is one of the important causes of long term care placement has also been reviewed in detail. A review of gastrointestinal symptoms which affect almost 90% of patient population has been given as well. A focused discussion of mechanisms involving the psychiatric and mood disturbances which have a negative impact on the quality of life of patients has also been provided. In addition to these symptoms, a synopsis of other non-motor symptoms has also been given so that reader can have familiarity with the diversity of non-motor symptoms of Parkinson's disease.

The relevant information is not only detailed but at the same time focused and is readily available to the reader. Health care professionals and other individuals working in the field of science can benefit to a great extent from this book.

Every effort has been made to present correct and up to date information in this book but medicine is a field with ongoing research and development, therefore readers may use other sources if the content of this book is found to be insufficient. Authors, editor, and publisher are not responsible for any errors, omissions, or consequences from the application of this information.

Dr. Abdul Qayyum Rana
Parkinson's Clinic of Eastern Toronto & Movement Disorders Center, Toronto, Canada

1

Cognitive Dysfunction in Parkinson's Disease

Sara Varanese[1], Bernardo Perfetti[2] and Alessandro Di Rocco[1]
[1]*New York University*
[2]*City College of New York*
USA

1. Introduction

With the progressive improvement in the management of the motor symptoms associated with Parkinson's disease, in the last decades the non-motor aspects of this disorder have gained growing attention by clinical and research communities. Cognitive functioning and its evolution are undoubtedly the most investigated non-motor aspects in PD due to their important implications in the diagnosis and treatment of the disorder as well as in the establishment of the disease functional outcomes. Despite the huge number of studies so far, the nature and the extent of cognitive decline are still poorly understood as well as their relation to disease type, duration and motor features. Heterogeneity has emerged as a key concept when describing the variety of cognitive deficits in PD and the diversity of their underlying neuro-pathophysiological mechanisms (Kehagia et al., 2010; Owen, 2004). Nonetheless, evaluation of the cognitive decline associated with PD is essential for good clinical and pharmacological management of the disease course.

Community-based studies of dementia in patients with Parkinson's disease (PD) have reported prevalence between 28% and 44%. However, longitudinal studies estimating the proportion of patients with PD who will eventually develop dementia reported a 4-year prevalence of dementia of at least 51.6% and an 8-year prevalence of 78% (Williams-Gray et al., 2006). The cumulative incidence of dementia increases with age, with a risk of dementia of 65% by the age of 85 years (Mayeux et al., 1990).

It has been widely assumed that cognitive deficits are only a feature of late-stage PD. Recent studies, however, reveal that subtle cognitive abnormalities that are not clinically apparent, mainly involving the executive functions, occur from the earliest stages of the disease (Foltynie et al., 2004a; Levin & Katzen, 2005) In this regard, two global cognitive profiles have been used to define the type of deficits found in PD, namely mild cognitive impairment and dementia.

The first is an umbrella definition and has been used to characterize the variety of impairments affecting patients without global and extensive cognitive decline. Disorders can involve one or more cognitive domains among which executive/attention, memory and visuospatial are the most common. Usually, mild cognitive impairment is found in the early and middle stages of disease course and is associated with older age at assessment and at disease onset, as well as to male gender, depression and more severe motor symptoms (Aarsland et al., 2011). Dementia instead is more common in the late stage of the disease and is often preceded by early cognitive impairments. It is characterized by a global cognitive deterioration that involves different domains and which can sensibly lower patients' quality of life. The profile of dementia described in PD is characterized by a subcortical quality (Emre, 2003), similar to dementia with Lewy bodies, and different from Alzheimer's disease (AD; Aarsland et al., 2003; Varanese et al., 2010).

Among the cognitive deficits described, the most well defined are impairments in executive functions. Similarly to those occurring in patients with frontal lesions, these include planning difficulties, inefficient cognitive strategies in problem solving and set shifting, altered goal-directed behavior. These impairments are though to represent a dysfunction of frontostriatal circuitry (Owen et al., 1992). It has been suggested that these two general cognitive profiles might be the behavioral reflections of different pathophysiological mechanisms mediated by distinct neurotransmitters and pathways (chatecholaminergic and cholinergic). In particular, the early deficits are often seen as a consequence of dopaminergic loss and the corresponding modification of the frontostriatal circuitry functioning whereas dementia seems to involve more cholinergic-dependent cortical dysfunction (Kehagia et al., 2010; Owen, 2004).

The etiopathological process underlying the cognitive disturbances in PD, however, is still not completely understood, although several morphological and neurochemical changes are now well recognized.

Alpha-synuclein-positive cortical Lewy body deposition is the key pathological finding in several post-mortem studies (Aarsland et al., 2005; Apaydin et al., 2002; Mattila et al., 2000). In order to avoid including patients with classical Lewy bodies dementia, these studies selected patients that have developed dementia at least 4 years after the diagnosis of PD.

Apaydin and colleagues found that diffuse or transitional Lewy body pathology was the primary substrate in 12 of the 13 patients enrolled in the study (1 patients was excluded due to primary PSP pathology, rather than PD). The mean Lewy body counts were approximately 10-fold higher among the PD patients who developed dementia. Although neocortical Lewy body counts were significantly correlated with the counts of senile plaques and neurofibrillary tangles in this group, suggesting a possible overlapping between these two pathologies, only one patient met the pathological criteria for an „intermediate probability of AD".

Aarsland and colleagues reported similar findings in a post-mortem study involving 22 PD patients, 18 of which diagnosed with dementia. Lewy body was the only pathology observed in demented PD patients, and was significantly associated with the rate of MMSE scores over a period of at least 4 years before death.

The pattern of distribution of Lewy bodies has also been investigated as an important contributor to the cognitive abnormalities observed in PD. Kovari and colleagues found that Lewy bodies density in the entorhinal and anterior cingulate cortices were significantly associated with clinical dementia rating scores, suggesting that Lewy body formation in limbic areas might be crucial for the development of dementia in PD (Kovari et al., 2003). This finding further supports the key role of the Lewy body deposition in the limbic area for the development of dementia in PD.

One of the studies that better clarified the correlation between the cerebral Lewy bodies' distribution and the development of cognitive symptoms in PD is certainly the work from Braak and colleagues (Braak et al., 2005). Their study involved 88 patients diagnosed with PD, who were assigned to one of the six hierarchical stages of PD at post-mortem analysis, based on the topographical distribution pattern of Lewy bodies. The main finding of the study was the correlation between increasing neuropathological stages and decreasing MMSE score, demonstrating a clear relationship between cognitive impairment and α-synuclein pathology. This specific relationship has also been confirmed in studies involving autosomal dominant forms of PD, were abnormalities in the α-synuclein genotype is associated with early-onset PD with dementia (Farrer et al., 2004; Singleton et al., 2003).

One of the most recent hypotheses suggests that the development of dementia in PD simply represents a shift toward dementia with Lewy bodies, being PD and DLB part of the same disease spectrum whereas the clinical distinction of the two conditions only reflects quantitative and temporal differences in the cerebral Lewy bodies' distribution. Evidence in supports of this hypothesis is provided by some imaging studies. Burton and colleagues have examined the pattern of cerebral atrophy in 57 patients with PD with and without dementia, and compared with controls and patients with Alzheimer's disease and dementia with Lewy bodies. PD patients with dementia were found to have significantly reduced grey matter volume in the occipital lobes bilaterally compared with cognitively intact PD patients, while no volumetric difference was observed between PD patients with dementia and DLB, and significantly less temporal lobe atrophy compared to AD was observed (Burton et al., 2004). Similarly, a study involving single photon emission computed tomography (SPECT) and MRI showed that perfusion deficit in PDD and DLB did not differ, involving in both cases the prenucleus and the inferior lateral parietal regions; this finding was clearly different from the perfusion deficit in the midline parietal region, thus more anterior, observed in AD (Firbank et al., 2003).

The understanding of the pathophysiology of the cognitive disorders in PD derives not only from neuropathological and neuroimaging studies, but also from neurochemical studies. The understanding of neurochemical changes actually provide obvious target for therapeutic interventions. Several neurotransmitter systems have been implicated in the development of cognitive disorders in PD, including dopaminergic, noradrenegirc, serotoninergic and cholinergic.

Dopaminergic deficits have been mainly correlated with executive, visuospatial and fluency deficits (Stern & Langston, 1985; Stern et al., 1990). This relationship is not surprising given that the medial substantia nigra projects to the caudate nucleus, which in turn send input to the frontostriatal circuitry, thought to subserve associative functions (Alexander et al., 1986). However, if dopaminergic deficits do play a major role in cognitive dysfunction in PD, one would expect that levodopa improves these symptoms. Although certain aspects of cognition, like speed information processing and spatial working memory, certainly improve following levodopa therapy (Lange et al., 1992), Williams-Gray and colleagues did not find any major functional impact on the dementia in PD (Williams-Gray et al., 2006) and other functions, like reversal learning, may actually worse (Cools et al., 2001). One possible explanation for the lack of a clear therapeutic benefit from levodopa is that intrinsic factors contribute to the level of dopamine in the prefrontal cortex, not only low level being insufficient, but also very high levels being toxic to the cognitive function. Among these intrinsic factors a major role seems to be played by the catechol-O-methyltransferase (COMT) Va158Met polymorphism. Patients with low-activity COMT genotypes shows increased prefrontal dopaminergic activity and impaired performance in problem solving tasks, with further worsening when the same patients are exposed to levodopa (Foltynie et al., 2004b). Williams-Gray and colleagues also identified that the microtubule-associated protein tau (*MAPT*) H1/H2 gene is an independent predictor of dementia risk (odds ratio =

12.1), with the H1 versus H2 haplotype being associated with a 20% increase in transcription of 4-repeat tau in Lewy body disease brains (Williams-Gray et al., 2009). In their study the *COMT* genotype had no effect on dementia, but had a significant impact on Tower of London performance, a frontostriatally based executive task, which was dynamic, such that the ability to solve this task changed with disease progression. This work suggests that the dementing process in Parkinson's disease is predictable and related to tau while frontal-executive dysfunction evolves independently with a more dopaminergic basis and better prognosis.

The lack of benefit from the levodopa is also motivated by the key involvement of other impaired neurotransmitter systems. While limited evidence exists for noradrenergic and serotoninergic deficits (Cash et al., 1987; Scatton et al., 1983), much stronger evidence exists to support the theory that cholinergic deficits play a major role in the etiology of cognitive deficits in PD. Indeed, cellular loss in the nucleus basalis of Meynert has been demonstrated and associated not only with cortical cholinergic deficits, but also with different levels of cognitive impairment including dementia. (Dubois et al., 1983; Perry et al., 1985). This evidence represents so far the strongest substrate for the treatment approach to the cognitive symptoms in PD.

2. Dysexecutive syndrome

The most common described cognitive deficits in non-demented PD are the impairments in executive functions. In clinical setting, this set of deficits is also known under the term of dysexecutive syndrome. Generally speaking, the main feature of this syndrome is a disruption of goal-directed behaviors that has a negative impact on daily activities especially when patients have to deal with novel situation (Lezak, 1995). In this regard, impairments of executive functions in PD closely resemble the neuropsychological symptoms following frontal lobe lesions, which involve cognitive skills like planning, problem solving, attention shifting, the developing of new and efficient strategies and working memory. This similarity, together with some neuroimaging and pharmacological evidence, suggested that the dysexecutive syndrome in PD might reflect a disruption of the dopaminergic system and of the corresponding frontostriatal circuitry (Kehagia et al., 2010; Owen, 2004). In addition to pure executive disorders, some investigations reported visuospatial and memory deficit that have been often addressed, though, as a consequence of the executive dysfunction (Dubois & Pillon, 1997; Varanese et al., 2011).

The concept of executive functions has a neuropsychological genesis and was introduced to account for a wide range of deficits, classically those associated with dysfunction of the frontal lobe. It postulates the existence of a set of mental skills devoted to the organization and supervision of disparate cognitive processes and to coordinate the exploitation of goal-directed behavior. Executive functions are thus fundamental for an individual to engage successfully in purposive, self-serving behavior. Such a high-level control is needed in daily life, especially in those situations in which the automatic and habitual behavior does not adequately fit the context demands. For instance, executive functions are recruited when a person has to face novel problems (e.g. learning to ride a motorbike), when has to override the interfering effects of irrelevant information (e.g. paying attention to the road despite the surrounding landscape) when mental planning is necessary before action execution (e.g. deciding which way to go at a crossing) when attention is divided among multiple tasks (e.g. talking at the phone while driving) when the individual has to prioritize among different goals (e.g. which move comes first in a chess game). Even if largely investigated, there is an extensive theoretical debate on the nature and number of executive processes. The first issue is whether a unique and single definition of executive functions can account for the variety of disorders associated with executive disruption. Different theories(Norman & Shallice, 1986) postulate the existence of a single high-level executive process that controls and organizes the functioning of lower level abilities in the service of the ongoing task. In the model proposed by Norman and Shallice (1986) for instance, the "supervisory attentional system" is responsible for the biasing of "schema" which can be roughly described as more routine and automatic behaviors. Baddeley and Hitch (1986) on the other hand, proposed the Working Memory model that consists of a high-level central executive component and a set of lower level subsidiary memory storages and buffers.

Differently from these models, executive processes might be also though as a set of distinct and partially independent skills that could be specifically recruited on the basis of task-goals. This set includes some cognitive abilities like flexibility and set shifting, complex motor programming, planning and problem solving, and self-monitoring.

The theoretical debate about the nature and number of executive functions (single versus multifaceted system) acquires a particular importance when assessing the dysexecutive syndrome in PD. A number of studies have reported dissociation between distinct executive components affected by PD as well as dissociation between low- and high-level functioning deficits. Even more interesting are the data showing that the extent of executive impairments and the cognitive domain involved might vary as a function of motor disorder (Owen, 2000). For instance, when tested with a spatial working memory task, medicated and non-medicated patients performed differently, with only the former showing significant deficits (Owen et al., 1992). Furthermore, it has been found that a group of PD patients showed impaired performance at spatial working memory test while normal performance in verbal working memory task (Bradley et al., 1989).

In the attempt to characterize this variability, some authors got to the conclusion that executive deficits associated with PD could be better described in terms of the involvement of high- versus low-level functioning that, in turn, seems to be related to the disease progression. Specifically, it has been suggested that high-level processing dysfunction might occur earlier during disease course, whereas impairments of low-level processes are associated with later stages of PD. Some results from a set of studies using verbal and spatial working memory tasks come in support of this hypothesis (Lewis et al., 2003a; Lewis et al., 2003b; Owen et al., 1993; Owen et al., 1992). Owen and colleagues manipulated the degree of attentional control involvement by varying some basic characteristics of a spatial task. In a first version of the test, in order to place selectively significant demands on memory processes, the authors had patients with PD remembering sequences of color-changing boxes presented on a computer screen. In a second version of the task, subjects were presented with a number of colored boxes and instructed to search for blue tokens hidden inside some of these boxes. An important rule was to avoid boxes in which a token was already found. Similarly to the first version this task involves spatial memory processes. However, in addition to that, it also recruits attentional control needed for the active manipulation and reorganization of relevant contents held in working memory and for the development of efficient searching strategies. Notably, the authors revealed important differences in the performance among patients and between tasks, which correlated with disease stages. In particular, medicated subjects who were experiencing more severe clinical symptoms performed poorly at the first task in which low level of attentional control was required. At the same test, patients with mild disease, who were either medicated or non-medicated, performed normally. However, these groups' differences disappeared when subjects were tested with more complex spatial search task. Medicated patients with either severe or mild disease performed poorly as compared to control. In addition, the non-medicated patients showed a trend toward impairment (Owen et al., 1993; Owen et al., 1992).

The distinction between low- versus high-level processing involvement is crucial for the understanding of the possible pathological mechanisms underlying PD cognitive decline and for the identification of the corresponding neural substrates. Several studies, have suggested that low and high-level processes might recruit partially distinct anatomical areas within the brain, and in particular within the prefrontal cortex. In normal subjects, PET and fMRI investigations revealed that the active manipulation of working memory contents as well as the identification of strategies based upon task goals load on the mid-dorsolateral frontal cortex. On the other hand, lower level functioning such as encoding and retrieval of information engage more ventral frontal regions (Owen, 2000).This evidence led to the description of the lateral frontal cortex as separated in two distinct systems, each supporting different aspects of executive processing in connections to posterior association areas. Briefly, the ventrolateral frontal cortex is the first station through which information coming from posterior regions accesses the frontal lobe to be integrated for further processing. It is thus considered to be critical for a variety of low-level memory processes. Conversely, the mid-dorsolateral frontal cortex is assumed to be a second-step station responsible for higher processes such as manipulation and monitoring of information held in memory. Based on this evidence, the dissociation between high- and low-level types of impairment seen in PD might reflect a different involvement of the two regions within frontal cortex during the disease progression. It is likely that PD might affect early a specific component of the executive system that is the one requiring attention control and that involve the mid-dorsolateral area. On the other hand, dysfunction of the ventrolateral cortex and, in turn, impairments of more basic mnemonic processes, might occur late in the pathology in parallel with the development of more severe motor symptoms.

Taken together, these findings point at the frontostriatal circuitry as a probable pathophysiological mechanism underlying the cognitive deficits in PD. The different anatomical and cytoarchitectonical prefrontal regions receive fibers from the distinct regions of the basal ganglia in a highly topographical manner (Alexander et al., 1986). It has been suggested that the executive impairments in PD might be a consequence of the interruption of the normal flow of information through these frontostriatal "highways" owe to the dopamine depletion associated with the disease. The dissociation between low and high-level executive impairments and the parallel progression of cognitive and motor symptoms reflect the spatiotemporal progression of dopamine loss in the striatum, which progressively affects distinct regions and their afferents to different frontal areas. Besides the frontostriatal circuitry, also the dopamine depletion within the prefrontal cortex itself might play an important role in the pattern of executive disorders observed in PD (Scatton et al., 1983)

The dopamine-dependent hypothesis has been put under investigation with a number of studies. First, it has been shown that dopaminergic enhancement has a restorative effect on a variety of executive processes such as flexibility during problem solving task, attention switching (Cools et al., 2003), working memory (Costa et al., 2009; Lewis et al., 2005) and

response inhibition (Gauggel et al., 2004). However, on the other hand, dopaminergic restoration has been associated with worsening of performance on a set of cognitive processes mainly involving feedback related learning. For instance dopaminergic overdose has been linked to increased impulsivity and abnormal betting in a gambling setting (Cools et al., 2003). Moreover, differently from unmedicated patients, subjects under dopaminergic treatment showed impulsive responding and failure to switch to a newly rewarded stimulus when the currently selected one is no longer associated with reward (reversal learning). The dual opposite effects of dopamine enhancement on cognitive functioning has been interpreted as a reflection of the different degree of dopamine depletion among the striatal regions. In fact, whereas dopaminergic dosing for adequate treatment of motor symptoms restores striatal dorsal regions functioning and ameliorates high-level cognitive processes, conversely it has deleterious effect on cognitive functions depending on less depleted striatal regions (ventral) and on the corresponding cortical projections (orbitofrontal cortex).
Besides these pharmacological studies, PET and fMRI works have investigated the contribution of the frontostriatal circuitry to PD executive impairments by examining the patterns of cortical and subcortical activations during executive tasks (Dagher et al., 2001; Lewis et al., 2003a; Mattay et al., 2002). The obtained results are inconsistent in terms of the specific frontal versus striatal contribution. However, besides those differences that are probably due to methodological issues, they generally confirmed the important role of the dopamine depletion in cognitive impairments associated with PD and the distinction between high and low level executive processes. These are to key concepts and have important implications in the neuropsychological evaluation of the dysexecutive syndrome in the daily practice.

3. Neuropsychological assessment of the dysexecutive syndrome

As previously reported, there is still a lack of consensus on a clear definition of executive functions. Some theories postulate the existence of a single system in which a putative central attention process coordinates and organizes the ongoing behavior by controlling low-level and subsidiary skills. On the other hand, executive functions have been described as set of partially independent, high-level functions that can be singularly disrupted by either selective lesions or system disease. As consequence of this theoretical debate, developing clinical instruments able to assess deficits of the executive functions have proved to be very difficult.
Nonetheless, when executive functions have been investigated in the normal population through a variety of tests, large individual differences were found, even within the same executive tasks. In addition, the weak correlations observed among individual performance at different executive tests suggested that the underlying cognitive processes might share little variance (Miyake et al., 2000a; Spitoni et al., 2002). These data have been generally interpreted as a convincing argument in favor of a separation of executive components, leading also to a revision of the "unique" system theories (Baddeley, 1996; Carlesimo et al., 2001; Klauer & Zhao, 2004).
This probable separation of executive components must be taken into account during neuropsychological evaluations in daily practice. In order to assess adequately executive functioning, a multidimensional approach seems to be fundamental. In this regard, there is need of tools able to scan and tap a variety of distinct abilities and capable of detecting the complexity of executive system (in terms of low- versus high level functioning). However, as pointed out by some authors (Miyake et al., 2000b), many of the classical executive tests adopted for clinical evaluation, do not have clear construct validity and seem to measure

different skills at the same time. For instance, the Wisconsin Card Sorting Test (WCST; Heaton et al., 1993) measures "mental set shifting" and the associated tendency to perseveration, "problem solving" and "abstract reasoning" abilities. In spite of the real difficulty to distinguish between the different capacities required to solve its demands, this test continues to be used as a measure of executive functions. Similarly, the Tower of London test (TOL; Shallice, 1982), is thought to be sensitive to a variety of impairments among which are "attention, "problem solving", "planning" and "cognitive inhibition" deficits.

Traditional executive tests have been used to investigate the dysexecutive syndrome in PD. Patients who do not have a global cognitive dysfunction showed poor performance when tested with the WCST, the Trail Making test (TMT) and the TOL (Bowen et al., 1975; Hietanen & Teravainen, 1986; Owen et al., 1992; Perfetti et al., 2010; Varanese et al., 2011; Vingerhoets et al., 2003). For instance, when compared to age matched control subjects, patients with PD showed poorer ability to find new categories (Varanese et al., 2011; Vingerhoets et al., 2003) in the WCST and a greater tendency to perseverate (Perfetti et al., 2010), lesser planning skill at the TOL (Owen et al., 1992; Perfetti et al., 2010). Verbal fluency and visuospatial memory also resulted impaired (Cooper et al., 1991; Owen et al., 1992) as well as inhibition of response (Petrova et al., 2010).

However, in light of the considerations mentioned above these traditional instruments might not be capable in detecting and precisely characterized the type of dysexecutive syndrome associated with PD. The first argument in favor of this hypothesis is that the traditional instruments might fail in distinguishing between different executive components as they often tap a variety of executive abilities without a clear distinction between them and between high and low-level functioning. In fact, based upon the results showing that high-level functioning might be early impaired in PD, performance at traditional tests might be globally disrupted by such a condition. Second, the presence of everyday problems in dysexecutive patients may not (necessary) fit with the scores resulting from a structured testing assessment like that provided by traditional measures. It has been reported that individual patients could perform well on these measures even if showing obvious and deleterious symptoms in less structure environment, suggestive of a more complex disorganization of everyday behavior (Eslinger & Damasio, 1985; Shallice & Burgess, 1991). In traditional neuropsychological testing, since instructions are explicit and task initiation is prompted by the examiner, success may be highly characterized which, in turns, might cause a failure in detecting executive dysfunction (Burgess et al., 2006). In order to overcome the limits of traditional executive measures and put the hypothesis mentioned above under investigation, we recently adopted an ecological neuropsychological battery to assess executive dysfunction in PD. Specifically, we administered a set of traditional executive tests and the Behavioral Assessment of Dysexecutive Syndrome (BADS; Wilson et al., 1996) battery to a group of non-demented PD patients and a sample of demographically matched control subjects. The BADS was purposely developed with the intent of measuring a wide range of executive impairments and to predict everyday problems (ecological approach) by assessing capacities that are normally involved in everyday activities through six different subtests. Moreover, the BADS takes into account the complexity of the high-level executive functioning by loading onto organizational skills and task-goals management capabilities. It requires participants to plan activities over long time intervals and, most importantly, to prioritize among competitive demands. Taken together these features make the BADS a less structure test (open-ended) and thus a good candidate for detecting subtle executive disorders associated with PD.

The results obtained in our study support the use of such a multidimensional approach. We showed that the PD sample generally performed less well then control subjects in almost the administered tests. However, when we compared the sensitivity of the different adopted tools in predicting group membership, we revealed that the BADS total score and the "modified six elements" sub-score were the best predictors. Figure 1 summarizes part of the results. The figure displays the executive tests' z-scores of the PD sample computed on the basis of normal subjects' performance.

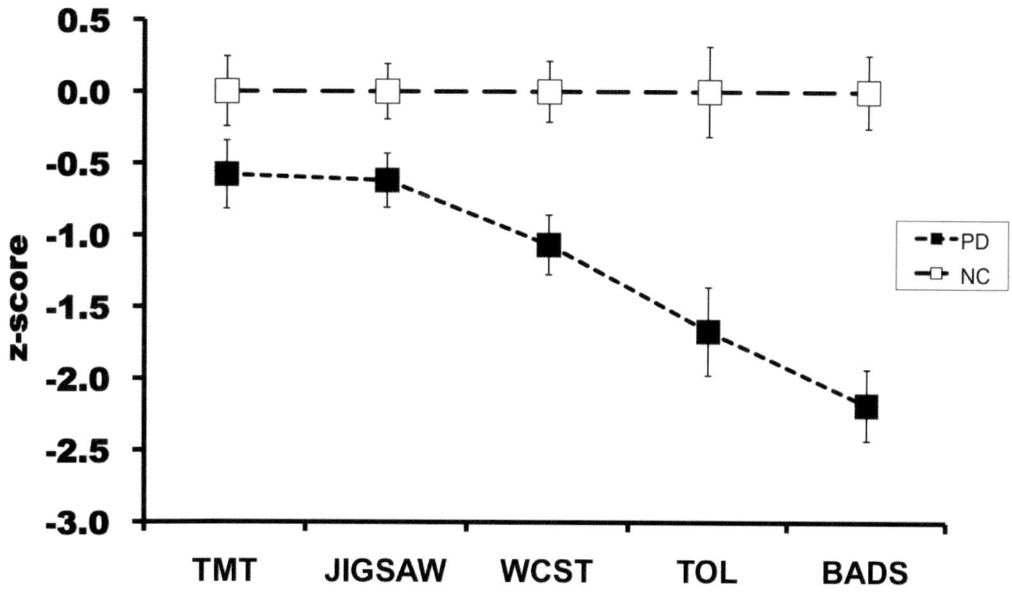

Fig. 1. Profile plots of the Z scores at the different administered tests, computed on the basis of normal subjects' performance. TMT, Trail Making Test; WCST, Wisconsin Card Sorting Test; TOL, Tower of London Test; BADS, Behavioural Assessment of the Dysexecutive Syndrome; JIGSAW, Jigsaw Puzzle Test; PD, Parkinson's Disease; NC, Normal Control

These results are in agreement with the hypothesized distinction between low- and high-level executive functioning in PD. The modified six elements subtest is a task that makes strong demands on the high-level functioning. Subject has to plan, organize and monitor the ongoing behavior over long period of time while concurrently remembering and carrying out a specific goal. It is an open-ended (less structured) task that strongly loads on subject's organizational skills making it sensitive to the disruption of goal-directed behavior. These results support and bolster the idea that, in early PD, impairment of executive functioning mainly involves the high attentional control causing a loss of the organizational skills. In addition, they support the use of a multidimensional approach during neuropsychological evaluation of patients with PD.
Evidence in line with these conclusions comes from an investigation conducted by Varanese and colleagues (2010). The authors were interested in studying the relation between apathy and cognitive profile in non-demented individuals with PD. The study is a good example of a multidimensional approach through the use of traditional executive tests. Apathy was associated with the presence of executive disorders that was detected and characterized by the identification of an underlying core deficit among the different administered tests (see table 1

for partial results). The authors reported that apathy patients showed a selective deficit in the free recalling of words at the California Verbal Learning Test (CVLT-II; Delis et al., 2002) and poor ability to find new categories at the WCST. Rather than a primary memory disorder the low score in free recalling was interpreted as an impairment of poor strategy implementation at the encoding and recalling stages. This interpretation was supported by the fact that, in the CVLT-II, the words to be retained can be more efficiently encoded and recalled by using a semantic strategy. Moreover, the lower number of categories identified by the apathetic patients at the WCST bare this conclusion. In summary, the main impairment associated with apathy in PD involved the ability to abstract reasoning and developing new strategies for the accomplishment of task goals. In other words PD patients were affected by a disruption of organizational skills and goal-directed behavior.

Domain	Test	Measure	PD-A	PD-NA	Sig.
recall	CVLT-II	**total free recall**	**22.8 (5.8)**	**28 (3.7)**	**0.000***
	CVLT-II	**short delay free**	**5.9 (2.3)**	**7.4 (1.2)**	**0.001***
	CVLT-II	**long delay free**	**5 (2.2)**	**7.2 (1.5)**	**0.000***
	CVLT-II	**long delay cued**	**5.1 (2.1)**	**7.4 (1.9)**	**0.000***
recognition	CVLT-II	**delayed recognition**	**8 (0.8)**	**8.6 (0.6)**	**0.01***
learning	CVLT-II	total learning slope	3 (1.2)	2.8 (1.1)	0.55
attention	D-KEFS	visual scanning	35.9 (17.4)	33.2 (12.4)	0.5
	Dsy		44.9 (16.5)	51.4 (15.2)	0.08
speed info processing	D-KEFS	number sequence	0.4 (0.9)	0.3 (0.5)	0.6
		letter sequence	0.6 (1)	0.2 (0.4)	0.1
		motor speed	52.4 (32)	45 (22.5)	0.6
executive functions	WCST-64	**total correct**	**34.9 (10.8)**	**45.6 (11.2)**	**0.000***
		perseverative responses	14.9 (7.9)	12.1 (11.5)	0.33
		categories completed	**1.6 (1.3)**	**3.2 (1.7)**	**0.000***
	D-KEFS	number-letter	2.5 (1.5)	1.7 (1)	0.09

P <0.05, FDR corrected. D-KEFS=Delis-Kaplan Executive Function system; CVLT-II=California Verbal Learning Test–II; WCST-64= Wisconsin Card Sorting Test-64 cards version; DSy= Digit symbol

Table 1. All values represent mean (SD). Between-groups comparisons have been investigating using univariate analysis of variance for each variable, with age, disease duration and Led as covariates and group membership (apathy vs. No apathy) as fixed factor (ANCOVA).

4. Dementia

Dementia in patients with Parkinson's disease (PDD) is usually defined as a subcortical pattern of cognitive impairment (i.e. deficits in attention, executive functions, visuospatial and constructional abilities), where the core features is represented by an impairment of cognitive functions, that leads to deficits in planning, sequencing, execution of goal-direct behavior, and typically in the maintenance of new sequence patterns after the shift from a previously learned sequence of movement (Emre, 2003). Memory is also impaired, with prevalent involvement of working and episodic memory, and procedural learning (Pillon et al., 1993) but differently from the amnesic syndrome of AD, these deficits in PD lies in retrieval rather than storage of information. Although also described in other forms of dementia, visuospatial impairment is more severe in PDD patients (Huber et al., 1989), and it has been suggested that impaired performance in visuospatial tasks may be related to problems with sequential organization of behavior, thus expressing a frontal executive dysfunction rather than pure parieto-occipital pathology (Stern et al., 1983). Attention is compromised with presence of attentive fluctuations (Ballard et al., 2002).

Psychotic symptoms are frequently associated with dementia in PD, with a prevalence ranging between 25 and 30% (Ravina et al., 2007). Visual hallucinations are the most prevalent manifestation of psychosis, and they can range from simple illusions or flashes of light or vague feelings of presence or passage of humans and animals, to the complex formed visions of animals and people more commonly observed.

Hence, PDD can be difficult to discriminate from DLB, and the temporal course is the main distinction.

4.1 Cognitive fluctuations

As previously discussed it has been hypothesized that subgroups with different cognitive profiles exist within PDD, suggesting that frontosubcortical changes are the main contributing factor for dementia in some patients while, in others, cortical and hippocampal changes may predominate (Aarsland et al., 2003). Varanese and colleagues identified the occurrence of cognitive fluctuations (FC) as the clinical variable associated with a DLB pattern of impairment in PDD. This study enrolled 27 PDD, 33 DLB, 18 AD patients and 20 healthy control subjects. Based on the presence or absence of FC, PDD patients were divided in two subgroups and their performance at the Dementia Rating Scale 2 (DRS-2) was compared with the performance of the other groups. The authors found that PDD patients with FC had a pattern of cognitive impairments similar to DLB, which involved prevalently the attention and initiation/perseveration domains, and which was significantly more pronounced compared to the pattern exhibited by PDD patients without FC (Varanese et al., 2010).

FC is described as an interruption in the ongoing flow of awareness or attention that impacts on functional abilities and appears as a fluctuation in the level of arousal and cognitive performance (Bradshaw et al., 2004; Serrano & Garcia-Borreguero, 2004), and it is also known to be associated with episodes of disturbed consciousness. Byrne and colleagues reported the case of one patient who had day-to-day changes of the MMSE, and the case of another patient who experienced confusional episodes that varied from being mute and unable to stand without assistance to being capable of carrying on a conversation (Byrne et al., 1989); Gibb and colleagues described episodes of stupor in a patient affected by DLB who appeared alert and responsive to commands out of these episodes (Gibb et al., 1987).

The most widely used instrument to detect the FC in the clinical setting is the Clinician Assessment of Fluctuation scale (CAF) (Walker et al., 2000a). This is a short scale developed to provide a quantitative score of the FC, based upon the clinician's interpretation of caregiver responses to the two key items that made up the scale: "Does the patient ever have spontaneous impaired alertness and concentration –i.e. appears drowsy but awake, looks dazed, is not aware of what's going on?" (clear examples demonstrating impaired consciousness with variations in performance/cognition are required to receive a positive rating); "Has the level of confusion experienced by the patient tended to vary recently from day to day or week to week? For example, becoming worse, then perhaps improving for a while?" (significant fluctuation is regarded as present if distinct examples of differences in performance/cognition can be given on at least two occasion over the month). If a positive rating of FC is present (two positive answers to question 1 and 2), a severity rating should be made on a 1 to 4 scale for the frequency of FC (where 1 = ≤ 1 per month, 2 = monthly-weekly, 3 = weekly-daily, 4 = ≥ daily), and on a 0 to 4 scale for duration of FC (where 0 = seconds, 1 = ≤ 5 minutes, 2 = 5 minutes-1 hour, 3 = ≥ 1 hour, 4 = ≥ 1 day). The two partial scores (frequency and duration) are multiplied together to produce a severity score from 0 to 12, 0 representing no fluctuating cognition, and 12 representing severe fluctuating cognition (a score of 16 would signify a continuous clouded state, which, by definition, would denote no fluctuation).

Bradshaw and colleagues showed that item one of CAF ("does the patient ever have spontaneous impaired alertness and concentrations – i.e. appears drowsy but awake, looks dazed, is not aware of what's going on?") is not enough specific in detecting FC in DLB, as AD caregivers response is often positive; but verbatim descriptions of FC in DLB have particular qualitative characteristics that differ from those obtained in AD patients: DLB caregivers frequently provided descriptions that suggested a lapse in the stream of awareness or attention reflecting that patient lost the ability to engage in meaningful cognitive or physical activity, while AD caregivers described periods of confusion characterized by repetitiveness in conversation or forgetfulness in relation to a recent event as a result of memory failure (Bradshaw et al., 2004).

Qualitative caregiver's description provides clear differences in the nature of the FC.

In our personal case study, caregivers usually described FC as a lapse in the stream of awareness or attention, sometimes reflecting confabulatory or delusional quality (17 patients, 89,47%: "sometimes he seems to be blank, and I must shake him to have a response", "she seems to be drowsy", "she seems to be confused", "he has temporary lapses and can't focus properly", "he seems to have some black out", "sometimes she says something senseless, than suddenly come back clear", "he seems to be not aware of what is around him", "he cannot concentrate on what he is doing", "she detaches", "sometimes he says that there are extra people staying at home, than he comes back clear", "sometimes we can talk over with him, sometimes doesn't understand a word"); only in two case (12.51%) FC appeared as episodes of forgetfulness ("sometimes she cannot find something at home because she don't remember where she put it, so she wonder around confused"; "some days he asks me the same question 10 times in 10 minutes"). The caregiver provided descriptions of the FC that reflected deficit in attention or awareness in a significant percentage of cases ($p<0.001$).

The evaluation of FC in the diagnosis of DLB causes the greatest difficulty in clinical practice because assessment methods, as the CAF largely rely on clinical experience and inter-rater

reliability is reported to be low (Litvan et al., 1998; Mega et al., 1996). Furthermore it is frequently difficult for raters to reach agreement on differentiating episodes of mild fluctuation in consciousness from diurnal hypersomnia, frequently observed in dementia (Lopez et al., 1999).
The EEG is a useful tool to detect FC, providing a measure of cortical arousal useful to define and stage levels of human awareness as well as levels of variability in the frequency of cortical rhythms. At the EEG FC are represented as slow activity and epoch-by-epoch fluctuation in the mean frequency (Barber et al., 2000; Briel et al., 1999; Onofrj et al., 2003; Walker et al., 2000b). In a study focused on EEG in AD, DLB and PDD, Bonanni and colleagues have recently shown that around 20% of PDD patients at onset exhibit FC and that only those with FC displayed the EEG alterations typically observed in DLB (pre-alpha activity and variability in the mean frequency), but the rate of PDD exhibiting FC significantly increased after two years of follow up (Bonanni et al., 2008).

5. Therapeutic management

The pharmacological management of the cognitive symptoms represents a major challenge e in PD.
Due to the paucity of evidence-based therapeutic options, the traditional approach has been widely based on withdrawal of medications known to worse the cognitive functioning. Any attempt should be made to avoid benzodiazepines and anitmuscaric antidepressants. Antiparkinsonian medications are also know to affect the cognitive functions and a gradual withdrawal should be considered for those medications with higher cognitive adverse effect but lower motor benefit, like anticholinergics, amantadine, selegiline and eventually dopamine-agonists.
Another important step, when dealing with a patient presenting with symptoms of confusion, is to exclude all the identifiable and removable triggering factors. The most frequent of these occurring in PD patients are concomitant infections, dehydration, subdural hematoma and electrolyte imbalance. Their treatment often is sufficient to improve the cognitive worsening.
There is now emerging evidence to support the efficacy of a specific class of drug, originally developed as a treatment for Alzheimer's disease: cholinesterase inhibitors.
These drugs enhance the cholinergic transmission by preventing the catabolism of acetylcholine released in the presynaptic neurons. The use of these compounds is certainly justified by the key role of disruption of the cholinergic system among the neurochemical changing involved in the development of dementia in PD, as discussed previously.
Rivastigmine, donepezil and galantamine are the three drugs of this class available, and they have different pharmacological properties that may reflect a different profile of efficacy and safety. It is well known, for instance, that rivastigmine inhibit both the acetylcholinesterase and the butirrylcholinesterase, leading to a greater efficacy (Poirier, 2002).
The beneficial effect of cholinesterase inhibitors, particularly donepezil and rivastigmine, on the cognitive function was originally suggested in preliminary open label studies, without any associated significant deterioration in motor function in the majority of the patients.
In more recent years evidence from large placebo-controlled trials conducted on rivastigmine and donepezil further highlighted the safety and efficacy of these compounds.

5.1 Rivastigmine

Rivastigmine was investigated in the "Exelon in Parkinson's Disease Dementia Study"(EXPRESS). This 24-week study involved 541 patients randomized to receive either rivastigmine or placebo in a double blind design. As per inclusion criteria patients had to be diagnosed with PD according to the UKPDS criteria and developed dementia at least 2 years after the diagnosis of PD, in order to reduce the chance of including patients with Lewy bodies disease. The rivstigmine dose ranged between 3 and 12 mg/day. The primary outcome measures of the study were the Alzheimer's disease Assessment scale (ADAS-cog) and the Alzheimer's disease Cooperative study - Clinician's Global Impression of Change (ADCS-CGIC). Although the improvement in the ADAS-cog was very modest (2.1 points in 70-point scale) in the rivastigmine group, the placebo group worsened of 0.7 points leading to a significant difference between the two groups ($p<0.001$). The improvement in the ADCS-CGI was, instead, clinically meaningful in 19.8% of patients receiving rivastigmine compared to 14.5% of patient receiving placebo ($p=0.007$). Hence rivastigmine produced a clinically relevant improvement in almost 20% of patient.
The drug was well tolerated, with 72.7% of patients completing the study. The adverse events were predominantly cholinergic and, among these, nausea was the most frequent one occurring in the 29% of patients. Although the UPDRS motor score did not significantly change at the end of the study, 27% of patients in the rivastigmine arm reported worsening of parkinsonian symptoms. Due to the limited duration of the trial data on safety and tolerability are certainly limited, although the 24-week open label extension study has not shown further safety and tolerability issues (Emre et al., 2004).

5.2 Donepezil

Donepezil was investigated in two small placebo-controlled trials.
The first trial involved 14 patients randomized to receive either donepezil 5-10 mg or placebo for 10 weeks in a double blind crossover design. The investigators reported an improvement of 2.1 scores in the MMSE compared to the placebo group ($p=0.013$), with no change in the UPDRS scores at the end of the study. However, although this trial suggested that donepezil can improve cognition in patients with PD without worsening of motor function, the study results are limited by the small sample size and by the crossover design, as no washout period was allowed between the two stages of the trial (Aarsland et al., 2002).
The second study involved 16 patients randomized to receive donepezil 2.5-10 mg or placebo for 18 weeks. This study showed improvement in only one outcome measure, the dementia rating scale, in the donepezil arm compared to the placebo arm (p0.03), however the improvement consisted in less than 3 points on a mean score of 22, thus the clinical meaningfulness of this change is very limited. Furthermore the study raised concerns about the tolerability of the drug, which was limited to a mean dose of 6.4 mg/day (Leroi et al., 2004).
In conclusion, rivastigmine should be the first-line cholinesterase inhibitor in patients with PD and dementia, as it is the only agent supported by evidence from a large scale randomized controlled trial.

5.3 Wakefulness-promoting medications

Modafinil and armodafinil are central nervous system stimulants, which exert their effect through activation of the orexin-containing neurons in the hypothalamus, prefrontal cortex and anterior cingulate cortex.

Modafinil has been shown to ameliorate excessive daytime sleepiness in patients with Parkinson's disease (Adler et al., 2003) as well as wakefulness, vigilance and attention in narcolepsy (Hirshkowitz et al., 2007) and in healthy volunteers (Wong et al., 1999). Modafinil has been associated with improvements in cognitive performance in healthy volunteers and in patients with attention-deficit hyperactivity disorder and schizophrenia, implying that it may be useful in cognitively impaired patients with PD with or without associated daytime sleepiness.

We have been investigating the use of waking-promoting agents (modafinil and armodafinil) as treatment for FC and cognitive dysfunction typical of PDD/DLB in two preliminary studies.

In a retrospective observation conducted in a group of six PDD patients who received modafinil or armodafinil for excessive daytime sleepiness and showed concomitant improvement in their cognitive skills. The evaluation was conducted through CGI scales (severity-S and improvement-I) extracted by two independent raters based upon the treating physician notes over a follow up period ranging between 18 and 66 months. The inter-rater reliability reached a kappa measure of 0.69. Four patients with stable medications over the follow up period were included in the final analysis, while three were excluded due to concomitant use of cognitive enhancers or other medications that could potentially have an impact on cognitive abilities. All the four patients showed improvement in their cognitive status that translated in improved social interactions and that was sustained over the entire follow up period. Interestingly, the greatest improvement was observed in those patients with more compromised cognitive status at baseline. The figure below summarizes the improvement observed:

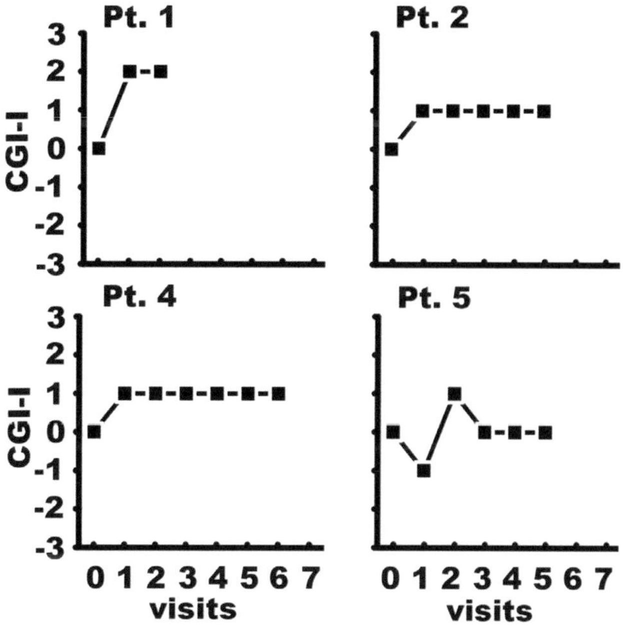

The interval between visits is six months.

Fig. 2. CGI-I ratings: 3=very much improved; 2=much improved; 1=minimally improved; 0=no change; -1=minimally worse; -2=much worse; -3= very much worse.

Based on the retrospective observation, we have collected preliminary behavioral data in a sample of 9 patients with PDD on their pre- and post-dose performance at vigilance and attention-computerized tests. For this one-day experiment, the patients received armodafinil 150 mg, and were tested twice, before and after the dose. They had to perform two different computerized tests, whose main outcome is reaction time (RT). The first test is a detection task assessing exogenous attention, in which the patient has to respond quickly to the appearance of a stimulus on the left or right side of the pc screen that can be either or not preceded by a brief blinking image (match or non-match trial); the second test is a classical psychomotor vigilance task (PVT), based on simple cued reaction time, in which the patient has to stop a counter appearing at random intervals on the pc screen. A preliminary analysis of the individual performances pre- and post dose showed that administration of armodafinil is followed by reduction in RT in both the detection task and the PVT; furthermore in the post-dose performances there is a consistent and relevant decrement in the standard deviation, which we consider a marker of cognitive stability during the test, thus reflecting a reduction in spontaneous fluctuations of attention occurring during the test performance. As in the case of the clinical series described above, we observed the greatest effect of armodafinil in the more cognitively compromised patient (pt. 2): this patient greatly improved in the PVT performance (she was unable to perform the detection task due to fatigue at baseline). The table below provides an example of patients' performance before and after the drug (means are expressed in milliseconds):

				pre-dose			post-dose		
Pt	age	MMSE	DRS-2	detection match mean RT (SD)	Detection nonmatch mean RT (SD)	PVT mean RT (SD)	detection match mean RT (SD)	Detection nonmatch mean RT (SD)	PVT mean RT (SD)
1	88	26	121	420.46 (149)	423.48 (150.57)	531.87 (250.77)	399.97 (123.02)	407.73 (133.60)	516.82 (191.29)
2	78	19	94	NA	NA	736.02 (364.56)	NA	NA	627.12 (292.74)
3	76	24	119	464.4 (191.58)	468.08 (130.90)	351.24 (90.24)	392.34 (96.09)	423.51 (110.37)	328.25 (70.11)

6. Conclusion

Contrary to James Parkinson's original description that intellect was preserved, it is now clear that subtle cognitive deficits occur in PD from the earliest stage of disease and a substantial proportion of patients eventually develop dementia. Although the underlying pathophysiology is not fully understood, evidence from post-mortem, neurochemical and neuroimaging studies suggests that the altered mechanisms leading to dementia in PD are similar to those described in DLB. Most likely the two syndromes represents a continuum within the spectrum of the alpha-synuclein pathology.

Early cognitive impairment, mainly in the form of dysexecutive syndrome, occurs in a significant proportion of patients even in the early stages of disease. The evaluation of this cognitive change represents a major challenge in the clinical setting, as traditional neuropsychological tools may fail to detect the subtle impairments even when they clearly impact on the patient's quality of life by decreasing the pre-disease executive abilities. More

ecological instruments, able to characterize patient's executive behavior in a less structured environment and closely resembling the daily routine, may provide a key contribution to the early detection of the dysexecutive syndrome in PD. Recognizing patients with dysexecutive syndrome may have important prognostic implications. It has been suggested, indeed, that the frontal-executive dysfunction evolves independently from dementia, relies on a more dopaminergic basis and has a better prognosis.
The underlying mechanisms of overt dementia in PD are still poorly understood. It is well established, however, that clinical manifestations of dementia in PD resemble very close the peculiarity of DLB. Among his cognitive fluctuations represent one of the core symptoms, with their frequency and severity progressively increasing during the course of the disease.
The most obvious therapeutic strategy in the treatment of dementia associated with PD is to target the cholinergic deficits. The available evidence, although limited, suggests that cholinesterase inhibitors may have a dual efficacy in ameliorating both cognitive and behavioral symptoms. However, their tolerability seems variable, with peripheral cholinergic adverse events often preventing therapeutic doses being reached. Due to the proposed mechanism of altered activation system, wakefulness promoting medications, like modafinil and armodafinil, may be able to improve cognition by improving alertness and certainly warrant more extensive investigations to determine their beneficial role in the treatment of dementia in in PD.

7. Acknowledgment

The authors acknowledge Cephalon for supporting the study on armodafinil by kindly providing the investigational drug. We are sincerely grateful to all the patients who volunteered in the authors' own works presented here with their enthusiasm and support. The first author is grateful to Mrs. Jamika Singleton Garvin for her administrative assistance and exceptional organization of the authors' own studies cited. The second author wishes to thank Fiscellus Mons for the valuable support and inspiration.

8. References

Aarsland, D.; Bronnick, K. & Fladby, T. (2011). Mild Cognitive Impairment in Parkinson's Disease, *Curr Neurol Neurosci Rep*, pp., ISSN 1534-6293

Aarsland, D.; Laake, K.; Larsen, J.P. & Janvin, C. (2002). Donepezil for cognitive impairment in Parkinson's disease: a randomised controlled study, *J Neurol Neurosurg Psychiatry*, Vol.72, No.6, pp. 708-712, ISSN 0022-3050

Aarsland, D.; Litvan, I.; Salmon, D.; Galasko, D.; Wentzel-Larsen, T. & Larsen, J.P. (2003). Performance on the dementia rating scale in Parkinson's disease with dementia and dementia with Lewy bodies: comparison with progressive supranuclear palsy and Alzheimer's disease, *J Neurol Neurosurg Psychiatry*, Vol.74, No.9, pp. 1215-1220, ISSN 0022-3050

Aarsland, D.; Perry, R.; Brown, A.; Larsen, J.P. & Ballard, C. (2005). Neuropathology of dementia in Parkinson's disease: a prospective, community-based study, *Ann Neurol*, Vol.58, No.5, pp. 773-776, ISSN 0364-5134

Adler, C.H.; Caviness, J.N.; Hentz, J.G.; Lind, M. & Tiede, J. (2003). Randomized trial of modafinil for treating subjective daytime sleepiness in patients with Parkinson's disease, *Mov Disord*, Vol.18, No.3, pp. 287-293, ISSN 0885-3185

Alexander, G.E.; DeLong, M.R. & Strick, P.L. (1986). Parallel organization of functionally segregated circuits linking basal ganglia and cortex, *Annu Rev Neurosci*, Vol.9, pp. 357-381, ISSN 0147-006X

Apaydin, H.; Ahlskog, J.E.; Parisi, J.E.; Boeve, B.F. & Dickson, D.W. (2002). Parkinson disease neuropathology: later-developing dementia and loss of the levodopa response, *Arch Neurol*, Vol.59, No.1, pp. 102-112, ISSN 0003-9942

Baddeley, A. (1996). The fractionation of working memory, *Proc Natl Acad Sci U S A*, Vol.93, No.24, pp. 13468-13472, ISSN 0027-8424

Ballard, C.G.; Aarsland, D.; McKeith, I.; O'Brien, J.; Gray, A.; Cormack, F.; Burn, D.; Cassidy, T.; Starfeldt, R.; Larsen, J.P.; Brown, R. & Tovee, M. (2002). Fluctuations in attention: PD dementia vs DLB with parkinsonism, *Neurology*, Vol.59, No.11, pp. 1714-1720, ISSN 0028-3878

Barber, P.A.; Varma, A.R.; Lloyd, J.J.; Haworth, B.; Snowden, J.S. & Neary, D. (2000). The electroencephalogram in dementia with Lewy bodies, *Acta Neurol Scand*, Vol.101, No.1, pp. 53-56, ISSN 0001-6314

Bonanni, L.; Thomas, A.; Tiraboschi, P.; Perfetti, B.; Varanese, S. & Onofrj, M. (2008). EEG comparisons in early Alzheimer's disease, dementia with Lewy bodies and Parkinson's disease with dementia patients with a 2-year follow-up, *Brain*, Vol.131, No.Pt 3, pp. 690-705, ISSN 1460-2156

Bowen, F.P.; Kamienny, R.S.; Burns, M.M. & Yahr, M. (1975). Parkinsonism: effects of levodopa treatment on concept formation, *Neurology*, Vol.25, No.8, pp. 701-704, ISSN 0028-3878

Braak, H.; Rub, U.; Jansen Steur, E.N.; Del Tredici, K. & de Vos, R.A. (2005). Cognitive status correlates with neuropathologic stage in Parkinson disease, *Neurology*, Vol.64, No.8, pp. 1404-1410, ISSN 1526-632X

Bradley, V.A.; Welch, J.L. & Dick, D.J. (1989). Visuospatial working memory in Parkinson's disease, *J Neurol Neurosurg Psychiatry*, Vol.52, No.11, pp. 1228-1235, ISSN 0022-3050

Bradshaw, J.; Saling, M.; Hopwood, M.; Anderson, V. & Brodtmann, A. (2004). Fluctuating cognition in dementia with Lewy bodies and Alzheimer's disease is qualitatively distinct, *J Neurol Neurosurg Psychiatry*, Vol.75, No.3, pp. 382-387, ISSN 0022-3050

Briel, R.C.; McKeith, I.G.; Barker, W.A.; Hewitt, Y.; Perry, R.H.; Ince, P.G. & Fairbairn, A.F. (1999). EEG findings in dementia with Lewy bodies and Alzheimer's disease, *J Neurol Neurosurg Psychiatry*, Vol.66, No.3, pp. 401-403, ISSN 0022-3050

Burgess, P.W.; Alderman, N.; Forbes, C.; Costello, A.; Coates, L.M.; Dawson, D.R.; Anderson, N.D.; Gilbert, S.J.; Dumontheil, I. & Channon, S. (2006). The case for the development and use of "ecologically valid" measures of executive function in experimental and clinical neuropsychology, *J Int Neuropsychol Soc*, Vol.12, No.2, pp. 194-209, ISSN 1355-6177

Burton, E.J.; McKeith, I.G.; Burn, D.J.; Williams, E.D. & O'Brien, J.T. (2004). Cerebral atrophy in Parkinson's disease with and without dementia: a comparison with Alzheimer's disease, dementia with Lewy bodies and controls, *Brain*, Vol.127, No.Pt 4, pp. 791-800, ISSN 0006-8950

Byrne, E.J.; Lennox, G.; Lowe, J. & Godwin-Austen, R.B. (1989). Diffuse Lewy body disease: clinical features in 15 cases, *J Neurol Neurosurg Psychiatry*, Vol.52, No.6, pp. 709-717, ISSN 0022-3050

Carlesimo, G.A.; Perri, R.; Turriziani, P.; Tomaiuolo, F. & Caltagirone, C. (2001). Remembering what but not where: independence of spatial and visual working memory in the human brain, *Cortex*, Vol.37, No.4, pp. 519-534, ISSN 0010-9452

Cash, R.; Dennis, T.; L'Heureux, R.; Raisman, R.; Javoy-Agid, F. & Scatton, B. (1987). Parkinson's disease and dementia: norepinephrine and dopamine in locus ceruleus, *Neurology*, Vol.37, No.1, pp. 42-46, ISSN 0028-3878

Cools, R.; Barker, R.A.; Sahakian, B.J. & Robbins, T.W. (2001). Enhanced or impaired cognitive function in Parkinson's disease as a function of dopaminergic medication and task demands, *Cereb Cortex*, Vol.11, No.12, pp. 1136-1143, ISSN 1047-3211

Cools, R.; Barker, R.A.; Sahakian, B.J. & Robbins, T.W. (2003). L-Dopa medication remediates cognitive inflexibility, but increases impulsivity in patients with Parkinson's disease, *Neuropsychologia*, Vol.41, No.11, pp. 1431-1441, ISSN 0028-3932

Cooper, J.A.; Sagar, H.J.; Jordan, N.; Harvey, N.S. & Sullivan, E.V. (1991). Cognitive impairment in early, untreated Parkinson's disease and its relationship to motor disability, *Brain*, Vol.114 (Pt 5), pp. 2095-2122, ISSN 0006-8950

Costa, A.; Peppe, A.; Dell'Agnello, G.; Caltagirone, C. & Carlesimo, G.A. (2009). Dopamine and cognitive functioning in de novo subjects with Parkinson's disease: effects of pramipexole and pergolide on working memory, *Neuropsychologia*, Vol.47, No.5, pp. 1374-1381, ISSN 0028-3932

Dagher, A.; Owen, A.M.; Boecker, H. & Brooks, D.J. (2001). The role of the striatum and hippocampus in planning: a PET activation study in Parkinson's disease, *Brain*, Vol.124, No.Pt 5, pp. 1020-1032, ISSN 0006-8950

Delis, D.; Kramer, J.; Kaplan, E. & Ober, B. (2002). *California verbal learning test second edition* Psychological Corporation, ISBN San Antonio, TX

Dubois, B. & Pillon, B. (1997). Cognitive deficits in Parkinson's disease, *J Neurol*, Vol.244, No.1, pp. 2-8, ISSN 0340-5354

Dubois, B.; Ruberg, M.; Javoy-Agid, F.; Ploska, A. & Agid, Y. (1983). A subcortico-cortical cholinergic system is affected in Parkinson's disease, *Brain Res*, Vol.288, No.1-2, pp. 213-218, ISSN 0006-8993

Emre, M. (2003). Dementia associated with Parkinson's disease, *Lancet Neurol*, Vol.2, No.4, pp. 229-237, ISSN 1474-4422

Emre, M.; Aarsland, D.; Albanese, A.; Byrne, E.J.; Deuschl, G.; De Deyn, P.P.; Durif, F.; Kulisevsky, J.; van Laar, T.; Lees, A.; Poewe, W.; Robillard, A.; Rosa, M.M.; Wolters, E.; Quarg, P.; Tekin, S. & Lane, R. (2004). Rivastigmine for dementia associated with Parkinson's disease, *N Engl J Med*, Vol.351, No.24, pp. 2509-2518, ISSN 1533-4406

Eslinger, P.J. & Damasio, A.R. (1985). Severe disturbance of higher cognition after bilateral frontal lobe ablation: patient EVR, *Neurology*, Vol.35, No.12, pp. 1731-1741, ISSN 0028-3878

Farrer, M.; Kachergus, J.; Forno, L.; Lincoln, S.; Wang, D.S.; Hulihan, M.; Maraganore, D.; Gwinn-Hardy, K.; Wszolek, Z.; Dickson, D. & Langston, J.W. (2004). Comparison of kindreds with parkinsonism and alpha-synuclein genomic multiplications, *Ann Neurol*, Vol.55, No.2, pp. 174-179, ISSN 0364-5134

Firbank, M.J.; Colloby, S.J.; Burn, D.J.; McKeith, I.G. & O'Brien, J.T. (2003). Regional cerebral blood flow in Parkinson's disease with and without dementia, *Neuroimage*, Vol.20, No.2, pp. 1309-1319, ISSN 1053-8119

Foltynie, T.; Brayne, C.E.; Robbins, T.W. & Barker, R.A. (2004a). The cognitive ability of an incident cohort of Parkinson's patients in the UK. The CamPaIGN study, *Brain*, Vol.127, No.Pt 3, pp. 550-560, ISSN 0006-8950

Foltynie, T.; Goldberg, T.E.; Lewis, S.G.; Blackwell, A.D.; Kolachana, B.S.; Weinberger, D.R.; Robbins, T.W. & Barker, R.A. (2004b). Planning ability in Parkinson's disease is influenced by the COMT val158met polymorphism, *Mov Disord*, Vol.19, No.8, pp. 885-891, ISSN 0885-3185

Gauggel, S.; Rieger, M. & Feghoff, T.A. (2004). Inhibition of ongoing responses in patients with Parkinson's disease, *J Neurol Neurosurg Psychiatry*, Vol.75, No.4, pp. 539-544, ISSN 0022-3050

Gibb, W.R.; Esiri, M.M. & Lees, A.J. (1987). Clinical and pathological features of diffuse cortical Lewy body disease (Lewy body dementia), *Brain*, Vol.110 (Pt 5), pp. 1131-1153, ISSN 0006-8950

Heaton, R.K.; Chelune, G.; Talley, J.; Kay, G. & Curtiss, G. (1993). *Wisconsin Card Sorting Test Manual. Revised and Expanded* Psychological Assessment Resources, Inc., ISBN FL

Hietanen, M. & Teravainen, H. (1986). Cognitive performance in early Parkinson's disease, *Acta Neurol Scand*, Vol.73, No.2, pp. 151-159, ISSN 0001-6314

Hirshkowitz, M.; Black, J.E.; Wesnes, K.; Niebler, G.; Arora, S. & Roth, T. (2007). Adjunct armodafinil improves wakefulness and memory in obstructive sleep apnea/hypopnea syndrome, *Respir Med*, Vol.101, No.3, pp. 616-627, ISSN 0954-6111

Huber, S.J.; Shuttleworth, E.C. & Freidenberg, D.L. (1989). Neuropsychological differences between the dementias of Alzheimer's and Parkinson's diseases, *Arch Neurol*, Vol.46, No.12, pp. 1287-1291, ISSN 0003-9942

Kehagia, A.A.; Barker, R.A. & Robbins, T.W. (2010). Neuropsychological and clinical heterogeneity of cognitive impairment and dementia in patients with Parkinson's disease, *Lancet Neurol*, Vol.9, No.12, pp. 1200-1213, ISSN 1474-4465

Klauer, K.C. & Zhao, Z. (2004). Double dissociations in visual and spatial short-term memory, *J Exp Psychol Gen*, Vol.133, No.3, pp. 355-381, ISSN 0096-3445

Kovari, E.; Gold, G.; Herrmann, F.R.; Canuto, A.; Hof, P.R.; Bouras, C. & Giannakopoulos, P. (2003). Lewy body densities in the entorhinal and anterior cingulate cortex predict cognitive deficits in Parkinson's disease, *Acta Neuropathol*, Vol.106, No.1, pp. 83-88, ISSN 0001-6322

Lange, K.W.; Robbins, T.W.; Marsden, C.D.; James, M.; Owen, A.M. & Paul, G.M. (1992). L-dopa withdrawal in Parkinson's disease selectively impairs cognitive performance in tests sensitive to frontal lobe dysfunction, *Psychopharmacology (Berl)*, Vol.107, No.2-3, pp. 394-404, ISSN 0033-3158

Leroi, I.; Brandt, J.; Reich, S.G.; Lyketsos, C.G.; Grill, S.; Thompson, R. & Marsh, L. (2004). Randomized placebo-controlled trial of donepezil in cognitive impairment in Parkinson's disease, *Int J Geriatr Psychiatry*, Vol.19, No.1, pp. 1-8, ISSN 0885-6230

Levin, B.E. & Katzen, H.L. (2005). Early cognitive changes and nondementing behavioral abnormalities in Parkinson's disease, *Adv Neurol*, Vol.96, pp. 84-94, ISSN 0091-3952

Lewis, S.J.; Cools, R.; Robbins, T.W.; Dove, A.; Barker, R.A. & Owen, A.M. (2003a). Using executive heterogeneity to explore the nature of working memory deficits in Parkinson's disease, *Neuropsychologia*, Vol.41, No.6, pp. 645-654, ISSN 0028-3932 0028-3932 (Linking)

Lewis, S.J.; Dove, A.; Robbins, T.W.; Barker, R.A. & Owen, A.M. (2003b). Cognitive impairments in early Parkinson's disease are accompanied by reductions in activity in frontostriatal neural circuitry, *J Neurosci*, Vol.23, No.15, pp. 6351-6356, ISSN 1529-2401 0270-6474 (Linking)

Lewis, S.J.; Slabosz, A.; Robbins, T.W.; Barker, R.A. & Owen, A.M. (2005). Dopaminergic basis for deficits in working memory but not attentional set-shifting in Parkinson's disease, *Neuropsychologia*, Vol.43, No.6, pp. 823-832, ISSN 0028-3932

Lezak, M. (1995). *Neuropsychological Assessment* Oxford unversity Press, ISBN 9780470747230, New York

Litvan, I.; MacIntyre, A.; Goetz, C.G.; Wenning, G.K.; Jellinger, K.; Verny, M.; Bartko, J.J.; Jankovic, J.; McKee, A.; Brandel, J.P.; Chaudhuri, K.R.; Lai, E.C.; D'Olhaberriague, L.; Pearce, R.K. & Agid, Y. (1998). Accuracy of the clinical diagnoses of Lewy body disease, Parkinson disease, and dementia with Lewy bodies: a clinicopathologic study, *Arch Neurol*, Vol.55, No.7, pp. 969-978, ISSN 0003-9942

Lopez, O.L.; Litvan, I.; Catt, K.E.; Stowe, R.; Klunk, W.; Kaufer, D.I.; Becker, J.T. & DeKosky, S.T. (1999). Accuracy of four clinical diagnostic criteria for the diagnosis of neurodegenerative dementias, *Neurology*, Vol.53, No.6, pp. 1292-1299, ISSN 0028-3878

Mattay, V.S.; Tessitore, A.; Callicott, J.H.; Bertolino, A.; Goldberg, T.E.; Chase, T.N.; Hyde, T.M. & Weinberger, D.R. (2002). Dopaminergic modulation of cortical function in patients with Parkinson's disease, *Ann Neurol*, Vol.51, No.2, pp. 156-164, ISSN 0364-5134

Mattila, P.M.; Rinne, J.O.; Helenius, H.; Dickson, D.W. & Roytta, M. (2000). Alpha-synuclein-immunoreactive cortical Lewy bodies are associated with cognitive impairment in Parkinson's disease, *Acta Neuropathol*, Vol.100, No.3, pp. 285-290, ISSN 0001-6322

Mayeux, R.; Chen, J.; Mirabello, E.; Marder, K.; Bell, K.; Dooneief, G.; Cote, L. & Stern, Y. (1990). An estimate of the incidence of dementia in idiopathic Parkinson's disease, *Neurology*, Vol.40, No.10, pp. 1513-1517, ISSN 0028-3878

Mega, M.S.; Masterman, D.L.; Benson, D.F.; Vinters, H.V.; Tomiyasu, U.; Craig, A.H.; Foti, D.J.; Kaufer, D.; Scharre, D.W.; Fairbanks, L. & Cummings, J.L. (1996). Dementia with Lewy bodies: reliability and validity of clinical and pathologic criteria, *Neurology*, Vol.47, No.6, pp. 1403-1409, ISSN 0028-3878

Miyake, A.; Emerson, M.J. & Friedman, N.P. (2000a). Assessment of executive functions in clinical settings: Problems and recommendations, *Semin Speech Lang*, Vol. 21, pp. 169-183, ISSN 0734-0478

Miyake, A.; Friedman, N.P.; Emerson, M.J.; Witzki, A.H.; Howerter, A. & Wager, T.D. (2000b). The unity and diversity of executive functions and their contributions to complex "Frontal Lobe" tasks: a latent variable analysis, *Cogn Psychol*, Vol.41, No.1, pp. 49-100, ISSN 0010-0285

Norman, W. & Shallice, T. (1986). Attention to action, In: *Consciousness and self regulation: Advances in research and theory, vol. 4.*, R. Davidson; G. Schwartz & D. Shapiro (Ed.)^(Eds.), pp. 1–18, Plenum, ISBN 9780306412141, New York

Onofrj, M.; Thomas, A.; Iacono, D.; Luciano, A.L. & Di Iorio, A. (2003). The effects of a cholinesterase inhibitor are prominent in patients with fluctuating cognition: a part 3 study of the main mechanism of cholinesterase inhibitors in dementia, *Clin Neuropharmacol*, Vol.26, No.5, pp. 239-251, ISSN 0362-5664

Owen, A.M. (2000). The role of the lateral frontal cortex in mnemonic processing: the contribution of functional neuroimaging, *Exp Brain Res*, Vol.133, No.1, pp. 33-43, ISSN 0014-4819

Owen, A.M. (2004). Cognitive dysfunction in Parkinson's disease: the role of frontostriatal circuitry, *Neuroscientist*, Vol.10, No.6, pp. 525-537, ISSN 1073-8584

Owen, A.M.; Beksinska, M.; James, M.; Leigh, P.N.; Summers, B.A.; Marsden, C.D.; Quinn, N.P.; Sahakian, B.J. & Robbins, T.W. (1993). Visuospatial memory deficits at different stages of Parkinson's disease, *Neuropsychologia*, Vol.31, No.7, pp. 627-644, ISSN 0028-3932

Owen, A.M.; James, M.; Leigh, P.N.; Summers, B.A.; Marsden, C.D.; Quinn, N.P.; Lange, K.W. & Robbins, T.W. (1992). Frontostriatal cognitive deficits at different stages of Parkinson's disease, *Brain*, Vol.115 (Pt 6), pp. 1727-1751, ISSN 0006-8950

Perfetti, B.; Varanese, S.; Mercuri, P.; Mancino, E.; Saggino, A. & Onofrj, M. (2010). Behavioural assessment of dysexecutive syndrome in Parkinson's disease without dementia: a comparison with other clinical executive tasks, *Parkinsonism Relat Disord*, Vol.16, No.1, pp. 46-50, ISSN 1873-5126

Perry, E.K.; Curtis, M.; Dick, D.J.; Candy, J.M.; Atack, J.R.; Bloxham, C.A.; Blessed, G.; Fairbairn, A.; Tomlinson, B.E. & Perry, R.H. (1985). Cholinergic correlates of cognitive impairment in Parkinson's disease: comparisons with Alzheimer's disease, *J Neurol Neurosurg Psychiatry*, Vol.48, No.5, pp. 413-421, ISSN 0022-3050

Petrova, M.; Raycheva, M.; Zhelev, Y. & Traykov, L. (2010). Executive functions deficit in Parkinson's disease with amnestic mild cognitive impairment, *Am J Alzheimers Dis Other Demen*, Vol.25, No.5, pp. 455-460, ISSN 1938-2731

Pillon, B.; Deweer, B.; Agid, Y. & Dubois, B. (1993). Explicit memory in Alzheimer's, Huntington's, and Parkinson's diseases, *Arch Neurol*, Vol.50, No.4, pp. 374-379, ISSN 0003-9942

Poirier, J. (2002). Evidence that the clinical effects of cholinesterase inhibitors are related to potency and targeting of action, *Int J Clin Pract Suppl*, No.127, pp. 6-19, ISSN 1368-504X

Ravina, B.; Marder, K.; Fernandez, H.H.; Friedman, J.H.; McDonald, W.; Murphy, D.; Aarsland, D.; Babcock, D.; Cummings, J.; Endicott, J.; Factor, S.; Galpern, W.; Lees, A.; Marsh, L.; Stacy, M.; Gwinn-Hardy, K.; Voon, V. & Goetz, C. (2007). Diagnostic criteria for psychosis in Parkinson's disease: report of an NINDS, NIMH work group, *Mov Disord*, Vol.22, No.8, pp. 1061-1068, ISSN 0885-3185

Scatton, B.; Javoy-Agid, F.; Rouquier, L.; Dubois, B. & Agid, Y. (1983). Reduction of cortical dopamine, noradrenaline, serotonin and their metabolites in Parkinson's disease, *Brain Res*, Vol.275, No.2, pp. 321-328, ISSN 0006-8993

Serrano, C. & Garcia-Borreguero, D. (2004). Fluctuations in cognition and alertness in Parkinson's disease and dementia, *Neurology*, Vol.63, No.8 Suppl 3, pp. S31-34, ISSN 1526-632X

Shallice, T. (1982). Specific impairments of planning, *Philos Trans R Soc Lond B Biol Sci*, Vol.298, No.1089, pp. 199-209, ISSN 0962-8436

Shallice, T. & Burgess, P.W. (1991). Deficits in strategy application following frontal lobe damage in man, *Brain*, Vol.114 (Pt 2), pp. 727-741, ISSN 0006-8950

Singleton, A.B.; Farrer, M.; Johnson, J.; Singleton, A.; Hague, S.; Kachergus, J.; Hulihan, M.; Peuralinna, T.; Dutra, A.; Nussbaum, R.; Lincoln, S.; Crawley, A.; Hanson, M.; Maraganore, D.; Adler, C.; Cookson, M.R.; Muenter, M.; Baptista, M.; Miller, D.; Blancato, J.; Hardy, J. & Gwinn-Hardy, K. (2003). alpha-Synuclein locus triplication causes Parkinson's disease, *Science*, Vol.302, No.5646, pp. 841, ISSN 1095-9203

Spitoni, G.; Antonucci, A.; Orsini, A.; D'Olimpio, F. & Cantagallo, A. (2002). A first step to assess different components of executive processes. *Proceedings of 3rd WorldCongress in Neurological Rehabilitation*, Venice, Italy, April 2-6

Stern, Y. & Langston, J.W. (1985). Intellectual changes in patients with MPTP-induced parkinsonism, *Neurology*, Vol.35, No.10, pp. 1506-1509, ISSN 0028-3878

Stern, Y.; Mayeux, R.; Rosen, J. & Ilson, J. (1983). Perceptual motor dysfunction in Parkinson's disease: a deficit in sequential and predictive voluntary movement, *J Neurol Neurosurg Psychiatry*, Vol.46, No.2, pp. 145-151, ISSN 0022-3050

Stern, Y.; Tetrud, J.W.; Martin, W.R.; Kutner, S.J. & Langston, J.W. (1990). Cognitive change following MPTP exposure, *Neurology*, Vol.40, No.2, pp. 261-264, ISSN 0028-3878

Varanese, S.; Perfetti, B.; Ghilardi, M.F. & Di Rocco, A. (2011). Apathy, but not depression, reflects inefficient cognitive strategies in Parkinson's disease, *PLoS One*, Vol.6, No.3, pp. e17846, ISSN 1932-6203

Varanese, S.; Perfetti, B.; Monaco, D.; Thomas, A.; Bonanni, L.; Tiraboschi, P. & Onofrj, M. (2010). Fluctuating cognition and different cognitive and behavioural profiles in Parkinson's disease with dementia: comparison of dementia with Lewy bodies and Alzheimer's disease, *J Neurol*, Vol.257, No.6, pp. 1004-1011, ISSN 1432-1459

Vingerhoets, G.; Verleden, S.; Santens, P.; Miatton, M. & De Reuck, J. (2003). Predictors of cognitive impairment in advanced Parkinson's disease, *J Neurol Neurosurg Psychiatry*, Vol.74, No.6, pp. 793-796, ISSN 0022-3050

Walker, M.P.; Ayre, G.A.; Cummings, J.L.; Wesnes, K.; McKeith, I.G.; O'Brien, J.T. & Ballard, C.G. (2000a). The Clinician Assessment of Fluctuation and the One Day Fluctuation Assessment Scale. Two methods to assess fluctuating confusion in dementia, *Br J Psychiatry*, Vol.177, pp. 252-256, ISSN 0007-1250

Walker, M.P.; Ayre, G.A.; Cummings, J.L.; Wesnes, K.; McKeith, I.G.; O'Brien, J.T. & Ballard, C.G. (2000b). Quantifying fluctuation in dementia with Lewy bodies, Alzheimer's disease, and vascular dementia, *Neurology*, Vol.54, No.8, pp. 1616-1625, ISSN 0028-3878

Williams-Gray, C.H.; Goris, A.; Foltynie, T.; Brown, J.; Maranian, M.; Walton, A.; Compston, D.A.; Sawcer, S.J. & Barker, R.A. (2006). Prevalence of the LRRK2 G2019S mutation in a UK community based idiopathic Parkinson's disease cohort, *J Neurol Neurosurg Psychiatry*, Vol.77, No.5, pp. 665-667, ISSN 0022-3050

Williams-Gray, C.H.; Goris, A.; Saiki, M.; Foltynie, T.; Compston, D.A.; Sawcer, S.J. & Barker, R.A. (2009). Apolipoprotein E genotype as a risk factor for susceptibility to and dementia in Parkinson's disease, *J Neurol*, Vol.256, No.3, pp. 493-498, ISSN 1432-1459

Wilson, B.A.; Alderman, N.; Burgess, P.; Emslie, H. & Evans, J.J. (1996). *Behavioural assessment of the dysexecutive syndrome: test manual* Thames Valley Test Company, ISBN Edmunds, England

Wong, Y.N.; Simcoe, D.; Hartman, L.N.; Laughton, W.B.; King, S.P.; McCormick, G.C. & Grebow, P.E. (1999). A double-blind, placebo-controlled, ascending-dose evaluation of the pharmacokinetics and tolerability of modafinil tablets in healthy male volunteers, *J Clin Pharmacol*, Vol.39, No.1, pp. 30-40, ISSN 0091-2700

2

Cognition and Gait Disturbances in Parkinson's Disease

Samo Ribarič
University of Ljubljana, Faculty of Medicine, Institute of Pathophysiology & University Clinical Centre Ljubljana, Departemnet of Neurology, Laboratory for Movement Disorders Slovenia

1. Introduction

Gait is a learned, complex and almost automatic task with limited involvement of cognitive control in healthy individuals until the onset of old age (Holtzer et al., 2006). These automatic and rhythmic motor activity patterns are generated by spinal networks of motor neurons and interneurons, also called the "central pattern generators" (Dietz, 2003). The activity of these spinal networks is modulated and initiated by the basal ganglia and the brainstem nuclei (Pahapill & Lozano, 2000). The basal ganglia and their two-way connections with cortical regions and cerebellum (Fig. 1) play a central role in both movement initiation and cognitive aspects, such as executive functioning (Yogev-Seligman et al., 2008). Pathological oscillatory activity in these networks, for example in Parkinson's disease (PD), is associated with gait disorders (Bartolić et al., 2010; Timmermann & Fink 2009).

Recent studies have established the importance of cognitive control on gait in older adults; gait slowing is more prevalent in people with cognitive impairment and slow gait in healthy older adults is associated with a higher risk of cognitive impairment, including dementia (Holtzer et al., 2006). Also a slow gait velocity has been associated with an increased risk of falls, hospitalization and mortality (Verghese et al., 2010). Therefore, with the progression of age related changes or neurodegenerative changes in the brain (*e.g.* in PD), previously automatic actions like gait become a "controlled" processes placing additional demands on the available shrinking cognitive resources. Under these circumstances, the performance of the cognitive task may only be preserved by diverting cognitive resources from the motor task.

In adults, the contribution of cognitive control to gait is evaluated by measuring the effect that a cognitive load (e.g. simultaneous talking or counting while walking) has on gait – *i.e.* the dual task (DT) paradigm (Srygley et al., 2009). The effect of DT on gait velocity (DT decrement) is related to impairments in executive function and attention. The extent of DT decrement varies from non-existent to detectable in healthy older adults, but can be significant in patients with PD (PPD). Therefore, the presence and extent of DT decrement in PPD depends on the patient's cognitive reserve and the complexity of gait pattern. Postural instability and gait disorders in PD are associated with a faster rate of cognitive decline and should be considered as risk factors for developing Parkinson's disease with dementia

(Korczyn, 2001). The assessment of DT decrement is important for detecting the early stages of cognitive impairment in PPD, when isolation of specific cognitive factors which impact mobility is still possible, since progression of the disease leads to global cognitive impairment (Holtzer et al., 2006). The interference of the attention-demanding task (*e.g.* simultaneous talking or counting while walking) with gait suggests that both tasks rely on the same functional subsystem (*i.e.* executive function and attention).

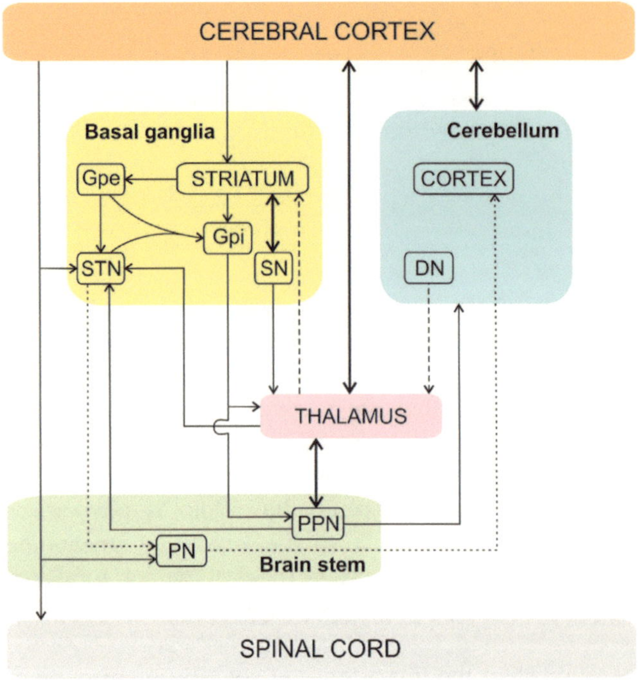

Fig. 1. Major connections of basal ganglia with brain structures. Abbreviations: DN (dentate nucleus), Gpe (external segment of the globus pallidus), Gpi (internal segment of the globus pallidus, PPN (pedunculopontine nucleus), PN (pontine nucleus), SN (substantia nigra), STN (subthalamic nucleus). Doted lines mark the connections between cerebellum and basal ganglia. SN is anatomically part of the brainstem and functionally part of the basal ganglia. The STN is anatomically part of the subthalamus but functionally part of the basal ganglia. The basal ganglia and the cerebellum form multisynaptic loops with the cerebral cortex. Recently, a disynaptic projection between the output nuclei of the cerebellum (the DN) and the input stage of basal ganglia processing (the striatum) was identified (Hoshi et al., 2005) and a return pathway from the STN projecting to the cerebellar cortex (via the PN) was also described (Bostan et al., 2010). These disynaptic connections between the basal ganglia and the cerebellum could have functional importance for human movement and cognition.

Cognitive motor interference in PPD is clinically important since assessment and monitoring of a person's DT performance contributes to assessment of the patient's everyday motor ability, to informed goal setting and to treatment planning (Morris et al., 2010). The level of DT interference, and the precise conditions and task combinations under which it occurs, may vary between patients and over time. Motor tasks performed under DT conditions provide a better index of the patient's functional everyday ability than a motor task performed under a single task condition since everyday activities often involve concurrent cognitive and motor components (Yogev-Seligman et al., 2008). To summarize, understanding the nature, prevalence, and prognosis of DT decrements is important for assessment and rehabilitation of the PPD.

2. Dual tasking and gait

Gait is a complex form of motor behavior that is influenced by mental processes under normal and pathological conditions. The contribution of cognition to gait is particulary evident in PPD with gait disorders who have a reduced ability to perform multiple tasks simultaneously, either because the central processing abilities have become too limited, or because patients fail to properly prioritize their balance control over other less important tasks (Bloem et al., 2006; Yogev-Seligman et al., 2008).

The higher cognitive processes, that use and modify information from different brain regions to modulate and produce behavior, are collectively known as executive function (Yogev-Seligman et al., 2008). The executive function (EF) integrates cognitive and behavioral components necessary for effective, goal-directed actions and for the control of intentional resources thus enabling the human being to manage independent daily activities (Stuss & Alexander, 2000; Stuss & Levine, 2002). The major components of EF are intentional behavior, self-awareness, planning, action monitoring, attention with DT and response inhibition (Stuss et al., 2000). The anterior parts of the frontal lobes deal with aspects of self-regulation (*e.g.* inhibition and self-awareness) and the dorsal parts deal with reasoning processes. Impairment of one or more of EF components reduces the ability to walk efficiently and safely (Yogev-Seligman et al., 2008). For example, poor self-awareness of limitations, an aspect of impaired volition, increases the risk of falling in elderly patients with dementia (van Iersel et al., 2006) or a reduced capacity to perform DT predisposes the PPD and gait disorders to freezing of gait and falls (see Section 3 for details). The concept that a specific component of the EF can be linked to a discrete brain region is a simplification since neuroimaging studies attempting to localize the activity of EF report inconsistent findings (Alvarez & Emory, 2006; Stuss & Alexander, 2000). This would suggest that connections amomg the frontal lobes and other cortical and subcortical brain regions are as important to the EF as discrete regions of the frontal lobes and that information sharing between brain regions depends on the specific task that is dealt with by the EF. For example, different EF tasks activate different frontal and parietal areas and also other areas of the brain (Collette et al., 2006). A practical implication of these facts is that patients without frontal lesions could, in theory, display clinical signs of impaired EF (Yogev-Seligman et al., 2008).

Age related changes to the frontal lobes (Craik & Grady, 2002) include lesions of diffused white matter, which might affect fronto-striatal circuits and impair EF (Buckner, 2004). White matter hyper-intensities on magnetic resonance imaging were associated with a decline of EF, but not with the level of general intelligence (Gunning-Dixon & Raz, 2003). Loss of dentritic branching in the prefrontal cortex is also associated with a decline in performance on EF tests (Burke & Barnes, 2006). Age-associated decline in dopaminergic activity in the frontal areas is also related to poorer performance on executive tasks (Burke & Barnes, 2006; Gunning-Dixon & Raz, 2003). EF is generally persevered in healthy and normal aging, with the exception of, for example attention, that shows a subtle decline (Yogev-Seligman et al., 2008). However, there is a great variability in frontal brain changes among aging individuals in terms of the magnitude, age when changes occur, and the influence of education and lifestyle (Buckner, 2004). Therefore cognitive evaluation should include the individual's ability to carry out independent daily activities that tax the EF.

The relationship between EF and gait performance, in 926 older adults with a normal cognitive function, was reported by Ble and coworkers (Ble et al., 2005). They evaluated the effect of DT, simultaneous walking over an obstacle course and solving a Trail Making Test (TMT) (*i.e.* testing cognitive flexibility), in non-demented older adults. Poor and moderate performance on the TMT was associated with decreased gait speed on the obstacle course, although the mean speeds in all three groups were within normal limits. The conclusion of the study was that EF is independently associated with tasks of lower extremity function that require high intentional demand (*i.e.* DT). Similar results were reported in a study that evaluated the association between gait velocity and cognitive function in 186 cognitively normal elders (Holtzer et al., 2006). Holtzer and coworkers reported on the associations between speed of processing, attention, memory, language and EF on the one hand and gait velocity on the other. EF and memory were correlated with gait speed under DT conditions but verbal IQ was not (Holtzer et al., 2006).

The effect of DT on gait is substantially larger in patients with stroke, Parkinson's disease or Alzheimer's disease than in healthy, age-matched groups (Yogev-Seligman et al., 2008). These pathological conditions of the brain are well known to degrade EF and to reduce the ability to divide attention (Albert, 1996; Baddeley et al., 2001; Bedard et al., 1998; Buckner, 2004; Dubois & Pillon, 1997). In addition, these patients have an altered, less automatic walking pattern suggesting a larger involment of EF in the execution of gait during normal daily activities (Baltadjieva et al., 2006; Giladi & Nieuwboer, 2008; Nakamura et al., 1996; Rochester et al., 2004; Schaafsma et al., 2003). Therefore, when the ability of the EF to perform dual tasking is overcome in PPD, this can be initially observed as a a slower gait speed, shorter strides, increased double support time, increased stride-to-stride variability (Yogev et al., 2005; Plotnik et al., 2008, 2009, 2011a,b) and ultimately as freezing of gait and falls.

DT elicited falls are not unique to PD. Lundin-Olsson and coworkers reported that older adults who could not "walk and talk" had a high incidence of falls, while those subjects who could walk and talk were much less prone to future falls (Lundin-Olsson et al., 1997). The participants in this study were able to walk with or without aids and able to follow simple instructions. The most common diagnoses in this group of older adults were dementia, depression and previous stroke (Lundin-Olsson et al., 1997).

The human brain has a default, posture first prioritization, presumably an evolutionary trait to reduce the risk of falls, which can be demonstrated in experimental conditions (Yogev-Seligman et al., 2008). Healthy young adults and healthy elderly tend to give priority to the stability of gait when walking and performing a cognitive task (Bloem et al., 2001a,b). Brain areas associated with prioritization between motor and cognitive demands are the prefrontal cortex and the anterior cingulate cortex (Dreher & Grafman, 2003; MacDonald et al., 2000). In healthy adults dual tasking while walking reduces the quality of the concurrent non-walking task, but the gait pattern and stability remain normal (Gerin-Lajoie et al., 2005; Lindenberger et al., 2000; Schrodt et al., 2004). In contrast to healthy adults, PPD disease have a weakened "posture first" strategy which makes them prone to perform all tasks simultaneously thus increasing their risk of falling in dual tasking situations (Bloem et al., 2001 a,b). An independent contributing factor that also increases the risk of falling in PPD is impaired motor learning (Bloem et al., 2001a,b; Harrington et al., 1990; Heindel et al., 1989; Soliveri et al., 1997).

Recently, it has been demonstrated that the DT effect is stronger in PPD who have a high risk of gait instability and fall, compared to patients with PPD with a lower risk (Plotnik et al., 2011a,b). The conclusion of this study was that specific cognitive capacities (executive function and attention) are impaired among PPD who tend to fall. In addition, the DT effects on gait were observed even when the patients responded to therapy - were in the "on" phase.

The relationship between DT, cognitive function and specific properties of gait (*i.e.* general mobility, gait variability and bilateral gait function) was investigated among PPD suffering from motor response fluctuations during the "on" state (Plotnik et al., 2011b). The authors concluded that the degree to which these gait parameters deteriorated during DT (compared to usual walking) was correlated with the baseline levels of impaired motor and cognitive capacities and that this relationship was conserved even during optimal medication.

3. Gait disorders in Parkinsons disease

Parkinson disease is a common disorder among older adults with an incidence rate of 16 to 19 per 100,000 per year. Worldwide, about 6 million people are currently living with this progressive neurological condition (Twelves et al., 2003). Gait disorders are a distinctive characteristic of PD; a slow, short stepped shuffling and forward-stooped gait with asymmetrical arm swing (Morris et al., 2010). Gait disorder includes difficulties with the execution of well-learned movement sequences (*e.g.* walking, turning, writing, and transfers) and some people with PD report freezing, falls, cognitive impairment, and autonomic disturbances (Simuni & Sethi, 2008) which affect quality of life and participation in societal roles (Visser et al., 2009).

The clinically observed differences between tremor-dominant and postural instability subtypes of PD are reflected in cerebral blood flow changes during single photon emission computed tomography. Patients with postural instability and gait difficulty had hypoperfusion in the anterior cingulate cortex and primary visual cortex that was not observed in the tremor-dominant group of PPD. The observed frontal reduction in perfusion in patients with gait disorders is consistent with the expected frontal executive function deficits in these patients (Yogev-Seligman et al., 2008).

A recent meta-analysis of falling in PD (pooled sample size 473 patients) reported that the average 3-month fall rate was 46% (Pickering et al., 2007). Even among patients without prior falls, the fall rate was considerable (21%). The conclusion of the study is that all of the patients with PD have a substantial risk of falling, even when they have not fallen previously. Maximal treatment with levodopa does not prevent the occurence of falls, consistent with the hypothesis that axial disability in late stage Parkinson's disease is largely doparesistant - due to extranigral and nondopaminergic brain lesions (Boonstra et al., 2008; Hely et al., 2008). Two explanations were given for the perseverence of fallls and an increased risk of fractures in levodopa treated patients with PD. Levodopa could cause adverse effects that predispose patients to falls (*e.g.* violent dyskinesias, drug-induced orthostatic hypotension) or patients on levodopa become more mobile and therefore more prone to falls (Boonstra et al., 2008). That patient mobility can predispose to falls is consistent with the fact that fall rates decrease with disease progression, probably because patients become increasingly immobilized (Pickering et al., 2007).

3.1 Freezing of gait

Gait disorders, especially episodic gait disorders are particularly incapacitating because patients cannot easily adjust their behavior to these paroxysmal walking problems (Snijders et al., 2007). An important and extremely debilitating gait disorder is freezing of gait (FOG). FOG occurs when patients with PD experience episodes during which they are either unable to start walking or while walking, suddenly fail to continue moving forward. Because FOG is sudden and unpredictable, it is an important cause of falls and injuries and is also independently associated with a decreased quality of life (Moore et al., 2007a). FOG is not unique to PD and is a more common and an earlier feature in other parkinsonian syndromes (*e.g.* primary progressive freezing of gait, multisystem atrophy, pure akinesia, vascular parkinsonism, progressive supranuclear palsy, or dementia of Lewy body type); for a review see Thanvi and coworkers (Thanvi & Treadwell, 2010). A comprehensive definition of FOG that includes its paroxysmal nature, association with gait disorders, and the influence of various external and internal stimuli is that FOG is "an episodic inability to generate effective stepping in the absence of any known cause other than Parkinsonism or high level gait disorders. It is most commonly experienced during turning and step initiation but also when faced with spatial constraint, stress, and distraction. Focused attention and external stimuli can overcome the episode" (Giladi & Nieuwboer, 2008).

About half of patients with PD experience FOG and risk factors include male gender and an akinetic-rigid subtype of PD (Macht et al., 2007; Lamberti et al., 1997). FOG tends to appear only under certain situations for example at gait initiation, approaching a destination, passing through a narrow passage or on turning (Thanvi & Treadwell, 2010). Distraction or dual tasking during such situations (*e.g.* talking while walking, counting backwards or carrying a glass of water while walking) increase the incidence of FOG. Paradoxically, an intense external stimulus such as an alarm bell may briefly ameliorate freezing and patients develop visual or audio cues (Bloem et al., 2004a) to overcome FOG attacks (*e.g.* stepping over objects or walking to a music or a beat). The severity of FOG varies from forward shuffling with small step, to trembling in place, to total akinesia in "off " period.

Patients tend to under report FOG episodes in the outpatient consultation unless they are specifically asked about it (Thanvi & Treadwell, 2010). Thefore a FOG specific questionnaire, comparing patients' ratings with those of the carers', may be a useful aid to for a more realistic asssesment of FOG occurance (Nieuwboer et al., 2009). Patients usually experience FOG as brief episodes lasting for a few seconds when their walking suddenly comes to a halt, and they feel as though their feet are "glued" to the floor. With increasingn severity of FOG the patient moves forward shuffling with small steps, trembles in place or in most severe cases patients cannot move forward at all. The two unique features of FOG in PD are that FOG is often worse during the "off" state and rarely occurs in "on" state. FOG is common in the akinetic rigid variety of PD but can also occur in the tremor predominant type of PD (Lamberti et al., 1997).

Hausdorff and coworkers demonstrated that the ability to regulate stride-to-stride timing during gait is severely impaired in FOG patients compared with other individuals with Parkinson's disease (Hausdorf et al., 2003). Therefore, analysis of stride-to-stride variability could be a useful method for identifying characteristics of gait that are closely linked to FOG an could predict its occurance. However, patients with PD that experience FOG also display premature muscle activation and termination patterns before a freezing episode, leading to an abnormally long stance phase (Nieuwboer et al., 2001, 2004). This altered timing suggests that a central timing deficit could predispose PPD to FOG (Almeida et al., 2007). Perceptual judgement deficits have been identified as a contributing factor to motor impairment in PD (Johnson et al., 2004). For example, PPD are unable to accurately evaluate self-motion in relation to upcoming obstacles (Almeida et al., 2005). Therefore, a central timing deficit could be the consequence of an altered perceptual processing capabilities (Almeida et al., 2010) in PPD that experience FOG. This mechanism could explain the occurance of FOG when PPD move through confined spaces.

PPD report feeling too large to pass through small spaces, even though they are aware that doorways are designed for human size (Lee & Harris, 1999). A recent study indirectly evaluated the influence of space perception on gait in individuals with Parkinson's disease who experience FOG, other Parkinson's disease patients (absent of FOG) and healthy age-matched participants (Almeida et al., 2010). Individuals with Parkinson's disease were tested while on dopaminergic medication. The objective was to evaluate the effect of doorway size on gait before reaching the doorway in these three groups of subjects. Almeida and coworkers reported (Almeida et al., 2010) that patiets with FOG, while approaching a narrow doorway, already exhibit alterations to gait (shortened step length, increased gait variability, increased base of support) indicative of an upcoming freezing episode. These changes were not evident in non-FOG individuals with Parkinson's disease, or healthy participants. The conclusion of the study was that indicators of freezing occurr when patients approach what they percive to be a confined space, suggesting that online perceptual processes must be interrupting the initial movement plan to pass through the doorway. Therefore, impaired perceptual ability could be an important factor contributing to FOG in PPD. Since PPD, that experience FOG, were most affected (in terms of step length and velocity) upon their first encounter with the doorway, practice (*i.e.* repeated passing through a doorway) could help PPD improve their spatial perception. Finally, FOG is difficult to elicit in a laboratory setting. Therefore it is important to consider whether patients categorized as non-freezers in a laboratory setting may experience of FOG within their home environment (Almeida et al., 2010).

3.2 Falls

At present, it is not possible to accuratly predict the occurence of falls in PPD. This is particulary true for prior nonfallers (Boonstra et al., 2008). The best available predictor of falling is two or more falls in the previous year. Fear of falling had a moderate sensitivity in predicting falls among prior nonfallers, suggesting that patients may sense their own instability before it can be detected on physical examination (Pickering et al., 2007). Fear of falling can be evaluated with the Activities-specific Balance Confidence (ABC) scale, which has been validated for use in Parkinson's disease (Peretz et al., 2006). Although fear of falling was also associated with prior falls in other studies, alternative determinants of falls were also reported rainging from impaired ambulation, impaired lower-limb motor planning to orthostasis (Bloem et al., 2004b; Dennison et al., 2007; Williams et al., 2006). Several methods were developed for the clinical and quantitative assessment of gait, FOG, postural instability and balance confidence (Dibble et al., 2006, 2008; Jacobs et al., 2006a, 2006b; Kegelmeyer et al., 2007; Moore et al., 2007b, 2008; Peppe et al., 2007; Peretz et al., 2006; Plotnik et al., 2007) but only a few studies are focused on predicting falls in PPD (Dibble et al., 2006; Jacobs et al., 2006a). The three key pathophysiological factors that seem to be relevant for the development of falls in PPD are turning, axial asymmetry and sensorimotor integration (Boonstra et al., 2008).

PPD often experience difficulty turning around (clinically described as en-bloc-turning), either while lying recumbent in bed or when standing upright. These turning problems are clinically relevant for PPD because falls are associated with hip fractures. Measuring the time during a 180^0 axial turn or counting the number of steps are simple and adequate methods for the assessment of turning (Huxham et al., 2006; Willems et al., 2007;) since PPD require more steps and also turn slower than controls. Alternative ambulatory monitors, that evaluate for example peak yaw and peak roll angular velocity of the trunk (Visser et al., 2007) — both are reduced in PD – are also available (Moore et al., 2008; Plotnik et al., 2007). Turning problems could be the consequence of poor interlimb coordination (Baltadjieva et al., 2006; Hausdorff et al., 2003) when the two legs have to move more "in phase" rather than "out of phase" as is usual during over ground straight walking. Another important factor that could contribute to difficulties in turning is axial stiffness and loss of intersegmental axial coordination. PPD have an increased resistance to passive axial rotations that was resistent to levodopa treatment in contrast to the limb movements, which appear to be controlled by separate dopaminergic neural systems (Baltadjieva et al., 2006; Wright et al., 2007).

Some PPD exhibited unsteadiness associated with orthostatic tremor of varying frequency (from 4 to 18 Hz) or orthostatic myoclonus; patients with fast tremor improved on clonazepam and patients with slow tremor or myoclonus improved on levodopa, and sometimes benefited further when clonazepam was added (Leu-Semenescu et al., 2007).

Idiopathic Parkinson's disease is by definition an asymmetrical disease. A study on 35 patients with Parkinson's disease who were not yet treated with any antiparkinsonian medication showed that asymmetries in gait (detected with simple pressure-sensitive insoles) are also present in the early stage of PD and are not merely a side effect of medication or a late disease complication (Baltadjieva et al., 2006). Gait assymetry could be detected even though stride-to-stride variability (previously thought to be one of the most sensitive measures of gait changes in Parkinson's disease) was normal in these early PPD. In addition, subtle asymmetries in balance control can be detected in Parkinson's disease by carefully analyzing the independent contribution of both legs to stance control, even before these changes are visually detected on clinical examination (van der Kooij et al., 2007).

Disturbed motor programming of postural corrections within the basal ganglia is not the only cause for postural instability in PD, since some motor deficits are at least partially due to central proprioceptive disturbances (Boonstra et al., 2008). When PPD were standing on a supporting platform and perturbed under conditions where they were dependent on proprioceptive feedback to maintain balance, they swayed abnormally, but were still able to partially correct this with visual feedback (Vaugoyeau et al., 2007). Compared to controls, the switch from proprioceptive-dependent to vision-dependent balance control is slower in PPD, suggesting an inappropriate changing between different sensory modalities (Brown et al., 2006). Further evidence that proprioceptive disturbances could contribute to gait disorders was provided by two studies that evaluated the response of PPD to tendon vibration and to a functional reach task. The response to tendom vibration was exaggerated and does not habituate well in patients with advanced PD (Valkovic et al., 2006). When PPD we asked to extend the arm forward as far as possible, with both feet fixed at the floor they tended to overestimate their limits of stability (Kamata et al., 2007). Therefore proprioceptive disturbances could produce a distorted body scheme and thus explain some changes in gait, for example the stooped posture of patients with Parkinson's disease, of which they are often subjectively unaware (Boonstra et al., 2008).

In human, the normal response to an imminent fall is stretching out the arms and taking compensatory steps. PPD have difficulties initiating a compensatory step (Jacobs et al., 2006a,b,c; King et al., 2008). The failure to initiate a compensatory step could be due to impairment of anticipatory postural adjustments; normally a lateral weight shift precedes a contralateral limb swing (King et al., 2008). Visual cues facilitate the initiation of compensatory stepping in PPD and initiation is inhibited when patients are unable to see their legs (Jacobs et al., 2006a,b,c; Mille et al., 2007). The importance of cuing in PPD is discussed under Section 4.4 Physical Therapy.

4. Treatment of gait disorders in Parkinsons disease

One of the most serious complications of FOG is falls. Although FOG and falls usually occur in the later stages of PD they are typically an early feature of atypical parkinsonian syndromes (Thanvi & Treadwell, 2010). The unpredictable and episodic nature of occurrence of FOG and falls poses a serious challenge to the patients, carers and the physicians. Frequent falls lead to injuries (*e.g.* fractures), fear of falling, restriction of mobility, and social isolation (Thanvi & Treadwell, 2010). FOG is often associated with cognitive and speech impairment, incontinence and falls. Therefore, it is best managed with a multidisciplinary team approach (Thanvi & Treadwell, 2010).

There is no universally effective therapy available to treat FOG (Thanvi & Treadwell, 2010). In PD, "off" period FOG responds initially well to interventions aimed at improving "on" time, though with increasing disease severity it becomes treatment refractory (like other L-dopa resistant features such as axial symptoms and postural disturbances). DT and very stressful conditions (*e.g.* crossing a busy road at a point not marked with a zebra crossing) increase the probability of FOG, whereas focused attention strategies (*e.g.* visual, auditory or sensory cueing), and a moderate amount of emotional stress can improve FOG (Thanvi & Treadwell, 2010). Patients often use a type of focused attention strategy to improve their freezing, and physiotherapists exploit them for gait training.

4.1 Dopaminergic drugs

FOG in patients with PD is considered dopamine resistant. Although the proportion of PD patients with motor disability increases with time, these deficits do not become unresponsive to levodopa (Clissold et al., 2006). The "off" phase FOG does respond to treatment with dopaminergic drugs. The "off" FOG is more common and often more severe than "on" freezing (Thanvi & Treadwell, 2010). L-dopa was shown to reduce "off " freezing (Lee et al., 2005) or reduce the frequency of the "off " period FOG (Schaafsma et al., 2003). Patients treated with L-dopa are less likely to have FOG compared with those who received placebo (Parkinson Study Group 2003). Dopaminergic receptor agonists also improve motor symptoms and increase "on" time in fluctuating PD patients. Apomorphine improves postural stability of PPD by decreasing rigidity (Bartolić et al. 2005). When compared to patients treated with ropinirole (Rascol et al., 2000) or pramipexole (Parkinson Study Group, 2001), L-dopa treated patients had less frequent episodes of FOG. L-dopa may adversely affect gait or balance control. One study (Almeida et al., 2007) showed that timing of gait to an external stimulus was worse in medicated patients compared with patients who had withdrawn from medication, presumably due to drug-induced dyskinesias.

4.2 Monoamine oxidase B inhibitors

Compared to placebo, Selegiline reduces the frequency of FOG in PPD (Giladi et al., 2001). This effect was also shown in the late stages of PD (Zuňiga et al., 2006). Similar observations were reported for Rasagiline when used as an adjunct to L-dopa (Giladi et al., 2004, as cited in Thanvi & Treadwell, 2010).

4.3 Miscellaneous drugs

L-Threo-DOPS, a norepinephrine precursor, has been shown to improve FOG in one study, (Narabayashi et al., 1987) but not in the other (Quinn et al., 1984). Improved gait and balance in advanced PD was achived with Atomoxetine (Jankovic, 2009) but these results have to be evaluated in controlled trials.

Methylphenidate, a central nervous system stimulator traditionally used for treating attention-deficit hyperactivity disorder, can decrease fall risks in community dwelling older adults, presumably by increasing availability of striatal dopamine or by improving attention (Ben-Itzhak et al., 2008). Trials have also shown that methylphenidate improves gait and FOG in PPD (Devos et al., 2007; Pollak et al., 2007).

4.4 Physical therapy

Adherence to a regular exercise regimen may be the most difficult challenge for the physical therapist and the patient (Morris et al., 2010). The development and progression of non-motor signs of PD (depression, apathy, and lack of initiative) also has a significant negative effect on patient complience to the exercise regimen (Morris et al., 2010). The efficacy of physical therapy is evaluated by gait-related outcomes including assessment of kinematics of gait (*e.g.* stride length), assessment of functional factors (*e.g.* walk distance over a defined time interval, ability to climb stairs or raise from chair), and assessment of factors associated with postural control that are closely related to gait (*e.g.* incidence of FOG or falls). Physical therapay of PPD has three objectives: strategy training, management of secondary sequelae and promotion of physical activities (Morris et al., 2010).

4.4.1 Strategy training

The first objective is to teach the patient how to move more easily and to maintain postural stability by using cognitive strategies that target the primary motor control deficit in the basal ganglia, brain stem, and motor cortex. The two forms of stategy training are compensatory strategies to bypass the defective basal ganglia and learning strategies to improve performance through practice (Morris et al., 2010). The theoretical rationale for using cognitive strategies is that the use of executive function of the frontal cortex, to regulate movement size or timing by consciously thinking about the desired movement, enables people with PD to compensate for the neurotransmitter imbalance in the basal ganglia.

Some of the first evidence that movement strategies can compensate for hypokinesia and thus assist people with PD to balance, move and walk more easily was provided by Morris and colleagues (Morris et al., 2000, 2006, 2009). For example, external cues, such as white lines on the floor or a rhythmical beat provided by a metronome or music, enable elderly people with moderate to severe PD to walk with longer steps and at a more normal stepping rate. Cueing is an established therapy for gait training of patients with PD. Theoretically, external cues could reduce attentional loads by reducing the need to prepare and plan a movement, but this hypothesis requires further testing (Boonstra et al., 2008). The effect of visual cues on FOG was first reported in 1967 (Martin, 1967) and several following studies reported transient beneficial effects of cueing in single or limited sessions (Cubo et al., 2003; Dibble et al., 2004; Dietz et al., 1990). For example, a three week home physiotherapy programme based on rhythmical cueing on gait and gait related activity in PPD reported significant improvements in gait and FOG questionnaire scores in the treatment group. Unfortunately, the effects were short-lived and disappeared by the 12 week follow-up (Nieuwboer et al., 2007). A recent study reported greater benefits with treadmill training plus auditory and visual cues than rehabilitation with cues but no treadmill training (Frazzitta et al., 2009). Apart from the transient beneficial effect of cueing an additional concern is that cueing strategies, even when effective in the lab under carefully controlled "single task" conditions, may not benefit patients in daily life complex situations, that typically requiring patients to deal with multiple tasks simultaneously (Boonstra et al., 2008). Two studies have shown that some, but not all, cueing strategies benefit patients in daily life complex situations. Auditory cues improved walking speed during a DT situation, whereas somatosensory cues had no effect, and visual cues had a negative effect. Rhythmic auditory cues had no effect in a single task situation (*i.e.* normal walking) (Baker et al., 2007; Rochester et al., 2007). The explanation for the latter result was that the participants were challenged more during the DT, or that patients relied more on external information during the complex tasks (Rochester et al., 2007).

Virtual reality represents a new and promising cueing strategy. A recent paper reported on the effects of 6 weeks of treadmill training (TT) with virtual reality (VR) on the mobility of PPD (Mirelman et al., 2011). The results of this study indicate that intensive and progressive TT with VR is viable for PPD and may significantly improve physical performance and gait beyond the previously reported improvements of TT alone (Mirelman et al., 2011). By promoting the development of new motor and cognitive strategies for obstacle navigation, training with TT + VR positively affected complex gait conditions such as walking with DT, obstacle negotiation, and even certain aspects of cognitive function (attention and memory) (Mirelman et al., 2011). In addition, the negative effects of drug therapy on gait became smaller after training with TT + VR and were significantly better than those observed after intensive TT alone (Mirelman et al., 2011). In summary, this study contributes to the growing body of evidence that suggests that motor and cognitive improvement may be achievable among older adults with PD (Li et al., 2010; Verghese et al., 2010). However, larger scale, randomized controlled studies are needed to firmly establish efficacy and the long-term retention effects of TT with VR on cognitive, motor function, and fall risk in patients with PD (Mirelman et al., 2011).

PPD with moderate postural instability, and a preserved cognitive function, walk with long, fast steps simply by focusing their attention on walking with long steps, even when floor markers are absent (Morris et al., 2009). Learning strategies to improve gait through practice (*e.g.* mentally rehearsing the desired movement pattern before the action is performed) are based on the theory that the ability to move normally is not lost in PD. Instead, there is an activation problem that can be overcome through targeted physical therapy together with optimal pharmacotherapy (Morris et al., 2010). The ability to learn a new motor skill is present in the early stages of PD. For example, the capacity to learn new upper-limb movement sequences was retained in people in the early to middle stages of PD (Behrman et al., 2000) and an increased multiple-task walking speed in people with mild PD could be achived with a multiple-task gait training program that combined walking with cognitive and manual activity practice (Canning et al., 2008). A recent study by Brauer and co-workers (Brauer et al., 2010) confirmed the assumption that PPD can be trained to walk with long steps under dual task conditions.

To summarize, physical therapy should be adjusted to the progression of PD. For patients with a mild to moderate gait disorder and conserved cognitive capacity, the aim of physical therapy is to maximize motor skill learning by high intensity, variable, distributed practice regimens with regular booster sessions over the longer term. For patinets with advanced gait disorders or cognitive impairment the recommned physical therapy would be repetition of a given movement or action sequence, avoidance of multitasking, use of external cues and reminders, and segmentation of actions into simple components (Dubois & Pillon, 1997; Morris et al., 2010).

4.4.2 Management of secondary sequelae

The second objective of physical therapy, management of secondary sequelae, is concerned with the management of secondary pathological conditions affecting the musculoskeletal and cardiorespiratory systems that occur as a result of deconditioning, reduced physical activity, advanced age, and comorbid conditions (Morris et al., 2010). Some of the changes in the musculoskeletal and cardiorespiratory systems of patients in the advanced stages of PD are also due to concurrent age related changes. Therefore studies that aim to develop physical training stategies specific for PPD should include age mached controls. Management of secondary pathological conditions (*e.g.* weakness, loss of range, loss of range of motion of axial structures, or reduced aerobic capacity) alone can improve balance, gait, and function in PPD without influencing the primary central nervous system disorder affecting the basal ganglia (Schenkman & Butler, 1989; Schenkman et al., 2000). For example, loss of lower-extremity strength contributes to gait disorders, falls, and functional decline in older people (Chandler et al., 1998; Falvo et al., 2008). Such loss of lower-extremity strength can be compensated by an appropropriate physical training programme as demonstrated by Dibble and coworkers (Dibble & Lange, 2006) who showed that a high-intensity eccentric quadriceps muscle strengthening program increased quadriceps muscle volume, improved 6-minute walk distance, and improved stair descent time. PPD have a less efficient muscle work and thus less efficient movement than age mached controls. Adults with PD used as much as 20% more oxygen to perform bicycling tasks than did the people without PD (Protas et al., 1996) and people with PD consume more oxygen than people without PD at every walking speed from 1 to 4 mph (Christiansen et al., 2009). Aerobic conditioning programs can improve the efficiency of maximum oxygen consumption, movement and kinematics of gait (Bergen et al., 2002; Burini et al., 2006; Schenkman et al., 2008). To sustain the benefits of physical therapy, individuals should continue exercising at least a few times per week as part of their daily routine. Patients in the early stages of PD should be reassessed by a physical therapist at least annually and more often in later stages of the disease to progress their exercise program (Morris et al., 2010).

A combination of physical impairments (*e.g.* FOG), cognitive dysfunction (*e.g.* depression and dementia), and fatigue predispose PPD toward a sedentary lifestyle (van Eijkeren et al., 2008). Regular physical activity of PPD is vital, since physical activity has positive effects in preventing the well known complications of immobility (*e.g.* an increased risk of cardiovascular disease, type-2 diabetes mellitus, osteoporosis and obesity). Osteoporosis

prevention is particularly important for PPD because they have an increased risk of falling (Pickering et al., 2007) and for fall-related fractures (Genever et al., 2005; Melton et al., 2006). Exercise may also slow down the progression of cognitive decline (Yaffe et al., 2001; van Gelder et al., 2004) or dementia (Laurin et al., 2001). Also, animal studies suggest that physical activity could slow down disease progression in PD (Tillerson et al., 2003). Therefore, it is vital to develop a reliable strategy to stimulate an active lifestyle in PD.
PPD can participate in exercise classes and improve their physical fitness but have difficulty in sustaining their active lifestyle (Keus et al., 2007). **Nordic walking** (*i.e.* Polestriding) is rapidly gaining popularity as a way to improve physical fitness in PD (van Eijkeren et al., 2008). Nordic walking combines simplicity and accessibility of walking with a full body walking workout that can burn significantly more calories without having to walk faster, due to the incorporation of many large body muscles. A practical advantage is that Nordic walking can be done year round in any climate (van Eijkeren et al., 2008). Two recent studies in PPD demonstrated short-term beneficial effects of Nordic walking on walking speed and stride length, as well as on UPDRS motor scores and quality of life (Baatile et al., 2000; Reuter et al., 2006). The long term effects of Nordic walking were evaluated in a study by Eijkeren et al. (van Eijkeren et al., 2008). The results of this study show that a 6-week Nordic walking program is associated with an improved walking speed, a faster TUG test, and increased timed walking distance and an improved quality of life in PPD even 5 months after training (van Eijkeren et al., 2008). Althogh all three studies are preliminary their encouraging results justify a large scale, randomized clinical trial.

4.4.3 Promotion of physical activities

The final, third objective of thysical theray, is the promotion of physical activities that assist the person in making lifelong changes in exercise and physical activity habits as well as preventing FOG and falls (Morris et al., 2010). Because of the chronic, progressive nature of PD, sustained exercise is vital to maintain the benefits of physical therapy by integrating physical activity into the patient's daily life. This is supported by follow-up data from human exercise interventions that have demonstrated a gradual return to baseline abilities after the supervised intervention was terminated (Mooris et al., 2009; Schenkman et al., 1998; Ellis et al., 2005). Research suggests that exercise not only enables people to maintain functional ability but could also have a neuroprotective effect. Tillerson and coworkers (Tillerson et al., 2003) reported that motorized treadmill running twice daily for 10 days enhanced motor performance and brain neurochemistry in 2 different rat models of PD. Also Dobrossy and Dunnett (Dobrossy & Dunnet, 2003) reported that rats that received motor training after striatal lesions or striatal grafts showed partial recovery in spontaneous movements and skilled motor performance. Research on human subjects suggests that high-intensity exercise can normalize corticomotor excitability in the early stages of PD (Fisher et al., 2008).

4.5 Deep brain stimulation

The internal globus pallidus (GPi) and the subthalamic nucleus (STN) are the most common targets for deep brain stimulation in the treatment of PPD (Thanvi & Treadwell, 2010). L-dopa induced dyskinesias and fluctuations are treated with stimulation of the GPi and STN stimulation is used to treat PD motor symptoms (*e.g.* tremor). Some of the effect of STN stimulation may act *via* "downward" projections onto the pedunculopontine nucleus (Gan et al., 2007).

Bilateral STN stimulation is an effective treatment for PD, for symptoms of the upper and lower limbs that responded well to levodopa preoperatively (Boonstra et al., 2008). The effects of STN stimulation on axial motor signs are less clear because of the differences in surgical techniques, candidates selected for surgery and outcome measures used (Boonstra et al., 2008). There are increasing concerns that deep brain stimulation of the STN may worsen axial mobility either as an immediate adverse effect of surgery, or as a longterm complication (Boonstra et al., 2008). After a 3-year follow-up of 36 patients with Parkinson's disease, STN stimulation had improved the United Parkinson's Disease Rating Scale (UPDRS) motor score and gait score but dopa-unresponsive axial signs had worsened in some patients (Gan et al., 2007). Another study, investigating gait changes after STN stimulation, found that gait improved in half the patients, but had worsened in the others (Kelly et al., 2006). It has been suggested that variability in electrode placement can explain the inconsistent effects of STN stimulation on axial mobility across PPD (Boonstra et al., 2008). For example, misplaced electrodes could unintentionally stimulate the pedunculopontine nucleus (Tommasi et al., 2007) which, when stimulated at high frequencies, worsens gait and balance (Androulidakis et al., 2008; Stefani et al., 2007). This hypothesis was addressed in a study of patients with Parkinson's disease with severe postoperative gait disorders whose outcome measures (including UPDRS, a timed walking task and FOG) improved when the stimulator frequency settings (130Hz) were changed to 60 Hz (Moreau et al., 2008).

An alternative target for DBS in patients with advanced PD is the pedunculopontine nucleus (Stefani et al., 2007). The effect of simultaneous bilateral implantation of electrodes in both the STN and pedunculopontine nucleus was studied in a group of six PPD (Stefani et al., 2007). During the "on" state, pedunculopontine stimulation alone had a positive effect on the UPDRS items for gait and balance, whereas STN stimulation did not. The pedunculopontine stimulation improved axial symptoms directly postoperatively and this persisted for 6 months. An alternative explanation for these results, the unintentional stimulation of nucleus peripeduncularis (Yelnik, 2007), has been suggested.

5. Conclusion

There is a need for further studies that investigate the treatment of gait disorders in patients with Parkinson's disease since there is still no universally effective therapy available. Recent research has identified novel gait parameters for evaluating freezing of gait and falls, with the potential to contribute to the prevention and treatment of gait disorders, that still have to be validated in large scale, randomized clinical trials.

6. Acknowledgement

This work was supported by the Slovenian Research Agency of the Republic of Slovenia, Grant number P3-0171.

7. References

Albert, MS. Cognitive and neurobiologic markers of early Alzheimer disease. (1996). *Proceedings of the National Academy of Sciences of the United States of America*, Vol.93, pp. 13547-13551, ISSN 0027-8424

Almeida, QJ.; Frank, JS.; Roy, EA.; Jenkins, ME.; Spaulding, S.; Patla, AE.; & Jog, MS. (2005). An evaluation of sensorimotor integration during locomotion toward a target in Parkinson's disease. *Neuroscience*, Vol.134, No.1, pp. 283-293, ISSN 0306-4522

Almeida, QJ.; Frank, JS.; Roy, EA.; Patla, AE. & Jog, MS. (2007). Dopaminergic modulation of timing control and variability in the gait of Parkinson's disease. *Movement Disorders*, Vol.22, pp. 1735–1742, ISSN 0885-3185

Almeida, QJ. & Lebold, CA. (2010). Freezing of gait in Parkinson's disease: a perceptual cause for a motor impairment? *Journal of Neurology, Neurosurgery, and Psychiatry*, Vol.81, No.5, pp. 513-518, ISSN 0022-3050

Alvarez, JA. & Emory, E. (2006). Executive function and the frontal lobes: a meta-analytic review. *Neuropsychology Review*, Vol.16, pp. 17-42, ISSN 1040-7308

Androulidakis, AG.; Khan, S.; Litvak, V.; Pleydell-Pearce, CW.; Brown, P. & Gill, SS. (2008). Local field potential recordings from the pedunculopontine nucleus in a Parkinsonian patient. *Neuroreport*, Vo.19, pp. 59–62, ISSN 0959-4965

Baatile, J.; Langbein, WE.; Weaver, F.; Maloney, C. & Jost, MB. (2000). Effect of exercise on perceived quality of life of individuals with Parkinson's disease. Journal *of Rehabilitation Research and Development*, Vol.37, pp. 529–534, ISSN 0748-7711

Baddeley, AD.; Baddeley, HA.; Bucks, RS. & Wilcock, GK. (2001). Attentional control in Alzheimer's disease. *Brain: a Journal of Neurology*, Vol.124, pp. 1492-1508, ISSN 0006-8950

Baker, K.; Rochester, L. & Nieuwboer, A. (2007). The immediate effect of attentional, auditory, and a combined cue strategy on gait during single and dual tasks in Parkinson's disease. *Archives of Physical Medicine and Rehabilitation*, Vol.88, pp. 1593–1600, ISSN 0003-9993

Baltadjieva, R.; Giladi, N.; Gruendlinger, L.; Peretz, C. & Hausdorff, JM. (2006). Marked alterations in the gait timing and rhythmicity of patients with de novo Parkinson's disease. *The European Journal of Neuroscience*, Vol.24, pp. 1815–1820, ISSN 0953-816X

Bartolić, A.; Pirtosek, Z.; Rozman, J. & Ribaric, S. (2005). Postural stability of Parkinson's disease patients is improved by decreasing rigidity. *European Journal of Neurology*, Vol.12, No.2, pp. 156-159, ISSN 1351-5101

Bartolić, A.; Pirtosek, Z.; Rozman, J. & Ribaric, S. (2010). Tremor amplitude and tremor frequency variability in Parkinson's disease is dependent on activity and synchronisation of central oscillators in basal ganglia. *Medical Hypotheses*, Vol.74, No.2, pp. 362-365, ISSN 0306-9877

Bedard, MA.; el Massioui, F.; Malapani, C.; Dubois, B.; Pillon, B.; Renault, B. & Agid, Y. (1998). Attentional deficits in Parkinson's disease: partial reversibility with naphtoxazine (SDZ NVI-085), a selective noradrenergic alpha 1 agonist. *Clinical Neuropharmacology*, Vol.21, pp. 108-117, ISSN 0362-5664

Behrman, AL.; Cauraugh, JH. & Light, KE. (2000). Practice as an intervention to improve speeded motor performance and motor learning in Parkinson's disease. *Journal of the Neurological Sciences*, Vol.174, pp127–136, ISSN 0022-510X

Ben-Itzhak, R.; Giladi, N.; Gruendlinger, L. & Hausdorff JM. (2008). Can methylphenidate reduce fall risk in community-living older adults? A double-blind, single-dose cross-over study. *Journal of the American Geriatrics Society*, Vol.56, pp. 695–700, ISSN 0002-8614

Bergen, JL.; Toole, T.; Elliott, RG.; Wallace, B.; Robinson, K. & Maitland, CG. (2002). Aerobic exercise intervention improves aerobic capacity and movement initiation in Parkinson's disease patients. *NeuroRehabilitation*, Vol.17, pp. 1621–1628, ISSN 1053-8135

Ble, A.; Volpato, S.; Zuliani, G.; Guralnik, JM.; Bandinelli, S.; Lauretani, F.; Bartali, B.; Maraldi, C.; Fellin, R. & Ferrucci, L. (2005). Executive function correlates with walking speed in older persons: the InCHIANTI study. *Journal of the American Geriatrics Society*, Vol.53, No.3, (March), pp. 410-415, ISSN 0002-8614

Bloem, BR.; Valkenburg, VV.; Slabbekoorn, M. & van Dijk, JG. (2001a). The multiple tasks test. Strategies in Parkinson's disease. *Experimental Brain Research*, Vol.137, No.3-4, pp. 478-486, ISSN 0014-4819

Bloem, BR.; Valkenburg, VV.; Slabbekoorn, M. & Willemsen, MD. (2001b). The multiple tasks test: development and normal strategies. *Gait & Posture*, Vol.14, No.3, pp.191-202, ISSN 0966-6362

Bloem, BR. & Bhatia, KP. (2004a). Gait and balance in basal ganglia disorders. In: *Clinical disorders of balance, posture and gait*, AM. Bronstein, T. Brandt, JG. Nutt, MH. Woollacott, (Eds.), 173-206, London: Arnold; ISBN 0-340-80657-5

Bloem, BR.; Hausdorff, JM.; Visser, JE. & Giladi, N. (2004b). Falls and freezing of gait in Parkinson's disease: a review of two interconnected, episodic phenomena. *Movement Disorders*, Vol.19, pp. 871-884, ISSN 0885-3185

Bloem, BR.; Grimbergen, YA.; van Dijk, JG. & Munneke, M. (2006). The ''posture second'' strategy: a review of wrong priorities in Parkinson's disease. *Journal of the Neurological Sciences*, Vol.248, No.1-2, pp. 196–204, ISSN 0022-510X

Boonstra, TA.; van der Kooij, H.; Munneke, M. & Bloem, BR. (2008). Gait disorders and balance disturbances in Parkinson's disease: clinical update and pathophysiology. *Current Opinion in Neurology*, Vol.21, No.4, pp. 461-471, ISSN 1350-7540

Bostan, AC.; Dum, RP. & Strick, PL. (2010). The basal ganglia communicate with the cerebellum. *Proceedings of the National Academy of Sciences of the United States of America*, Vol.107, No.18, (May 4), pp. 8452-8456, ISSN 0027-8424

Brauer, SG. & Morris, ME. (2010). Can people with Parkinson's disease improve dual tasking when walking? *Gait Posture*, Vol.31, No.2, pp. 229-233, ISSN 0966-6362

Brown, LA.; Cooper, SA.; Doan, JB.; Dickin, DC.; Whishaw, IQ.; Pellis, SM. & Suchowersky, O. (2006). Parkinsonian deficits in sensory integration for postural control: temporal response to changes in visual input. *Parkinsonism & Related Disorders*, Vol.12, pp. 376–381, ISSN 1353-8020

Buckner, RL. (2004). Memory and executive function in aging and AD: multiple factors that cause decline and reserve factors that compensate. *Neuron*, Vol.44, pp.195-208, ISSN 0896-6273

Burini, D.; Farabollini, B. & Iacucci, S. (2006). A randomized controlled cross-over trial of aerobic training versus qigong in advanced Parkinson's disease. *Europa Medicophysica*, Vol.4, pp. 231–238, ISSN 0014-2573

Burke, SN. & Barnes, CA. (2006). Neural plasticity in the ageing brain. *Nature Reviews Neuroscience*, Vol.7, pp.30-40, ISSN 1471-003X

Canning, CG.; Ada, L. & Woodhouse, E. (2008). Multiple-task walking training in people with mild to moderate Parkinson's disease: a pilot study. *Clinical Rehabilitation*, Vol.22, pp. 226–233, ISSN 0269-2155

Chandler, J.; Duncan, PW.; Kochersberger, G. & Studenski, S. (1998). Is lower extremity strength gain associated with improvement in physical performance and disability in frail, community-dwelling elders? *Archives of Physical Medicine and Rehabilitation*, Vol.79, pp.24 -30, ISSN 0003-9993

Christiansen, CL.; Schenkman, ML.; Kohrt WM, et al. (2009). Energy expenditure in people with Parkinson's disease during treadmill walking, Presented at: *Combined Sections Meeting of the American Physical Therapy Association*; pp. 9-12, February Las Vegas, Nevada.

Clissold, BG.; McColl, CD.; Reardon, KR.; Shiff, M. & Kempster, PA. (2006). Longitudinal study of the motor response to levodopa in Parkinson's disease. *Movement Disorders*, Vol.21, pp. 2116–2121, ISSN 0885-3185

Collette, F.; Hogge, M.; Salmon, E. & Van der Linden, M. (2006). Exploration of the neural substrates of executive functioning by functional neuroimaging. *Neuroscience*, Vol.139, No.1, pp. 209-221, ISSN 0306-4522

Craik, FIM. & Grady, CL. (2002). Aging, memory, and frontal lobe functioning. In: *Principles of frontal lobe function*, D.T. Stuss, R.T. Knight (Eds.), Oxford University Press, p 528–540, New York

Cubo, E.; Moore, CG.; Leurgans, S. &, Goetz, CG. (2003). Wheeled and standard walkers in Parkinson's disease patients with gait freezing. *Parkinsonism & Related Disorders*, Vol.10, No.1, pp. 9-14, ISSN 1353-8020

Dennison, AC.; Noorigian, JV.; Robinson, KM.; Fisman, DN.; Cianci, HJ.; Moberg, P.; Bunting-Perry, L.; Martine, R.; Duda, J. & Stern, MB. (2007). Falling in Parkinson disease: identifying and prioritizing risk factors in recurrent fallers. *American Journal of Physical Medicine & Rehabilitation*, Vol.86, pp. 621–632, ISSN 0894-9115

Devos, D.; Krystkowiak, P.; Clement, F.; Dujardin, K.; Cottencin, O.; Waucquier, N.; Ajebbar, K.; Thielemans, B.; Kroumova, M.; Duhamel, A.; Destée, A.; Bordet, R. & Defebvre, L. (2007). Improvement of gait by chronic, high doses of methylphenidate in patients with advanced Parkinson's disease. *Journal of Neurology, Neurosurgery, and Psychiatry*, Vol.78, pp. 470–475, ISSN 0022-3050

Dibble, LE.; Nicholson, DE.; Shultz, B.; MacWilliams, BA.; Marcus, RL. & Moncur, C. (2004). Sensory cueing effects on maximal speed gait initiation in persons with Parkinson's disease and healthy elders. *Gait & Posture*, Vol.19, pp. 215-225, ISSN 0966-6362

Dibble, LE. & Lange, M. (2006). Predicting falls in individuals with Parkinson disease: a reconsideration of clinical balance measures. *Journal of Neurologic Physical Therapy*, Vol.30, pp. 60–67, ISSN 1557-0576

Dibble, LE.; Christensen, J.; Ballard, DJ. & Foreman, KB. (2008). Diagnosis of fall risk in Parkinson disease: an analysis of individual and collective clinical balance test interpretation. Physical Therapy, Vol.88, pp. 323–332, ISSN 0031-9023

Dietz, MA.; Goetz, CG. & Stebbins, GT. (1990). Evaluation of a modified inverted walking stick as a treatment for parkinsonian freezing episodes. *Movement Disorders*, Vol.5, pp. 243-247, ISSN 0885-3185

Dietz, V. (2003). Spinal cord pattern generators for locomotion. *Clinical Neurophysiology*, Vol.114, No.8, pp. 1379–1389, ISSN 1388-2457

Dobrossy, MD. & Dunnett, SB. (2003). Motor training effects on recovery of function after striatal lesions and striatal grafts. *Experimental Neurology*, Vol.184, pp. 274–284, ISSN 0014-4886

Dreher, JC. & Grafman, J. (2003). Dissociating the roles of the rostral anterior cingulate and the lateral prefrontal cortices in performing two tasks simultaneously or successively. *Cerebral Cortex*, Vol.13, pp. 329-339, ISSN 1047-3211

Dubois, B. & Pillon, B. (1997). Cognitive deficits in Parkinson's disease. *Journal of Neurology*, Vol.244, pp. 2-8, ISSN 0340-5354

Ellis, T.; Goede, CJ.; Feldman, R.; Wolters, EC.; Kwakkel, G. & Wagenaar, RC. (2005). Efficacy of a physical therapy program in patients with Parkinson's disease: a randomised control trial. *Archives of Physical Medicine and Rehabilitation*, Vol.4, pp. 626–632, ISSN 0003-9993

Falvo, MJ.; Schilling, BK. & Earhart, GM. (2008). Parkinson's disease and resistive exercise: rationale, review, and recommendations. *Movement Disorders*, Vol.23, pp. 1–11, ISSN 0885-3185

Fisher, BE.; Wu, AD.; Salem, GJ.; Song, J.; Lin, CH.; Yip, J.; Cen, S.; Gordon, J.; Jakowec, M.& Petzinger, G. (2008). The effect of exercise training in improving motor performance and corticomotor excitability in people with early Parkinson's disease. *Archives of Physical Medicine and Rehabilitation*, Vol.89, No.7, pp. 1221-1229, ISSN 0003-9993

Frazzitta, G; Maestri, R; Uccellini, D; Bertotti, G. & Abelli, P. (2009). Rehabilitation treatment of gait in patients with Parkinson's disease with freezing: a comparison between two physical therapy protocols using visual and auditory cues with or without treadmill training. *Movement Disorders*, Vol.24, pp.1139-1143, ISSN 0885-3185

Gan, J.; Xie-Brustolin, J.; Mertens, P.; Polo, G.; Klinger, H.; Mollion, H.; Benatru, I.; Henry, E.; Broussolle, E. & Thobois, S. (2007). Bilateral subthalamic nucleus stimulation in advanced Parkinson's disease: three years follow-up. *Journal of Neurology*, Vol.254, pp. 99–106, ISSN 0340-5354

Genever, RW.; Downes, TW. & Medcalf, P. (2005). Fracture rates in Parkinson's disease compared with age- and gender-matched controls: a retrospective cohort study. *Age and Ageing*, Vol.34, pp. 21–24, ISSN 0002-0729

Gerin-Lajoie, M.; Richards, CL. & McFadyen, BJ. (2005). The negotiation of stationary and moving obstructions during walking: anticipatory locomotor adaptations and preservation of personal space. *Motor Control*, Vol.9, pp. 242-269, ISSN 1087-1640

Giladi, N.; Gurevich, T.; Shabtai, H.; Paleacu, D. & Simon, ES. (2001). The effect of botulinum toxin injections to the calf muscles on freezing of gait in parkinsonism: a pilot study. *Journal of Neurology*, Vol.248, No.7, pp. 572-576, ISSN 0340-5354

Giladi, N. & Nieuwboer A. (2008). Understanding and treating freezing of gait in parkinsonism, proposed working definition, and setting the stage. *Movement Disorders*, Vol.23, (Suppl 2), pp. S423-5, ISSN 0885-3185

Gunning-Dixon, FM. & Raz, N. (2003). Neuroanatomical correlates of selected executive functions in middle-aged and older adults: a prospective MRI study. *Neuropsychologia*, Vol.41, pp. 1929-1941, ISSN 0028-3932

Harrington, DL.; Haaland, KY.; Yeo, RA. & Marder, E. (1990). Procedural memory in Parkinson's disease: impaired motor but not visuoperceptual learning. *Journal of Clinical and Experimental Neuropsychology*, Vol.12, pp. 323–339, ISSN 1380-3395

Hausdorff, JM.; Schaafsma, JD.; Balash, Y.; Bartels, AL.; Gurevich, T. & Giladi, N. (2003). Impaired regulation of stride variability in Parkinson's disease subjects with freezing of gait. *Experimental Brain Research*, Vol.149, pp. 187–194, ISSN 0014-4819

Heindel, WC.; Salmon, DP.; Shults, CW.; Walicke, PA. & Butters, N. (1989). Neuropsychological evidence for multiple implicit memory systems: a comparison of Alzheimer's, Huntington's, and Parkinson's disease patients. *The Journal of Neuroscience*, Vol.9, No.2, pp.582-587, ISSN 0270-6474

Hely, MA.; Reid, WG.; Adena, MA.; Halliday, GM. & Morris, JG. (2008). The Sydney multicenter study of Parkinson's disease: the inevitability of dementia at 20 years. *Movement Disorders*, Vol.23, pp.837–844, ISSN 0885-3185

Holtzer, R.; Verghese, J.; Xue, X. & Lipton, RB. (2006). Cognitive processes related to gait velocity: results from the Einstein Aging Study. *Neuropsychology*, Vol.20, No.2, pp. 215-223, ISSN 0894-4105

Hoshi, E., Tremblay, L., Féger, J., Carras, PL. & Strick, PL. (2005) The cerebellum communicates with the basal ganglia. *Nature Neuroscience*, Vol.8, No.11, pp1491-1493, ISSN 1097-6256

Huxham, F.; Gong, J.; Baker, R.; Morris, M. & Iansek, R. (2006). Defining spatial parameters for nonlinear walking. *Gait & Posture*, Vol.23, pp. 159–163, ISSN: 0966-6362

Jacobs, JV. & Horak, FB. (2006a). Abnormal proprioceptive-motor integration contributes to hypometric postural responses of subjects with Parkinson's disease. *Neuroscience*, Vol.141, pp. 999–1009, ISSN 0306-4522

Jacobs, JV.; Horak, FB.; Tran, VK. & Nutt, JG. (2006b). Multiple balance tests improve the assessment of postural stability in subjects with Parkinson's disease. *Journal of Neurology, Neurosurgery, and Psychiatry*, Vol.77, No.3, pp. 322-326, ISSN 0022-3050

Jacobs, JV.; Horak, FB.; Van, TK. & Nutt, JG. (2006c). An alternative clinical postural stability test for patients with Parkinson's disease. *Journal of Neurology*, Vol.253, pp. 1404–1413, ISSN 0340-5354

Jankovic, J. (2009). Atomoxetine for freezing of gait in Parkinson disease. *Journal of the Neurological sciences*, Vol.284, No.1-2, (September), pp. 177-178, ISSN 0022-510X

Johnson, AM.; Almeida, QJ.; Stough, C.; Thompson, JC.; Singarayer, R. & Jog, MS. (2004). Visual inspection time in Parkinson's disease: deficits in early stages of cognitive processing. *Neuropsychologia*, Vol.42, pp. 577-583, ISSN 0028-3932

Kamata, N.; Matsuo, Y.; Yoneda, T.; Shinohara, H.; Inoue, S. & Abe, K. (2007). Overestimation of stability limits leads to a high frequency of falls in patients with Parkinson's disease. *Clinical Rehabilitation*, Vol.21, pp. 357–361, ISSN 0269-2155

Kegelmeyer, DA.; Kloos, AD.; Thomas, KM. & Kostyk, SK. (2007). Reliability and validity of the tinetti mobility test for individuals with Parkinson disease. *Physical Therapy*, Vol.87, pp. 1369–1378, ISSN 0031-9023

Kelly, VE.; Samii, A.; Slimp, JC.; Price, R.; Goodkin, R. & Shumway-Cook, A. (2006). Gait changes in response to subthalamic nucleus stimulation in people with Parkinson disease: a case series report. *Journal of Neurologic Physical Therapy*, Vol.30, pp. 184–194, ISSN 1557-0576

Keus, SH.; Bloem, BR.; Hendriks, EJ.; Bredero-Cohen, AB. & Munneke, M. (2007). Evidence-based analysis of physical therapy in Parkinson's disease with recommendations for practice and research. *Movement Disorders*, Vol.22, pp. 451–460, ISSN 0885-3185

King, LA. & Horak, FB. (2008). Lateral stepping for postural correction in Parkinson's disease. *Archives of Physical Medicine and Rehabilitation*, Vol.89, pp. 492–499, ISSN 0003-9993

Korczyn, AD. (2001). Dementia in Parkinson's disease. *Journal of Neurology*, Vol.248 (Suppl 3), pp. III1-4, ISSN 0340-5354

Lamberti, P.; Armenise, S.; Castaldo, V.; de Mari, M.; Iliceto, G.; Tronci, P. & Serlenga, L. (1997). Freezing gait in Parkinson's disease. *European Neurology*, Vol.38, pp. 297-301, ISSN 0014-3022

Laurin, D.; Verreault, R.; Lindsay, J.; MacPherson, K. & Rockwood, K. (2001). Physical activity and risk of cognitive impairment and dementia in elderly persons. *Archives of Neurology*, Vol.58, pp. 498–504, ISSN 0003-9942

Lee, AC. & Harris, JP. (1999). Problems with perception of space in Parkinson's disease. *Neuro-Ophthalmology*, Vol.22, pp. 1-15, ISSN 0165-8107

Lee, MS.; Kim, HS. & Lyoo, CH. (2005). "Off" gait freezing and temporal discrimination threshold in patients with Parkinson disease. *Neurology*, Vol.64, pp. 670-674, ISSN 0028-3878

Leu-Semenescu, S.; Roze, E.; Vidailhet, M.; Legrand, AP.; Trocello, JM.; Cochen, V.; Sangla, S. & Apartis E. (2007). Myoclonus or tremor in orthostatism: an under-recognized cause of unsteadiness in Parkinson's disease. *Movement Disorders*, Vol.22, No.14, (October), pp. 2063–2069, ISSN 0885-3185

Li, KZ.; Roudaia, E.; Lussier, M.; Bherer, L.; Leroux, A. & McKinley, PA. (2010). Benefits of cognitive dual-task training on balance performance in healthy older adults. The Journals of Gerontology. Series A, *Biological Sciences and Medical Sciences*, Vol.65, No.12, pp. 1344-1352, ISSN 1079-5006

Lindenberger, U.; Marsiske, M. & Baltes, PB. (2000). Memorizing while walking: increase in dual-task costs from young adulthood to old age. *Psychology and Aging*, Vol.15, pp. 417-436, ISSN 0882-7974

Lundin-Olsson, L.; Nyberg, L. & Gustafson, Y. (1997). "Stops walking when talking" as a predictor of falls in elderly people. *Lancet*, Vol.349, No.9052, (March), pp. 617, ISSN 0140-6736

MacDonald, AW. 3rd.; Cohen, JD.; Stenger, VA. & Carter, CS. (2000). Dissociating the role of the dorsolateral prefrontal and anterior cingulate cortex in cognitive control. *Science*, Vol.288, pp. 1835-1838, ISSN 0036-8075

Macht, M.; Kaussner, Y.; Möller, JC.; Stiasny-Kolster, K.; Eggert, KM.; Krüger, HP. & Ellgring, H. (2007). Predictors of freezing in Parkinson's disease: a survey of 6,620 patients. *Movement Disorders*, Vol.22, No.7, 953-956, ISSN 0885-3185

Martin JP. (1967). *The basal ganglia and posture*. Pitman Medical, ASIN B0000CNL13, London

Melton, LJ. 3rd, Leibson, CL.; Achenbach, SJ.; Bower, JH.; Maraganore, DM.; Oberg, AL. & Rocca, WA. (2006). Fracture risk after the diagnosis of Parkinson's disease: influence of concomitant dementia. *Movement Disorders*, Vol.21, No.9, pp. 1361–1367, ISSN 0885-3185

Mille, ML.; Johnson, HM.; Martinez, KM.; Simuni, T. & Rogers, MW. (2007). Acute effects of a lateral postural assist on voluntary step initiation in patients with Parkinson's disease. *Movement Disorders*, Vol.22, No.1, pp. 20-27, ISSN 0885-3185

Mirelman, A.; Maidan, I.; Herman, T.; Deutsch, JE.; Giladi, N. & Hausdorff, JM. (2011). Virtual reality for gait training: can it induce motor learning to enhance complex walking and reduce fall risk in patients with Parkinson's disease? *The Journals of Gerontology*. Series A, Biological Sciences and Medical Sciences, Vol.66, No.4, (February), pp. 234-240, ISSN 1079-5006

Moore, O.; Peretz, C. & Giladi, N. (2007a). Freezing of gait affects quality of life of peoples with Parkinson's disease beyond its relationships with mobility and gait. *Movement Disorders*, Vol.22, pp. 2192–2195, ISSN 0885-3185

Moore, ST.; Macdougall, HG.; Gracies, JM.; Cohen, HS. & Ondo, WG. (2007b). Long-term monitoring of gait in Parkinson's disease. *Gait & Posture*, Vol.26, No.2, pp. 200–207, ISSN 0966-6362

Moore, ST.; MacDougall, HG. & Ondo, WG. (2008). Ambulatory monitoring of freezing of gait in Parkinson's disease. *Journal of Neuroscience Methods*, Vol.167, No.2, pp. 340–348, ISSN 0165-0270

Moreau, C.; Defebvre, L.; Destée, A.; Bleuse, S.; Clement, F.; Blatt, JL.; Krystkowiak, P. & Devos, D. (2008). STN-DBS frequency effects on freezing of gait in advanced Parkinson disease. *Neurology*, Vol.71, No.2, pp. 80-84, ISSN 0028-3878

Morris ME. (2000). Movement disorders in people with Parkinson disease: a model for physical therapy. *Physical Therapy*, Vol.80, pp. 578–597, ISSN 0031-9023

Morris, ME. (2006). Locomotor training in people with Parkinson disease. *Physical Therapy*, Vol.86, pp. 1426–1435, ISSN 0031-9023

Morris, ME.; Iansek, R. & Kirkwood, B. (2009). A randomized controlled trial of movement strategies compared with exercise for people with Parkinson's disease. *Movement Disorders*, Vol.24, pp. 64 –71, ISSN 0885-3185

Morris, ME.; Martin, CL. & Schenkman, ML. (2010). Striding out with Parkinson disease: evidence-based physical therapy for gait disorders. *Physical Therapy*, Vol.90, No.(2), pp. 280-288, ISSN 0031-9023

Nakamura, T.; Meguro, K. & Sasaki, H. (1996). Relationship between falls and stride length variability in senile dementia of the Alzheimer type. *Gerontology*, Vol.42, pp. 108-113, ISSN 0304-324X

Narabayashi, H.; Kondo, T.; Yokochi, F. & Nagatsu, T. (1987). Clinical effects of L-threo-3,4-dihydroxyphenylserine in cases of parkinsonism and pure akinesia. *Advances in Neurology*, Vol.45, pp. 593-602, ISSN: 0091-3952

Nieuwboer, A.; Dom, R.; De Weerdt, W.; Desloovere, K.; Fieuws, S. & Broens-Kaucsik, E. (2001). Abnormalities of the spatiotemporal characteristics of gait at the onset of freezing in Parkinson's disease. *Movement Disorders*, Vol.16, No.6, pp. 1066-1075, ISSN 0885-3185

Nieuwboer, A.; Dom, R.; De Weerdt, W.; Desloovere, K.; Janssens, L. & Stijn, V. (2004). Electromyographic profiles of gait prior to onset of freezing episodes in patients with Parkinson's disease. *Brain: a Journal of Neurology*, Vol.127, No. 7, pp.1650-1660, ISSN 0006-8950

Nieuwboer, A.; Kwakkel, G.; Rochester, I.; Jones, D.; van Wegen, E.; Willems, AM.; Chavret, F.; Hetherington, V.; Baker, K. & Lim, I. (2007). Cueing training in the home improves gait-related mobility in Parkinson's disease: the RESCUE trial. *Journal of Neurology, Neurosurgery, and Psychiatry*, Vol.78, pp. 134-140, ISSN 0022-3050

Nieuwboer, A.; Rochester, L.; Herman, T.; Vandenberghe, W.; Emil, GE.; Thomaes, T. & Giladi, N. (2009). Reliability of the new freezing of gait questionnaire: agreement between patients with Parkinson's disease and their carers. *Gait & Posture*, Vol.30, pp. 459-463, ISSN 0966-6362

Pahapill, PA. & Lozano, AM. (2000). The pedunculopontine nucleus and Parkinson's disease. *Brain*, Vol.123, pp. 767–783, ISSN 0006-8950

Parkinson Study Group. (2001). Dopamine transporter brain imaging to assess the effects of pramipexole vs levodopa on Parkinson disease progression. *JAMA*, Vol.287, No.13, pp. 1653-1661, ISSN 0098-7484

Parkinson Study Group. (2003). Does levodopa slow or hasten the rate of progression of Parkinson's disease? The results of the ELLDOPA trial. *Neurology*, Vol.60, No.5, (Suppl 1), pp. A80-A81, ISSN 0028-3878

Peppe, A.; Ranaldi, A.; Chiavalon, C.; Gasbarra, A.; Collepardo, A.; Romeo, R.; Pasqualetti, P. & Caltagirone, C. (2007). Global Mobility Task: index for evaluating motor impairment and motor rehabilitation programs in Parkinson's disease patients. *Acta Neurologica Scandinavica*, Vol.116, No.3, pp. 182–189, ISSN 0001-6314

Peretz, C.; Herman, T.; Hausdorff, JM. & Giladi, N. (2006). Assessing fear of falling: can a short version of the activities-specific balance confidence scale be useful? *Movement Disorders*, Vol. 21, pp. 2101–2105, ISSN 0885-3185

Pickering, RM.; Grimbergen, YA.; Rigney, U.; Ashburn, A.; Mazibrada, G.; Wood, B.; Gray, P.; Kerr, G. & Bloem, BR. (2007). A meta-analysis of six prospective studies of falling in Parkinson's disease. *Movement Disorders*, Vol.22, pp. 1892–1900, ISSN 0885-3185

Plotnik, M.; Giladi, N. & Hausdorff, JM. (2007). A new measure for quantifying the bilateral coordination of human gait: effects of aging and Parkinson's disease. *Experimental Brain Research*, Vol.181, pp. 561–570, ISSN 0014-4819

Plotnik, M. & Hausdorff, JM. (2008). The role of gait rhythmicity and bilateral coordination of stepping in the pathophysiology of freezing of gait in Parkinson's disease. *Movement Disorders* Vol.23 (Suppl 2), pp. S444-S450, ISSN 0885-3185

Plotnik, M.; Giladi, N. & Hausdorff, JM. (2009). Bilateral coordination of gait and Parkinson's disease: the effects of dual tasking. *Journal of Neurology, Neurosurgery, and Psychiatry*,Vol.80, No. 3, (March), pp. 347–350, ISSN 0022-3050

Plotnik, M.; Giladi, N.; Dagan, Y. & Hausdorff, JM. (2011a). Postural instability and fall risk in Parkinson's disease: impaired dual tasking, pacing, and bilateral coordination of gait during the "ON" medication state. *Experimental Brain Research*, Jan 30. [Epub ahead of print]

Plotnik, M.; Dagan, Y.; Gurevich, T.; Giladi, N. & Hausdorff, JM. (2011b). Effects of cognitive function on gait and dual tasking abilities in patients with Parkinson's disease suffering from motor response fluctuations. *Experimental Brain Research*, Vol.208, No.2, pp. 169–179, ISSN 0014-4819

Pollak, L.; Dobronevsky, Y.; Prohorov, T.; Bahunker, S. & Rabey, JM. (2007). Low dose methylphenidate improves freezing in advanced Parkinson's disease during off-state. *Journal of Neural Transmission. Supplementum*, Vol.72, pp. 145–148, ISSN 0303-6995

Protas, EJ.; Stanley, RK.; Jankovic, J. & MacNeill, B. (1996). Cardiovascular and metabolic responses to upper- and lower-extremity exercise in men with idiopathic Parkinson's disease. *Physical Therapy*, Vol.76, pp. 34–40, ISSN 0031-9023

Quinn, N.; Perlmutter, J. & Marsden, CD. (1984). Acute administration of L-Threo-DOPS does not affect the freezing phenomenon in parkinsonian patients. *Neurology*, Vol.34, pp. 149A, ISSN 0028-3878

Rascol, O.; Brooks, DJ.; Korczyn, AD.; De Deyn, PP.; Clarke, CE. & Lang, AE. (2000). A five-year study of the incidence of dyskinesia in patients with early Parkinson's disease who were treated with ropinirole or levodopa. *The New England journal of medicine*, Vol.342, pp. 1484-1491, ISSN 0028-4793

Reuter, I.; Leone, P.; Schwed, M. & Oechsner, M. (2006). Effect of Nordic walking in Parkinson's disease. *Movement Disorders*, Vol.21, pp. S567, ISSN 0885-3185

Rochester, L.; Hetherington, V.; Jones, D.; Nieuwboer, A.; Willems, AM.; Kwakkel, G. & Van Wegen, E. (2004). Attending to the task: interference effects of functional tasks on walking in Parkinson's disease and the roles of cognition, depression, fatigue, and balance. *Archives of Physical Medicine and Rehabilitation*, Vol.85, pp. 1578-1585, ISSN 0003-9993

Rochester, L.; Nieuwboer, A.; Baker, K.; Hetherington, V.; Willems, AM.; Chavret, F.; Kwakkel, G.; Van Wegen, E.; Lim, I. & Jones, D. (2007). The attentional cost of external rhythmical cues and their impact on gait in Parkinson's disease: effect of cue modality and task complexity. *Journal of Neural Transmission*, Vol.114, pp. 1243–1248, ISSN 0300-9564

Schaafsma, JD.; Giladi, N.; Balash, Y., Bartels, AL., Gurevich, T. & Hausdorff, JM. (2003). Gait dynamics in Parkinson's disease: relationship to Parkinsonian features, falls and response to levodopa. *Journal of the Neurological Sciences*, Vol.212, pp. :47-53, ISSN 0022-510X

Schenkman, ML. & Butler, RB. (1989). A model for multisystem evaluation treatment of individuals with Parkinson's disease. *Physical Therapy*, Vol.69, pp. 932–944, ISSN 0031-9023

Schenkman, ML.; Cutson, TM.; Kuchibhatla, M.; Chandler, J.; Pieper, CF.; Ray, L. & Laub, KC. (1998). Exercise to improve spinal flexibility and function for people with Parkinson's disease: a randomized, controlled trial. *Journal of the American Geriatrics Society*, Vol.46, pp. 1207–1216, ISSN 0002-8614

Schenkman, ML.; Morey, M. & Kuchibhatla, M. (2000). Spinal flexibility and balance control among community-dwelling adults with and without Parkinson's disease. *The*

Journals of Gerontology. Series A, Biological Sciences and Medical Sciences, Vol.55, pp. M441–M445, ISSN 1079-5006

Schenkman, ML.; Hall, D., Kumar, R. & Kohrt, WM. (2008). Endurance exercise training to improve economy of movement of people with Parkinson disease: three case reports. *Physical Therapy,* Vol.88, pp. 63–76, ISSN 0031-9023

Schrodt, LA.; Mercer, VS.; Giuliani, CA. & Hartman, M. (2004). Characteristics of stepping over an obstacle in community dwelling older adults under dual-task conditions. *Gait & Posture* Vol.19, pp. 279-287, ISSN 0966-6362

Simuni, T. & Sethi, K. (2008). Nonmotor manifestations of Parkinson's disease. Annals of *Neurology,* Vol.64 (Suppl 2), pp. S65–S80, ISSN 0364-5134

Snijders, AH.; van de Warrenburg, BP.; Giladi, N. & Bloem, BR. (2007). Neurological gait disorders in elderly people: clinical approach and classification. *Lancet Neurology,* Vol.6, pp. 63–74, ISSN 1474-4422

Soliveri, P.; Brown, RG.; Jahanshahi, M.; Caraceni, T. & Marsden, CD. (1997), Learning manual pursuit tracking skills in patients with Parkinson's disease. *Brain: a Journal of Neurology,* Vol.120, pp. 1325–1337, ISSN 0006-8950

Srygley, JM.; Mirelman, A.; Herman, T.; Giladi, N. & Hausdorff, JM. (2009). When does walking alter thinking? Age and task associated findings. *Brain Research,* Vol.1253, pp. 92-99, ISSN 0006-8993

Stefani, A.; Lozano, AM.; Peppe, A.; Stanzione, P.; Galati, S.; Tropepi, D.; Pierantozzi, M.; Brusa, L.; Scarnati, E. & Mazzone, P. (2007). Bilateral deep brain stimulation of the pedunculopontine and subthalamic nuclei in severe Parkinson's disease. *Brain: a Journal of Neurology,* Vol.130, pp. 1596–1607, ISSN 0006-8950

Stuss, DT. & Alexander, MP. (2000). Executive functions and the frontal lobes: a conceptual view. *Psychological Research,* Vol.63, pp. 289-298, ISSN 0340-0727

Stuss, DT. & Levine, B. (2002). Adult clinical neuropsychology: lessons from studies of the frontal lobes. *Annual Review of Psychology,* Vol.53, pp. 401-433, ISSN 0066-4308

Thanvi, B. & Treadwell, SD. (2010). Freezing of gait in older people: associated conditions, clinical aspects, assessment and treatment. *Postgraduate Medical Journal,* Vol.86, No.1018, pp. 472-477, ISSN 0032-5473

Tillerson, JL.; Caudle, WM.; Reveron, ME. & Miller, GW. (2003). Exercise induces behavioral recovery and attenuates neurochemical deficits in rodent models of Parkinson's disease. *Neuroscience,* Vol.119, pp. 899–911, ISSN 0306-4522

Timmermann, L. & Fink, GR. (2009). Modulating pathological oscillatory activity in Parkinson's disease: What's the rhythm? *Experimental Neurology,* Vol.215, No.2, pp. 209-211, ISSN 0014-4886

Tommasi, G.; Lopiano, L.; Zibetti, M.; Cinquepalmi, A.; Fronda, C.; Bergamasco, B.; Ducati, A. & Lanotte, M. (2007). Freezing and hypokinesia of gait induced by stimulation of the subthalamic region. *Journal of the Neurological Sciences,* Vol.258, pp. 99–103, ISSN 0022-510X

Twelves, D.; Perkins, KS. & Counsell, C. (2003). Systematic review of incidence studies of Parkinson's disease. *Movement Disorders,* Vol.18, No.1, pp.19-31, ISSN 0885-3185

Valkovic, P.; Krafczyk, S. & Botzel, K. (2006). Postural reactions to soleus muscle vibration in Parkinson's disease: scaling deteriorates as disease progresses. *Neuroscience Letters*, Vol.401, pp. 92–96, ISSN 0304-3940

van der Kooij, H.; van Asseldonk, EH.; Geelen, J.; van Vugt, JP. & Bloem, BR. (2007). Detecting asymmetries in balance control with system identification: first experimental results from Parkinson patients. *Journal of Neural Transmission*, Vol.114, pp. 1333–1337, ISSN 0300-9564

van Eijkeren, FJ.; Reijmers, RS.; Kleinveld, MJ.; Minten, A., Bruggen, JP. & Bloem, BR. (2008). Nordic walking improves mobility in Parkinson's disease. *Movement Disorders*, Vol.23, No.15, pp. 2239-2243, ISSN 0885-3185

van Gelder, BM.; Tijhuis, MA.; Kalmijn, S., Giampaoli, S.; Nissinen, A. & Kromhout, D. (2004). Physical activity in relation to cognitive decline in elderly men: the FINE Study. *Neurology*, Vol.63, pp. 2316–2321, ISSN 0028-3878

van Iersel, MB.; Verbeek, AL.; Bloem, BR.; Munneke, M., Esselink, RA. & Rikkert, MG. (2006). Frail elderly patients with dementia go too fast. *Journal of Neurology, Neurosurgery, and Psychiatry*, Vol.77, pp. 874-876, ISSN 0022-3050

Vaugoyeau, M., Viel, S.; Assaiante, C.; Amblard, B. & Azulay, JP. (2007). Impaired vertical postural control and proprioceptive integration deficits in Parkinson's disease. *Neuroscience* Vol.146, pp. 852–863, ISSN 0306-4522

Verghese, J.; Mahoney, J.; Ambrose, AF.; Wang, C. & Holtzer, R. (2010). Effect of cognitive remediation on gait in sedentary seniors. *The Journals of Gerontology. Series A, Biological Sciences and Medical Sciences*, Vol.65, No.12, pp. 1338-1343, ISSN 1079-5006

Visser, JE.; Voermans, NC.; Oude Nijhuis, LB.; van der Eijk, M.; Nijk, R.; Munneke, M. & Bloem, BR. (2007). Quantification of trunk rotations during turning and walking in Parkinson's disease. *Clinical Neurophysiology*, Vol.118, pp. 1602–1606, ISSN 1388-2457

Visser, M.; Verbaan, D.; van Rooden, S.; Marinus, J.; van Hilten, J. & Stiggelbout, A. (2009). A longitudinal evaluation of health-related quality of life of patients with Parkinson's disease. *Value Health*, Vol.12, pp. 392–396, ISSN 1098-3015

Willems, AM.; Nieuwboer, A.; Chavret, F.; Desloovere, K.; Dom, R.; Rochester, L.; Kwakkel, G.; van Wegen, E. & Jones, D. (2007). Turning in Parkinson's disease patients and controls: the effect of auditory cues. *Movement Disorders*, Vol.22, pp. 1871–1878, ISSN 0885-3185

Williams, DR.; Watt, HC. & Lees, AJ. (2006). Predictors of falls and fractures in bradykinetic rigid syndromes: a retrospective study. *Journal of Neurology, Neurosurgery, and Psychiatry*, Vol.77, pp. 468–473, ISSN 0022-3050

Wright, WG.; Gurfinkel, VS.; Nutt, J.; Horak, FB. & Cordo, PJ. (2007). Axial hypertonicity in Parkinson's disease: direct measurements of trunk and hip torque. *Experimental Neurology*, Vol.208, pp. 38–46, ISSN 0014-4886

Yaffe, K.; Barnes, D.; Nevitt, M.; Lui, LY. & Covinsky, K. (2001). A prospective study of physical activity and cognitive decline in elderly women: women who walk. *Archives of Internal Medicine*, Vol.161, pp. 1703–1708, ISSN 0730-188X

Yelnik, J. (2007). PPN or PPD, what is the target for deep brain stimulation in Parkinson's disease? *Brain: a Journal of Neurology*, Vol.130, (Pt6), pp. 1596-607, ISSN 0006-8950

Yogev, G.; Giladi, N.; Peretz, C.; Springer, S.; Simon, ES, & Hausdorff, JM. (2005). Dual tasking, gait rhythmicity, and Parkinson's disease: which aspects of gait are attention demanding? *The European Journal of Neuroscience*, Vol.22, pp. 1248-1256, ISSN 0953-816X

Yogev-Seligmann, G.; Hausdorff, JM. & Giladi, N. (2008). The role of executive function and attention in gait. *Movement Disorders*, Vol.23, No.3, pp. 329-342, ISSN 0885-3185

Zúñiga, C.; Lester, J.; Cersósimo, MG.; Díaz, S. & Micheli, FE. (2006). Treatment of primary progressive freezing of gait with high doses of selegiline. *Clinical Neuropharmacology*, Vol.29, pp. 20-21, ISSN 0362-5664

3

Nocturnal Disturbances in Patients with Parkinson's Disease

Keisuke Suzuki, Tomoyuki Miyamoto, Masayuki Miyamoto, Masaoki Iwanami and Koichi Hirata
Department of Neurology, Center of Sleep Medicine, Dokkyo Medical University School of Medicine
Japan

1. Introduction

Sleep disturbances are common problems in patients with Parkinson's disease (PD) caused by various factors including nocturnal motor symptoms, psychiatric symptoms, dementia, medication use and circadian cycle disruptions as well as comorbidity with sleep apnea syndrome (SAS), restless legs syndrome (RLS) and rapid eye movement sleep behavior disorder (RBD) (Table 1). As impaired sleep quality and sleep fragmentation due to nighttime problems are associated with daytime motor dysfunction and have a negative impact on the quality of life of the patient (Gómez-Esteban et al., 2010), an intensive and detailed evaluation of nighttime problems is warranted. Patients often may be unaware of sleep disturbances and even neurologists have been reported to fail to recognize sleep disorders in approximately 40% of PD patients (Shulman et al., 2002). Here, we review sleep disorders in patients with PD, mainly focusing on nighttime problems.

2. Sleep disturbances related to Parkinson's disease itself

Impaired sleep architecture and sleep-wakefulness systems are observed in PD as disease related changes. Insomnia in patients with the early stage of disease or in untreated patients may be associated with disease-related sleep disturbances rather than sleep disturbances caused by other factors including motor dysfunction, medication use, neuropsychiatric symptoms and cognitive dysfunction, though non-motor symptoms can occur in the early phase of the disease. Polysomnography (PSG) recordings yield altered sleep structure that is characterized by a reduction in The percentage of slow wave sleep and a decrease in the amount of REM sleep (Petit et al., 2004) caused by the degeneration of cholinergic neurons in the basal forebrain, noradrenergic neurons in the locus ceruleus and serotoninergic neurons in the raphe nucleus (N.J. Diederich & Comella, 2003).
Serotonin, acetylcholine and noradrenalin play a role in maintaining wakefulness, and thus, disturbances lead to excessive daytime sleepiness. In some patients with PD, excessive daytime sleepiness and sudden onset of sleep episodes have been associated with a short sleep latency and sleep onset REM period recorded by the multiple sleep latency test (Arnulf et al., 2002). Similar features are observed in narcolepsy, a sleep disorder characterized by severe daytime sleepiness caused by loss of orexin neurons. Loss of orexinergic neurons in the

posterior portion of the lateral hypothalamus (Fronczek et al., 2007) and the reduction of the A10 dopaminergic group in the ventral tegmental area (Rye, 2004) have also been implicated in impaired wakefulness in PD. Further study is required to examine whether impairment of the orexin system accounts for excessive daytime sleepiness in PD and whether decreased orexin levels reflect disease-related changes or secondary compensatory changes resulting from dopaminergic dysfunctions (Baumann et al., 2008; Compta et al., 2009).

Impairment of sleep architecture
Involvement of the cholinergic, serotoninergic and noradrenergic systems reduces REM and slow-wave sleep
Impairment of the arousal system (orexin, serotonin, noradrenalin, acetylcholine and dopamine)
Nocturnal motor symptoms
(wearing-off phenomenon, rigidity, akinesia, tremor, medication-related dyskinesia and dystonia)
Psychiatric symptoms including depression and psychosis
Nightmares and vivid dreams
Hallucinations
Cognitive dysfunction
Nocturia
Pain
Medication use
Sleep apnea syndrome
REM sleep behavior disorder
Restless legs syndrome
Periodic limb movement disorder

Table 1. Multifactorial causes associated with sleep disorders in PD

3. Dopamine and sleep

Dopamine has a role in regulating the sleep-wake cycle (Rye & Jankovic, 2002). Biphasic effects of dopaminergic stimulation on sleep have been reported based on animal studies. High doses of D2 agonists reduce slow-wave sleep and REM sleep and increase wakefulness mediated via postsynaptic receptors, whereas low doses of D2 stimulants increase slow wave sleep and induce sleep mediated via presynaptic receptors (Monti et al., 1988). A D1 receptor agonist suppresses the amount of REM sleep in dose-dependent manner and enhanced wakefulness, while D1 antagonists increase REM sleep (Trampus et al., 1991). The study by Qu et al. examined the mechanism by which modafinil increases wakefulness. They found that the pretreatment of D2 receptor knockout mice with a D1 receptor antagonist completely abolished the arousal effects of modafinil, strongly indicating that dopaminergic D1 and D2 receptors are essential for the wakefulness induced by modafinil (Qu et al., 2008). The involvement of dopamine systems in the mesocorticolimbic and striatal systems in conjunction with dopaminergic therapy further complicates the role of dopamine in PD sleep disturbances.

4. Nocturnal motor problems

Nocturnal disturbances have been reported in up to 98% of patients with PD (Lees et al., 1988). Disturbances include rigidity, tremor, dystonia, akinesia, nightmares, hallucinations, muscle cramps and nocturia. These symptoms result in frequent nocturnal awakenings that contribute to sleep maintenance insomnia, a common form of insomnia in PD (Chaudhuri et al., 2002; Factor et al., 1990; Lees et al., 1988; Suzuki et al., 2007; Tandberg et al., 1998). Sleep onset insomnia can be seen in PD, but it does not seem to account for the majority of insomnia in PD when compared with age-matched controls. In a community-based sleep study, sleep onset insomnia, sleep maintenance insomnia and early awakening were observed in 31.8%, 38.9% and 23.4% of PD patients compared with 22%, 12% and 11% of healthy controls, respectively (Tandberg et al., 1998). The frequency of sleep onset insomnia was not significantly different between the groups. Identification of the nature of nocturnal motor symptoms and the appropriate treatment (e.g., an increase or reduction in the amount of dopaminergic drugs) can improve nocturnal disturbances. A further tool is necessary for assessing nighttime disabilities related to PD. Although PSG is considered to be the gold standard in the assessment of sleep disorders because it provides information about the patient's actual sleep status, including sleep efficiency, sleep latency and sleep structure and can detect SAS, RBD or RLS, several questionnaires have been developed to address insomnia or daytime sleepiness in the general population (the Pittsburgh Sleep Quality Index, or the Epworth sleepiness scale, ESS) (Buysse et al., 1989; Johns, 1991).

4.1 Parkinson's disease sleep scale

Chaudhuri et al. developed the Parkinson's disease sleep scale (PDSS) (Chaudhuri et al., 2002), a visual analogue scale that assesses 15 PD-related nocturnal symptoms of nocturnal disability in PD. This scale is now regarded as a recommended, reliable scale (Högl et al., 2010). The scale includes the following: overall quality of night's sleep (item 1); sleep onset and maintenance insomnia (items 2 and 3); nocturnal restlessness (items 4 and 5); nocturnal psychosis (items 6 and 7); nocturia (items 8 and 9); nocturnal motor symptoms (items 10-13); sleep refreshment (item 14); and daytime dozing (item 15). It has been validated and used extensively in a number of countries with high reliability (Abe et al., 2005; Margis et al., 2009; Martinez-Martin et al., 2004; Suzuki et al., 2007; Wang et al., 2008). Their study found that patients with advanced disease had more severe nocturnal disabilities when compared to patients with early or moderate disease. Our multicenter study also revealed more severe nocturnal disturbances measured by PDSS in patients with advanced PD [Hoehn & Yahr (H&Y), stage IV] when compared to those with early and moderate PD (H&Y, stages I -III). The characteristics of sleep disturbances in PD were distinguishable from that in the control subjects (Figure 1A and B). Sleep disturbances were associated with disease duration, depressive symptoms and complications with dopaminergic treatment (dyskinesia and wearing off) (Suzuki et al., 2007). However, it has been shown that although nocturnal symptoms assessed by PDSS, such as nocturia, nighttime cramp, dystonia and tremor, were more severe in advanced PD patients, they could also be observed in untreated or early stage PD patients when compared with control subjects (Dhawan et al., 2006). This suggests that nocturnal disturbances can develop in the early stages of PD, even when the patients are untreated and exhibit only mild motor symptoms. Thus, nocturnal problems can be treated with dopaminergic treatments.

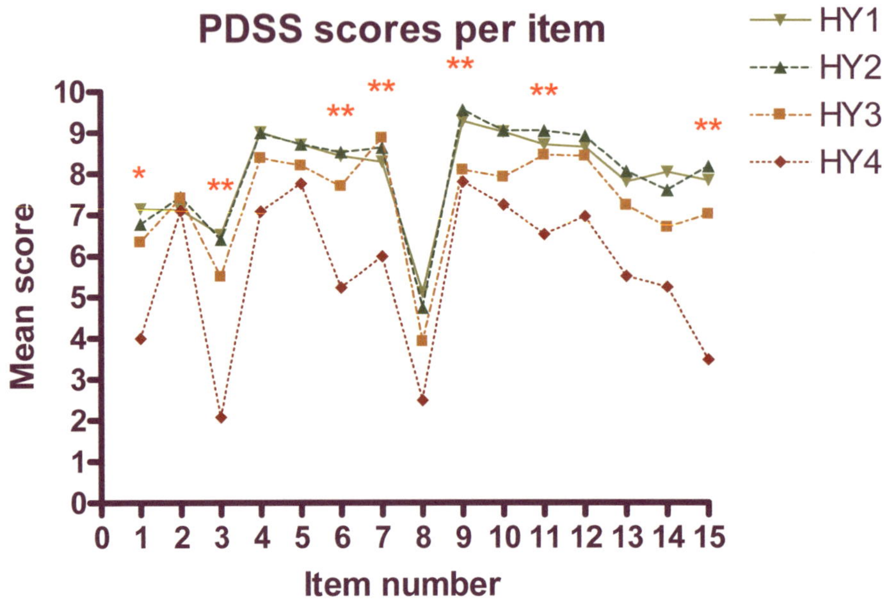

Fig. 1A. Profiles of the mean PDSS scores of each item according to the stage of the disease as defined by H&Y. There were highly significant differences between H&Y Stage 4 and H&Y Stages 1-3 for item 3 (sleep maintenance insomnia), item 6 (distressing dreams at night), item 11 (painful muscle cramp) and item 15 (falling asleep unexpectedly).

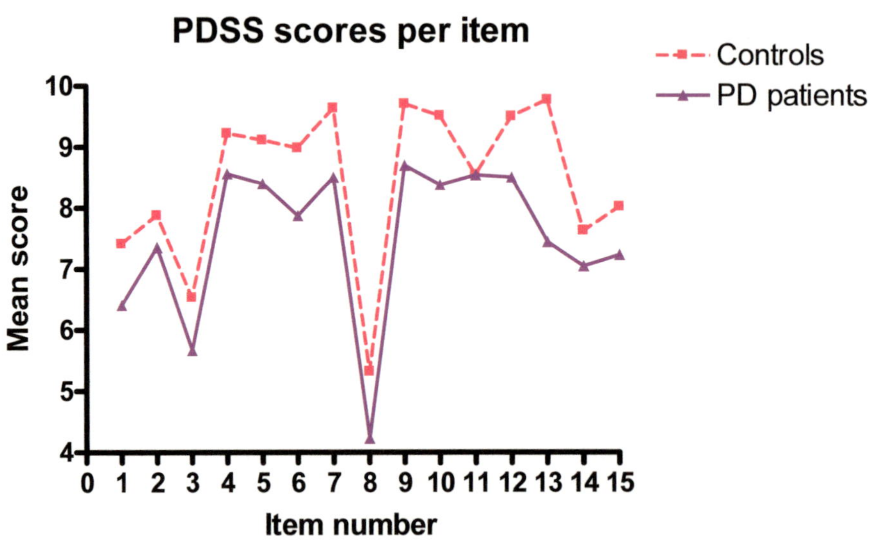

Fig. 1B. Profiles of mean PDSS scores for each item in PD and control patients. The most severe ratings in both groups were found for sleep maintenance insomnia (item 3) and nocturia (item 8). With the exception of item 2 (sleep onset insomnia), item 11 (painful muscle cramp) and item 14 (tiredness and sleepiness after waking in the morning), PDSS scores of patients with PD were significantly lower when compared to healthy subjects.

4.2 Parkinson's disease sleep scale-2

Importantly, the PDSS does not screen for sleep apnea syndrome (SAS). Recently, a modified version of PDSS, PDSS-2, has been published and is shown to have excellent validity and reliability (Trenkwalder et al., 2011b). The item regarding unexpected daytime sleepiness was removed because it can be caused by numerous factors in PD, and a new item to screen for SAS was added. Three aspects of sleep problems can be obtained by factor analysis: sleep-specific disturbance, such as sleep onset and the maintenance insomnia, unrestored sleep in the morning, getting up to pass urine and the overall quality of sleep; PD-specific nocturnal motor symptoms at night, such as akinesia, early morning dystonia, tremor during waking periods at night, periodic limb movements, restless behavior and motor symptoms probably due to RBD; and PD-specific nocturnal non-motor symptoms, such as hallucinations, confused states, pain, difficulty breathing with snoring and immobility. A recent study assessing the effect of rotigotine, a non-ergot dopamine agonist with 24-hour transdermal delivery, on early morning motor function and sleep have shown that rotigotine administration improved motor abilities as assessed by the Unified Parkinson Disease Rating Scale (UPDRS) motor score and sleep problems as assessed by PDSS-2 (Trenkwalder et al., 2011a). In clinical practice, the use of both ESS and PDSS-2 would be useful for assessing daytime sleepiness and nighttime problems in PD.

5. Motor symptoms at night

Importantly, disabling motor symptoms, such as akinesia, resting tremor and rigidity, occur not only during the daytime but also during the nighttime. Patients in the advanced stages of the disease are likely to have motor dysfunction throughout the day, but some patients, especially those in the early stages of the disease, may predominantly have nighttime motor problems (Dhawan et al., 2006). This is supported by the results of several studies showing a weak or nonexistent correlation between sleep disturbances and daytime motor symptoms (UPDRS motor score) (Chaudhuri & Martinez-Martin, 2004; Tandberg et al., 1998) and no correlation between nocturnal motor symptoms obtained by PDSS-2 and UPDRS motor score (Trenkwalder et al., 2011b). Kumar et al., however, found a patient's UPDRS motor score to be a significant determinant of sleep disturbances (Kumar et al., 2002).

Nocturnal motor symptoms can result in frequent awakenings at night, which sometimes can contribute to daytime sleepiness. In our previous study, however, PD patients with excessive daytime sleepiness (ESS $\geq$ 10) had similar PDSS scores, except for falling asleep unexpectedly (item 15), when compared to those without excessive daytime sleepiness (ESS $<$ 10), suggesting that excessive daytime sleepiness is more related to disease related changes and dopaminergic medication use than nocturnal disturbances (Suzuki et al., 2008).

When wearing off-related motor symptoms or the worsening of motor symptoms during the night are significant problems for a patient, providing continuous dopaminergic stimulation via a long-acting dopamine agonist at nighttime (Pahwa et al., 2007; Poewe et al., 2007), deep brain stimulation (Arnulf et al., 2000) or an overnight subcutaneous infusion of apomorphine (Reuter et al., 1999) has been reported to be beneficial. For hallucinations, psychosis or medication-related dyskinesia at night, however, reductions in the dose of dopaminergic agents and/or the addition of atypical antipsychotics may help. Amantadine or selegiline can cause frequent nocturnal awakenings, and reducing the dose or changing the time of the administration of these drugs to the morning may reduce nocturnal awakening.

6. Nocturia

Urinary bladder related symptoms, such as frequency, urgency and urge incontinence, are common in PD and can cause frequent nocturnal awakenings. Although nocturia is associated with the normal aging process, 80% of PD patients have had two or more episodes of nocturia per night that were caused by overflow incontinence and a spastic bladder (Lees et al., 1988). These symptoms are attributable to diffuse autonomic dysfunction in PD. Lewy bodies can be found in autonomic regulatory regions, including the hypothalamus, sympathetic (intermediolateral nucleus of the thoracic cord and sympathetic ganglia), and parasympathetic nervous systems (dorsal, vagal, and sacral parasympathetic nuclei) (Micieli et al., 2003). Furthermore, the emergence of lesions in the dorsal vagus nucleus and in other autonomic braintstem centers has been found before the manifestation of motor symptoms related to pathological changes in the substantia nigra (Braak et al., 2003).

Dopaminergic mechanisms also play a role in normal bladder control and overactive bladder. In animal studies, the stimulation of D1 receptors inhibits the micturition reflex, while the stimulation of D2 receptors facilitates the micturition reflex. Therefore, D2 depletion of dopaminergic neurons induces overactive bladder and D1 receptor agonists produce a dose dependent inhibition of the micturition reflex (Winge & Fowler, 2006). In PD models, the beneficial effect of concurrent activation of D1/D2 receptors rather than selective stimulation of D2 receptors has been reported (Yoshimura et al., 1998). Kuno et al. reported that switching from bromocriptine to pergolide improved nocturia, thereby improving sleep status in patients with PD (Kuno et al., 2004). Anticholinergic drugs, such as oxybutinin and tolterodine, are commonly used for detrusor hyperreflexia. The beneficial effect of subthalamic deep brain stimulation on detrusor hyperreflexia has been reported (Seif et al., 2004). When nocturia is related to wearing off symptoms, changing medications to a long-acting dopamine agonist before bedtime can be beneficial. A urologic examination is recommended to rule out underlying urologic diseases.

7. Pain

Pain has been reported in approximately 60% of PD patients (Barone et al., 2009) and is associated with sleep disorders and depressive symptoms (Goetz et al., 1987; Starkstein et al., 1991), in addition to tremor, rigidity, akinesia, dystonia and akathisia. A recent review classified pain into the following categories: musculoskeletal pain, radicular or neuropathic pain, dystonia-related pain, akathitic discomfort and primary central parkinsonian pain (Ford, 2010). Pain is thought to be mediated through medial and lateral pain pathways. However, the pathophysiology of pain perception is not yet well understood. The basal ganglia appear to have an important role for the relay of nociceptive information within the striatum and limbic system (Ford, 2010), and dopamine has been implicated in endogenous pain modulation systems (Potvin et al., 2009). Nocturnal pain is related to nocturnal awakening but not to all sleep disorders. Primary central parkinsonian, akathitic and dystonia-related pain may respond to dopaminergic treatment, and painful symptoms can worsen during wearing off periods. Thus, the appropriate evaluation of pain-related symptoms and managing wearing off-related symptoms during nighttime can improve pain-related sleep disturbances.

8. Hallucinations and psychosis

Hallucinations and psychosis affect 30 to 45% of PD patients treated with levodopa for a long period (Goetz, 1999). Among a wide spectrum of hallucinations, visual hallucinations are commonly seen. Sleep disturbances, daily doses of levodopa, older age, depression and cognitive impairment have been shown to increase the risk for hallucinations in PD patients (Goetz, 2010; Nausieda et al., 1982). A single photon emission computed tomography imaging study showed that PD patients with visual hallucinations had perfusion reductions in the bilateral inferior parietal lobule, inferior temporal gyrus, precuneus gyrus and occipital cortex (Matsui et al., 2006). A ten-year longitudinal study of sleep disorders and hallucinations in PD showed that visual hallucinations were associated with concurrent nightmares, vivid dreams and severe sleep fragmentation. At baseline, no sleep abnormalities at study entry predicted future development of hallucinations in PD patients not currently experiencing hallucinations (Goetz et al., 2010). When reductions in dopaminergic treatments are ineffective, administration of antipsychotics should be considered.

9. Depressive symptoms and nocturnal disturbances

A close link between depression and sleep disorders has been reported in PD (Borek et al., 2006; Happe et al., 2001). Both have a negative impact on the quality of life in PD patients (Gómez-Esteban et al., 2010; Rahman et al., 2008). In a recent systematic review, the prevalence of depression in PD patients varies, ranging from 2.7% to 89% (Reijnders et al., 2008). However, the exact details of nocturnal symptoms that contribute to depression in PD are not well studied. In our multi-center study, depressive symptoms (Zung Self-Rating Depression Scale, SDS score ≥ 40) were present in 64.9% of PD patients, and SDS scores were strongly correlated with PDSS scores (Figure 2A) (Suzuki et al., 2009). Using a regression model, PDSS scores and UPDRS Part I (mental state) were significant determinants of depressive symptoms. However, depressed PD patients showed greater disease severity and more severe motor dysfunction than non-depressed PD patients. Similarly, Chaudhuri and Martinez-Martin reported a significant correlation between PDSS score and depressive symptoms (Chaudhuri & Martinez-Martin, 2004). Compared to patients without depressive symptoms and controls, patients with depressive symptoms had significantly impaired scores in almost all PDSS items except item 2 (difficulty in initiating sleep) and item 11 (painful muscle clamp) (Figure 2B). Surprisingly, there were no significant differences between controls and non-depressed patients in PDSS sub-items, suggesting that depressive symptoms play a pivotal role in developing nocturnal disturbances. Upon detailed evaluation of nocturnal symptoms, early morning tremor and nocturnal dystonia were closely associated with depressive symptoms. This result is in line with the finding that depressive symptoms were exacerbated during periods of time in which patients experienced nocturnal wearing off-related (hypodopaminergic state) motor symptoms (Cummings, 1992). While depression can trigger motor fluctuations, such as the wearing off phenomenon (Lieberman, 2006). Raising awareness of depressive symptoms and the application of appropriate management techniques may improve both depression and sleep disorders in PD patients.

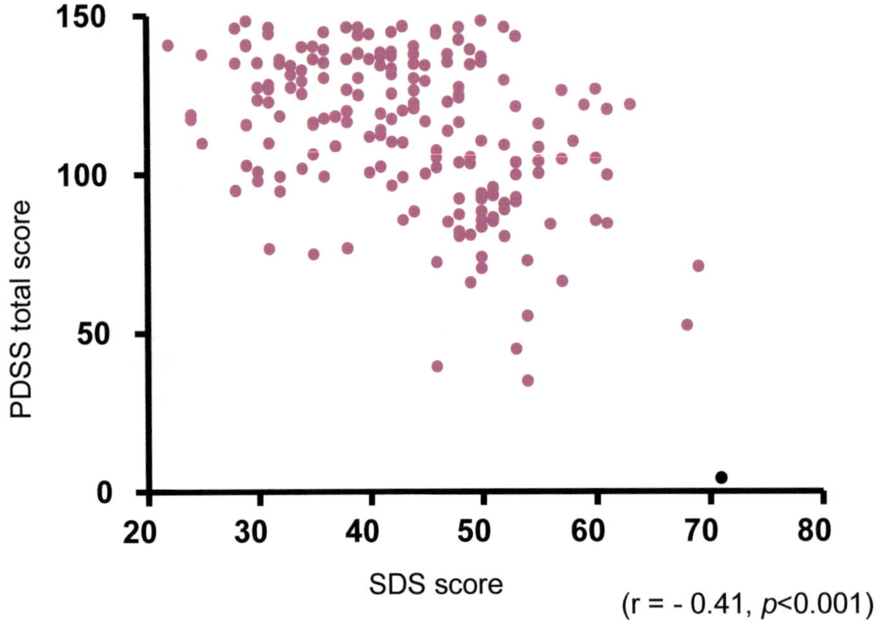

Fig. 2A. Correlation between PDSS total score and SDS score

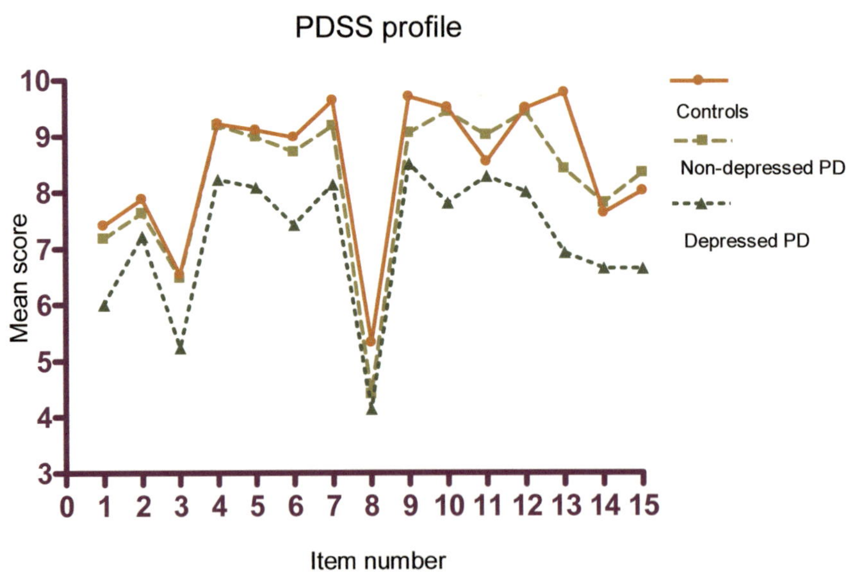

Fig. 2B. Profiles of mean PDSS scores of items in depressed PD (SDS ≥ 40), nondepressed PD (SDS < 40) patients and controls.

10. REM sleep behavior disorder (RBD)

REM sleep behavior disorder (RBD) is characterized by a loss of muscle atonia during REM sleep, enabling patients to act out dreams, often leading to injuries to themselves or their bed partner (Schenck et al., 1986). RBD is likely to affect older individuals and is predominantly seen in males (Olson et al., 2000). Animal studies show that lesions of the locus coeruleus perialpha in cats and the sublaterodorsal nucleus in rats caused REM sleep without atonia and with complex movements (Sastre & Jouvet, 1979). RBD was initially thought to be an idiopathic disorder; however, a study in 1996 by Schenck demonstrated that 38% of 29 patients with idiopathic RBD developed PD within 3.7 ± 1.4 years (Schenck et al., 1996). RBD is associated with neurodegenerative disorders, particularly with synucleinopathies, such as PD, multiple system atrophy and dementia with Lewy bodies (Olson et al., 2000; Postuma et al., 2009; Stiasny-Kolster et al., 2005). Moreover, nonmotor symptoms of PD, such as impaired visual and olfactory discrimination, cardiac sympathetic denervation and cognitive impairment, that often precede the onset of motor symptoms have been found in idiopathic RBD patients (Gagnon et al., 2006; Miyamoto et al., 2006; Miyamoto et al., 2010; Postuma et al., 2010b; Postuma et al., 2006). In RBD, substantia nigra hyperechogenicity (Iwanami et al., 2010) and decreased regional cerebral blood flow in the parietooccipital and limbic lobes and the cerebellar hemispheres (Hanyu et al., 2011) have been found to correspond with alpha syncleinopathies, including PD. As a possible prodromal phase of neurodegenerative diseases, a diagnosis of RBD is crucial for early intervention. Excessive tonic and phasic EMG activity during REM sleep is increased over time in patients with RBD (Iranzo et al., 2009). Postuma et al. reported that the severity of REM atonia loss during baseline PSG can predict the development of PD (Postuma et al., 2010a).

PD patients with RBD exhibited a nontremor predominant phenotype, increased frequency of falls and poor response to dopaminergic medications (Postuma et al., 2008b). However, the overall disease severity, quantitative motor testing and motor complications did not differ between the PD patients with and without RBD. Additionally, the presence of RBD in PD is associated with orthostatic hypotension and impaired color vision but not olfactory impairment (Postuma et al., 2008a). Interestingly, restored motor control (movements, speech and facial expressions) has been observed in PD and in multiple system atrophy patients with RBD during REM sleep (De Cock et al., 2011; De Cock et al., 2007). The mechanism for the improvement of parkinsonism during RBD was unclear but may be due to enhanced dopamine transmission.

RBD can be triggered by antidepressants. Clonazepam (0.5 to 1.5 mg) at bedtime is the most effective treatment for RBD patients. Melatonin (3-12 mg) at bedtime has been shown to ameliorate RBD (Aurora et al., 2010). Administration of 2.5 g of Yi-Gan San, an herbal medication, three times a day, alone or in conjunction with 0.25 mg clonazepam, has also been reported to be effective in the treatment of RBD (Shinno et al., 2008).

11. Restless legs syndromes (RLS)

Restless legs syndrome (RLS) is a sensorimotor disorder associated with an irresistible urge to move the legs, causing insomnia. Symptoms get worse at rest and become apparent in the evening and at nighttime. Some studies have demonstrated a higher rate of RLS comorbidity in PD when compared to the general population (Gómez-Esteban et al., 2007;

Peralta et al., 2010), while the other studies found no difference (Calzetti et al., 2009; Loo & Tan, 2008). Although the pathophysiology of RLS is unclear, central dopaminergic dysfunction has been implicated based on the estimated impairment of A11 dopaminergic nuclei in the hypothalamus and a favorable response to a dopamine agonist. This structure innervates preganglionic sympathetic neurons and the dorsal horn as well as serotoninergic pathways and motor neurons in the spinal cord (Walters & Rye, 2009). Iron deficiency also contributes to impairments in dopamine signaling in the brain. Low iron and ferritin levels in cerebrospinal fluid have been found in patients with RLS (Mizuno et al., 2005).

Caffeine, alcohol and some medications, including antihistamines, dopamine antagonists, tricyclic antidepressants and serotonergic reuptake inhibitors, can exacerbate or cause RLS (Ekbom & Ulfberg, 2009). Iron replacement therapy should be considered when serum ferritin levels are lower than 50 μg/L. Dopamine agonists, pramipexole and ropinirole, at bedtime are effective treatments for RLS.

In PD patients, however, nonmotor symptoms related to nondopaminergic systems (e.g., cognitive impairment, autonomic dysfunction, depression and sleepiness), but not motor symptoms, were found to be associated with RLS (Verbaan et al., 2010). Gómez-Esteban et al. found high prevalence of RLS in PD patients but found no difference in disease severity, UPDRS scores or quality of life between groups with or without RLS (Gómez-Esteban et al., 2007). Peralta et al. found a positive association between motor fluctuation, wearing off phenomenon, and RLS symptoms in PD patients but suggested wearing off-induced restlessness can be an "RLS-mimic" (Peralta et al., 2010).

Autopsy studies have shown increased substantia nigra iron levels in PD patients (Morris & Edwardson, 1994) and decreased substantia nigra iron levels in RLS patients (Connor et al., 2003). Interestingly, when comparing PD with and without RLS, transcranial sonography findings demonstrated that there were no significant differences in SN echogenicity, which is considered to reflect the amount of tissue iron content, between the two groups, whereas idiopathic RLS patients showed significant substantia nigra hypoechogenicity (Kwon et al., 2010). This suggests that the pathogenesis of RLS in PD and idiopathic RLS may involve different mechanisms.

12. Sleep apnea syndrome (SAS)

Previous studies reported a high incidence (approximately 40-60%) of sleep apnea syndrome (SAS) in PD patients (N. J. Diederich et al., 2005; Maria et al., 2003). Upper airway muscle dysfunction may have a role in the development of obstructive sleep apnea (Vincken et al., 1984). However, recent studies assessing the prevalence of SAS in PD revealed that the apnea-hypopnea index was not significantly different between PD patients and controls, and the rate of obstructive sleep apnea in PD were similar to that seen in the general population (De Cock et al., 2010; Trotti & Bliwise, 2010). These findings indicate that obstructive sleep apnea may be not a relevant issue in PD. Nocturnal stridor caused by vocal cord abductor dysfunction can develop in patients with PD but more frequently occurs in patients with multiple system atrophy (MSA) (Isozaki et al., 1995). It is important to screen for vocal cord abductor dysfunction with a laryngoscopy during sleep when nocturnal stridor occurs. Treatment, such as continuous positive airway pressure therapy or a tracheotomy, is effective. However, these treatments do not always prevent sudden death in patients with MSA, suggesting a mechanism such as central hypoventilation, other than upper airway obstruction, may play a role (Shimohata et al., 2008).

13. Conclusion

Sleep disturbances in PD are complicated by various factors. We reviewed the current literature regarding nighttime problems in PD. Appropriate evaluation and management of nocturnal motor and non-motor symptoms are essential to improve the patient's quality of life. Importantly, several symptoms are responsive to changes in the dose or timing of dopaminergic medications. Substantial research effort has been made to develop effective treatment for motor symptoms, however, treating non-motor symptoms remains a challenging issue.

14. Appendix

The Parkinson's Disease Sleep Scale (Chaudhuri et al., 2002)

1. The overall quality of your night's sleep is:
2. Do you have difficulty falling asleep each night?
3. Do you have difficulty staying asleep?
4. Do you have restlessness of legs or arms at night or in the evening causing disruption of sleep?
5. Do you fidget in bed?
6. Do you suffer from distressing dreams at night?
7. Do you suffer from distressing hallucination at night (seeing or hearing things that you are told do not exist)?
8. Do you get up at night to pass urine?
9. Do you have incontinence of urine because you are unable to move due to "off" symptoms?
10. Do you experience numbness or tingling of your arms or legs which wake you from sleep at night?
11. Do you have painful muscle cramps in your arms or legs whilst sleeping at night?
12. Do you wake early in the morning with painful posturing of arms or legs?
13. On waking do you experience tremor?
14. Do you feel tired and sleepy after waking in the morning?
15. Have you unexpectedly fallen asleep during the day?

Scores for a given individual item range from 0 to 10: 10 represents the best, 0 represents the worst score. For question 1: Awful = 0, Excellent = 10. For question 15: Frequently = 0, Never = 10. For the remainder of the questions: Always = 0, Never = 10.

15. References

Abe, K., Hikita, T., & Sakoda, S. (2005). Sleep disturbances in Japanese patients with Parkinson's disease--comparing with patients in the UK. *J Neurol Sci, 234*(1-2), 73-78.

Arnulf, I., Bejjani, B. P., Garma, L., Bonnet, A. M., Houeto, J. L., Damier, P., Derenne, J. P., & Agid, Y. (2000). Improvement of sleep architecture in PD with subthalamic nucleus stimulation. *Neurology, 55*(11), 1732-1734.

Arnulf, I., Konofal, E., Merino-Andreu, M., Houeto, J. L., Mesnage, V., Welter, M. L., Lacomblez, L., Golmard, J. L., Derenne, J. P., & Agid, Y. (2002). Parkinson's disease and sleepiness: an integral part of PD. *Neurology, 58*(7), 1019-1024.

Aurora, R. N., Zak, R. S., Maganti, R. K., Auerbach, S. H., Casey, K. R., Chowdhuri, S., Karippot, A., Ramar, K., Kristo, D. A., & Morgenthaler, T. I. (2010). Best practice guide for the treatment of REM sleep behavior disorder (RBD). *J Clin Sleep Med, 6*(1), 85-95.

Barone, P., Antonini, A., Colosimo, C., Marconi, R., Morgante, L., Avarello, T. P., Bottacchi, E., Cannas, A., Ceravolo, G., Ceravolo, R., Cicarelli, G., Gaglio, R. M., Giglia, R. M., Iemolo, F., Manfredi, M., Meco, G., Nicoletti, A., Pederzoli, M., Petrone, A., Pisani, A., Pontieri, F. E., Quatrale, R., Ramat, S., Scala, R., Volpe, G., Zappulla, S., Bentivoglio, A. R., Stocchi, F., Trianni, G., & Dotto, P. D. (2009). The PRIAMO study: A multicenter assessment of nonmotor symptoms and their impact on quality of life in Parkinson's disease. *Mov Disord, 24*(11), 1641-1649.

Baumann, C. R., Scammell, T. E., & Bassetti, C. L. (2008). Parkinson's disease, sleepiness and hypocretin/orexin. *Brain, 131*(Pt 3), e91.

Borek, L. L., Kohn, R., & Friedman, J. H. (2006). Mood and sleep in Parkinson's disease. *J Clin Psychiatry, 67*(6), 958-963.

Braak, H., Del Tredici, K., Rub, U., de Vos, R. A., Jansen Steur, E. N., & Braak, E. (2003). Staging of brain pathology related to sporadic Parkinson's disease. *Neurobiol Aging, 24*(2), 197-211.

Buysse, D. J., Reynolds, C. F., 3rd, Monk, T. H., Berman, S. R., & Kupfer, D. J. (1989). The Pittsburgh Sleep Quality Index: a new instrument for psychiatric practice and research. *Psychiatry Res, 28*(2), 193-213.

Calzetti, S., Negrotti, A., Bonavina, G., Angelini, M., & Marchesi, E. (2009). Absence of co-morbidity of Parkinson disease and restless legs syndrome: a case-control study in patients attending a movement disorders clinic. *Neurol Sci, 30*(2), 119-122.

Chaudhuri, K. R., & Martinez-Martin, P. (2004). Clinical assessment of nocturnal disability in Parkinson's disease: the Parkinson's Disease Sleep Scale. *Neurology, 63*(8 Suppl 3), S17-20.

Chaudhuri, K. R., Pal, S., DiMarco, A., Whately-Smith, C., Bridgman, K., Mathew, R., Pezzela, F. R., Forbes, A., Hogl, B., & Trenkwalder, C. (2002). The Parkinson's disease sleep scale: a new instrument for assessing sleep and nocturnal disability in Parkinson's disease. *J Neurol Neurosurg Psychiatry, 73*(6), 629-635.

De Cock, V.C., Abouda, M., Leu, S., Oudiette, D., Roze, E., Vidailhet, M., Similowski, T., & Arnulf, I. (2010). Is obstructive sleep apnea a problem in Parkinson's disease? *Sleep Med, 11*(3), 247-252.

Compta, Y., Santamaria, J., Ratti, L., Tolosa, E., Iranzo, A., Munoz, E., Valldeoriola, F., Casamitjana, R., Rios, J., & Marti, M. J. (2009). Cerebrospinal hypocretin, daytime sleepiness and sleep architecture in Parkinson's disease dementia. *Brain, 132*(Pt 12), 3308-3317.

Connor, J. R., Boyer, P. J., Menzies, S. L., Dellinger, B., Allen, R. P., Ondo, W. G., & Earley, C. J. (2003). Neuropathological examination suggests impaired brain iron acquisition in restless legs syndrome. *Neurology, 61*(3), 304-309.

Cummings, J. L. (1992). Depression and Parkinson's disease: a review. *Am J Psychiatry, 149*(4), 443-454.

De Cock, V. C., Debs, R., Oudiette, D., Leu, S., Radji, F., Tiberge, M., Yu, H., Bayard, S., Roze, E., Vidailhet, M., Dauvilliers, Y., Rascol, O., & Arnulf, I. (2011). The improvement of movement and speech during rapid eye movement sleep behaviour disorder in multiple system atrophy. *Brain, 134*(Pt 3), 856-862.

De Cock, V. C., Vidailhet, M., Leu, S., Texeira, A., Apartis, E., Elbaz, A., Roze, E., Willer, J. C., Derenne, J. P., Agid, Y., & Arnulf, I. (2007). Restoration of normal motor control in Parkinson's disease during REM sleep. *Brain, 130*(Pt 2), 450-456.

Dhawan, V., Dhoat, S., Williams, A. J., Dimarco, A., Pal, S., Forbes, A., Tobias, A., Martinez-Martin, P., & Chaudhuri, K. R. (2006). The range and nature of sleep dysfunction in untreated Parkinson's disease (PD). A comparative controlled clinical study using the Parkinson's disease sleep scale and selective polysomnography. *J Neurol Sci, 248*(1-2), 158-162.

Diederich, N. J., & Comella, C. L. (2003). Sleep disturbances in Parkinson's disease. In S. Chokroverty, W. A. Hening & A. S. Walters (Eds.), *Sleep and Movement Disorders.* (pp. 478–488). Philadelphia: Elsevier Science.

Diederich, N. J., Vaillant, M., Leischen, M., Mancuso, G., Golinval, S., Nati, R., & Schlesser, M. (2005). Sleep apnea syndrome in Parkinson's disease. A case-control study in 49 patients. *Mov Disord, 20*(11), 1413-1418.

Ekbom, K., & Ulfberg, J. (2009). Restless legs syndrome. *J Intern Med, 266*(5), 419-431.

Factor, S. A., McAlarney, T., Sanchez-Ramos, J. R., & Weiner, W. J. (1990). Sleep disorders and sleep effect in Parkinson's disease. *Mov Disord, 5*(4), 280-285.

Ford, B. (2010). Pain in Parkinson's disease. *Mov Disord, 25 Suppl 1*, S98-103.

Fronczek, R., Overeem, S., Lee, S. Y., Hegeman, I. M., van Pelt, J., van Duinen, S. G., Lammers, G. J., & Swaab, D. F. (2007). Hypocretin (orexin) loss in Parkinson's disease. *Brain, 130*(Pt 6), 1577-1585.

Gómez-Esteban, J. C., Tijero, B., Somme, J., Ciordia, R., Berganzo, K., Rouco, I., Bustos, J. L., Valle, M. A., Lezcano, E., & Zarranz, J. J. (2010). Impact of psychiatric symptoms and sleep disorders on the quality of life of patients with Parkinson's disease. *J Neurol.*

Gómez-Esteban, J. C., Zarranz, J. J., Tijero, B., Velasco, F., Barcena, J., Rouco, I., Lezcano, E., Lachen, M. C., Jauregui, A., & Ugarte, A. (2007). Restless legs syndrome in Parkinson's disease. *Mov Disord, 22*(13), 1912-1916.

Gagnon, J. F., Postuma, R. B., Mazza, S., Doyon, J., & Montplaisir, J. (2006). Rapid-eye-movement sleep behaviour disorder and neurodegenerative diseases. *Lancet Neurol, 5*(5), 424-432.

Goetz, C. G. (1999). Hallucinations in Parkinson's disease: the clinical syndrome. *Adv Neurol, 80*, 419-423.

Goetz, C. G. (2010). New developments in depression, anxiety, compulsiveness, and hallucinations in Parkinson's disease. *Mov Disord, 25 Suppl 1*, S104-109.

Goetz, C. G., Ouyang, B., Negron, A., & Stebbins, G. T. (2010). Hallucinations and sleep disorders in PD: ten-year prospective longitudinal study. *Neurology, 75*(20), 1773-1779.

Goetz, C. G., Wilson, R. S., Tanner, C. M., & Garron, D. C. (1987). Relationships among pain, depression, and sleep alterations in Parkinson's disease. *Adv Neurol, 45*, 345-347.

Högl, B., Arnulf, I., Comella, C., Ferreira, J., Iranzo, A., Tilley, B., Trenkwalder, C., Poewe, W., Rascol, O., Sampaio, C., Stebbins, G. T., Schrag, A., & Goetz, C. G. (2010). Scales to assess sleep impairment in Parkinson's disease: Critique and recommendations. *Mov Disord.*

Hanyu, H., Inoue, Y., Sakurai, H., Kanetaka, H., Nakamura, M., Miyamoto, T., Sasai, T., & Iwamoto, T. (2011). Regional cerebral blood flow changes in patients with idiopathic REM sleep behavior disorder. *Eur J Neurol. in press.*

Happe, S., Schrodl, B., Faltl, M., Muller, C., Auff, E., & Zeitlhofer, J. (2001). Sleep disorders and depression in patients with Parkinson's disease. *Acta Neurol Scand, 104*(5), 275-280.

Iranzo, A., Ratti, P. L., Casanova-Molla, J., Serradell, M., Vilaseca, I., & Santamaria, J. (2009). Excessive muscle activity increases over time in idiopathic REM sleep behavior disorder. *Sleep, 32*(9), 1149-1153.

Isozaki, E., Shimizu, T., Takamoto, K., Horiguchi, S., Hayashida, T., Oda, M., & Tanabe, H. (1995). Vocal cord abductor paralysis (VCAP) in Parkinson's disease: difference from VCAP in multiple system atrophy. *J Neurol Sci, 130*(2), 197-202.

Iwanami, M., Miyamoto, T., Miyamoto, M., Hirata, K., & Takada, E. (2010). Relevance of substantia nigra hyperechogenicity and reduced odor identification in idiopathic REM sleep behavior disorder. *Sleep Med, 11*(4), 361-365.

Johns, M. W. (1991). A new method for measuring daytime sleepiness: the Epworth sleepiness scale. *Sleep, 14*(6), 540-545.

Kumar, S., Bhatia, M., & Behari, M. (2002). Sleep disorders in Parkinson's disease. *Mov Disord, 17*(4), 775-781.

Kuno, S., Mizuta, E., Yamasaki, S., & Araki, I. (2004). Effects of pergolide on nocturia in Parkinson's disease: three female cases selected from over 400 patients. *Parkinsonism Relat Disord, 10*(3), 181-187.

Kwon, D. Y., Seo, W. K., Yoon, H. K., Park, M. H., Koh, S. B., & Park, K. W. (2010). Transcranial brain sonography in Parkinson's disease with restless legs syndrome. *Mov Disord, 25*(10), 1373-1378.

Lees, A. J., Blackburn, N. A., & Campbell, V. L. (1988). The nighttime problems of Parkinson's disease. *Clin Neuropharmacol, 11*(6), 512-519.

Lieberman, A. (2006). Depression in Parkinson's disease -- a review. *Acta Neurol Scand, 113*(1), 1-8.

Loo, H. V., & Tan, E. K. (2008). Case-control study of restless legs syndrome and quality of sleep in Parkinson's disease. *J Neurol Sci, 266*(1-2), 145-149.

Margis, R., Donis, K., Schonwald, S. V., Fagondes, S. C., Monte, T., Martin-Martinez, P., Chaudhuri, K. R., Kapczinski, F., & Rieder, C. R. (2009). Psychometric properties of the Parkinson's Disease Sleep Scale--Brazilian version. *Parkinsonism Relat Disord, 15*(7), 495-499.

Maria, B., Sophia, S., Michalis, M., Charalampos, L., Andreas, P., John, M. E., & Nikolaos, S. M. (2003). Sleep breathing disorders in patients with idiopathic Parkinson's disease. *Respir Med, 97*(10), 1151-1157.

Martinez-Martin, P., Salvador, C., Menendez-Guisasola, L., Gonzalez, S., Tobias, A., Almazan, J., & Chaudhuri, K. R. (2004). Parkinson's Disease Sleep Scale: validation study of a Spanish version. *Mov Disord, 19*(10), 1226-1232.

Matsui, H., Nishinaka, K., Oda, M., Hara, N., Komatsu, K., Kubori, T., & Udaka, F. (2006). Hypoperfusion of the visual pathway in parkinsonian patients with visual hallucinations. *Mov Disord, 21*(12), 2140-2144.

Micieli, G., Tosi, P., Marcheselli, S., & Cavallini, A. (2003). Autonomic dysfunction in Parkinson's disease. *Neurol Sci, 24 Suppl 1*, S32-34.

Miyamoto, T., Miyamoto, M., Inoue, Y., Usui, Y., Suzuki, K., & Hirata, K. (2006). Reduced cardiac 123I-MIBG scintigraphy in idiopathic REM sleep behavior disorder. *Neurology, 67*(12), 2236-2238.

Miyamoto, T., Miyamoto, M., Iwanami, M., Hirata, K., Kobayashi, M., Nakamura, M., & Inoue, Y. (2010). Olfactory dysfunction in idiopathic REM sleep behavior disorder. *Sleep Med, 11*(5), 458-461.

Mizuno, S., Mihara, T., Miyaoka, T., Inagaki, T., & Horiguchi, J. (2005). CSF iron, ferritin and transferrin levels in restless legs syndrome. *J Sleep Res, 14*(1), 43-47.

Monti, J. M., Hawkins, M., Jantos, H., D'Angelo, L., & Fernandez, M. (1988). Biphasic effects of dopamine D-2 receptor agonists on sleep and wakefulness in the rat. *Psychopharmacology (Berl), 95*(3), 395-400.

Morris, C. M., & Edwardson, J. A. (1994). Iron histochemistry of the substantia nigra in Parkinson's disease. *Neurodegeneration, 3*(4), 277-282.

Nausieda, P. A., Weiner, W. J., Kaplan, L. R., Weber, S., & Klawans, H. L. (1982). Sleep disruption in the course of chronic levodopa therapy: an early feature of the levodopa psychosis. *Clin Neuropharmacol, 5*(2), 183-194.

Olson, E. J., Boeve, B. F., & Silber, M. H. (2000). Rapid eye movement sleep behaviour disorder: demographic, clinical and laboratory findings in 93 cases. *Brain, 123*((Pt 2)), 331-339.

Pahwa, R., Stacy, M. A., Factor, S. A., Lyons, K. E., Stocchi, F., Hersh, B. P., Elmer, L. W., Truong, D. D., & Earl, N. L. (2007). Ropinirole 24-hour prolonged release: randomized, controlled study in advanced Parkinson disease. *Neurology, 68*(14), 1108-1115.

Peralta, V., Campos, M. S., De Jalon, E. G., & Cuesta, M. J. (2010). Motor behavior abnormalities in drug-naive patients with schizophrenia spectrum disorders. *Mov Disord, 25*(8), 1068-1076.

Petit, D., Gagnon, J. F., Fantini, M. L., Ferini-Strambi, L., & Montplaisir, J. (2004). Sleep and quantitative EEG in neurodegenerative disorders. *J Psychosom Res, 56*(5), 487-496.

Poewe, W. H., Rascol, O., Quinn, N., Tolosa, E., Oertel, W. H., Martignoni, E., Rupp, M., & Boroojerdi, B. (2007). Efficacy of pramipexole and transdermal rotigotine in advanced Parkinson's disease: a double-blind, double-dummy, randomised controlled trial. *Lancet Neurol, 6*(6), 513-520.

Postuma, R. B., Gagnon, J. F., Rompre, S., & Montplaisir, J. Y. (2010a). Severity of REM atonia loss in idiopathic REM sleep behavior disorder predicts Parkinson disease. *Neurology, 74*(3), 239-244.

Postuma, R. B., Gagnon, J. F., Vendette, M., Charland, K., & Montplaisir, J. (2008a). Manifestations of Parkinson disease differ in association with REM sleep behavior disorder. *Mov Disord, 23*(12), 1665-1672.

Postuma, R. B., Gagnon, J. F., Vendette, M., Charland, K., & Montplaisir, J. (2008b). REM sleep behaviour disorder in Parkinson's disease is associated with specific motor features. *J Neurol Neurosurg Psychiatry, 79*(10), 1117-1121.

Postuma, R. B., Gagnon, J. F., Vendette, M., Fantini, M. L., Massicotte-Marquez, J., & Montplaisir, J. (2009). Quantifying the risk of neurodegenerative disease in idiopathic REM sleep behavior disorder. *Neurology, 72*(15), 1296-1300.

Postuma, R. B., Lanfranchi, P. A., Blais, H., Gagnon, J. F., & Montplaisir, J. Y. (2010b). Cardiac autonomic dysfunction in idiopathic REM sleep behavior disorder. *Mov Disord, 25*(14), 2304-2310.

Postuma, R. B., Lang, A. E., Massicotte-Marquez, J., & Montplaisir, J. (2006). Potential early markers of Parkinson disease in idiopathic REM sleep behavior disorder. *Neurology, 66*(6), 845-851.

Potvin, S., Grignon, S., & Marchand, S. (2009). Human evidence of a supra-spinal modulating role of dopamine on pain perception. *Synapse, 63*(5), 390-402.

Qu, W. M., Huang, Z. L., Xu, X. H., Matsumoto, N., & Urade, Y. (2008). Dopaminergic D1 and D2 receptors are essential for the arousal effect of modafinil. *J Neurosci, 28*(34), 8462-8469.

Rahman, S., Griffin, H. J., Quinn, N. P., & Jahanshahi, M. (2008). Quality of life in Parkinson's disease: the relative importance of the symptoms. *Mov Disord, 23*(10), 1428-1434.

Reijnders, J. S., Ehrt, U., Weber, W. E., Aarsland, D., & Leentjens, A. F. (2008). A systematic review of prevalence studies of depression in Parkinson's disease. *Mov Disord, 23*(2), 183-189; quiz 313.

Reuter, I., Ellis, C. M., & Ray Chaudhuri, K. (1999). Nocturnal subcutaneous apomorphine infusion in Parkinson's disease and restless legs syndrome. *Acta Neurol Scand, 100*(3), 163-167.

Rye, D. B. (2004). The two faces of Eve: dopamine's modulation of wakefulness and sleep. *Neurology, 63*(8 Suppl 3), S2-7.

Rye, D. B., & Jankovic, J. (2002). Emerging views of dopamine in modulating sleep/wake state from an unlikely source: PD. *Neurology, 58*(3), 341-346.

Sastre, J. P., & Jouvet, M. (1979). [Oneiric behavior in cats]. *Physiol Behav, 22*(5), 979-989.

Schenck, C. H., Bundlie, S. R., Ettinger, M. G., & Mahowald, M. W. (1986). Chronic behavioral disorders of human REM sleep: a new category of parasomnia. *Sleep, 9*(2), 293-308.

Schenck, C. H., Bundlie, S. R., & Mahowald, M. W. (1996). Delayed emergence of a parkinsonian disorder in 38% of 29 older men initially diagnosed with idiopathic rapid eye movement sleep behaviour disorder. *Neurology, 46*(2), 388-393.

Seif, C., Herzog, J., van der Horst, C., Schrader, B., Volkmann, J., Deuschl, G., Juenemann, K. P., & Braun, P. M. (2004). Effect of subthalamic deep brain stimulation on the function of the urinary bladder. *Ann Neurol, 55*(1), 118-120.

Shimohata, T., Ozawa, T., Nakayama, H., Tomita, M., Shinoda, H., & Nishizawa, M. (2008). Frequency of nocturnal sudden death in patients with multiple system atrophy. *J Neurol, 255*(10), 1483-1485.

Shinno, H., Kamei, M., Nakamura, Y., Inami, Y., & Horiguchi, J. (2008). Successful treatment with Yi-Gan San for rapid eye movement sleep behavior disorder. *Prog Neuropsychopharmacol Biol Psychiatry, 32*(7), 1749-1751.

Shulman, L. M., Taback, R. L., Rabinstein, A. A., & Weiner, W. J. (2002). Non-recognition of depression and other non-motor symptoms in Parkinson's disease. *Parkinsonism Relat Disord, 8*(3), 193-197.

Starkstein, S. E., Preziosi, T. J., & Robinson, R. G. (1991). Sleep disorders, pain, and depression in Parkinson's disease. *Eur Neurol, 31*(6), 352-355.

Stiasny-Kolster, K., Doerr, Y., Moller, J. C., Hoffken, H., Behr, T. M., Oertel, W. H., & Mayer, G. (2005). Combination of 'idiopathic' REM sleep behaviour disorder and olfactory dysfunction as possible indicator for alpha-synucleinopathy demonstrated by dopamine transporter FP-CIT-SPECT. *Brain, 128*(Pt 1), 126-137.

Suzuki, K., Miyamoto, M., Miyamoto, T., Okuma, Y., Hattori, N., Kamei, S., Yoshii, F., Utsumi, H., Iwasaki, Y., Iijima, M., & Hirata, K. (2009). Correlation between depressive symptoms and nocturnal disturbances in Japanese patients with Parkinson's disease. *Parkinsonism Relat Disord, 15*(1), 15-19.

Suzuki, K., Miyamoto, T., Miyamoto, M., Okuma, Y., Hattori, N., Kamei, S., Yoshii, F., Utsumi, H., Iwasaki, Y., Iijima, M., & Hirata, K. (2008). Excessive daytime sleepiness and sleep episodes in Japanese patients with Parkinson's disease. *J Neurol Sci, 271*(1-2), 47-52.

Suzuki, K., Okuma, Y., Hattori, N., Kamei, S., Yoshii, F., Utsumi, H., Iwasaki, Y., Iijima, M., Miyamoto, T., Miyamoto, M., & Hirata, K. (2007). Characteristics of sleep disturbances in Japanese patients with Parkinson's disease. A study using Parkinson's disease sleep scale. *Mov Disord, 22*(9), 1245-1251.

Tandberg, E., Larsen, J. P., & Karlsen, K. (1998). A community-based study of sleep disorders in patients with Parkinson's disease. *Mov Disord, 13*(6), 895-899.

Trampus, M., Ferri, N., Monopoli, A., & Ongini, E. (1991). The dopamine D1 receptor is involved in the regulation of REM sleep in the rat. *Eur J Pharmacol, 194*(2-3), 189-194.

Trenkwalder, C., Kies, B., Rudzinska, M., Fine, J., Nikl, J., Honczarenko, K., Dioszeghy, P., Hill, D., Anderson, T., Myllyla, V., Kassubek, J., Steiger, M., Zucconi, M., Tolosa, E., Poewe, W., Surmann, E., Whitesides, J., Boroojerdi, B., & Chaudhuri, K. R. (2011a). Rotigotine effects on early morning motor function and sleep in Parkinson's disease: A double-blind, randomized, placebo-controlled study (RECOVER). *Mov Disord.*

Trenkwalder, C., Kohnen, R., Hogl, B., Metta, V., Sixel-Doring, F., Frauscher, B., Hulsmann, J., Martinez-Martin, P., & Chaudhuri, K. R. (2011b). Parkinson's disease sleep scale-validation of the revised version PDSS-2. *Mov Disord.*

Trotti, L. M., & Bliwise, D. L. (2010). No increased risk of obstructive sleep apnea in Parkinson's disease. *Mov Disord, 25*(13), 2246-2249.

Verbaan, D., van Rooden, S. M., van Hilten, J. J., & Rijsman, R. M. (2010). Prevalence and clinical profile of restless legs syndrome in Parkinson's disease. *Mov Disord, 25*(13), 2142-2147.

Vincken, W. G., Gauthier, S. G., Dollfuss, R. E., Hanson, R. E., Darauay, C. M., & Cosio, M. G. (1984). Involvement of upper-airway muscles in extrapyramidal disorders. A cause of airflow limitation. *N Engl J Med, 311*(7), 438-442.

Walters, A. S., & Rye, D. B. (2009). Review of the relationship of restless legs syndrome and periodic limb movements in sleep to hypertension, heart disease, and stroke. *Sleep, 32*(5), 589-597.

Wang, G., Cheng, Q., Zeng, J., Bai, L., Liu, G. D., Zhang, Y., Tan, Y. Y., Pan, J., Hong, Z., Wang, Y., & Chen, S. D. (2008). Sleep disorders in Chinese patients with Parkinson's disease: validation study of a Chinese version of Parkinson's disease sleep scale. *J Neurol Sci, 271*(1-2), 153-157.

Winge, K., & Fowler, C. J. (2006). Bladder dysfunction in Parkinsonism: mechanisms, prevalence, symptoms, and management. *Mov Disord, 21*(6), 737-745.

Yoshimura, N., Mizuta, E., Yoshida, O., & Kuno, S. (1998). Therapeutic effects of dopamine D1/D2 receptor agonists on detrusor hyperreflexia in 1-methyl-4-phenyl-1,2,3,6-tetrahydropyridine-lesioned parkinsonian cynomolgus monkeys. *J Pharmacol Exp Ther, 286*(1), 228-233.

4

Neuropsychological Deficits in Initial Parkinson's Disease

Raquel Rodriguez Fernandez[1] and Jose Antonio Muñiz Casado[2]
[1]*Faculty of Psychology. National University of Distance Education (UNED)*
[2]*Neurological Rehabilitation Center "Arco Iris" in Madrid*
Spain

1. Introduction

Parkinson's disease (PD), is a neurodegenerative illness, producing movement disorders, although it is also associated to cognitive deficit and emotional and behavioral alterations (Fuiza & Mayán, 2005; Vera-Cuesta et al., 2006), being prominent the presence of neuropsychological deficits among the majority of PD patients.

The neuropsychological disorders can be observed from the very initial phases of the illness, nevertheless, the results obtained from studies of these deficits are often confusing and little clear. These contradictory results are due to diverse factors, which mainly are: the heterogeneity of the samples used in the studies, the absence of consensus during the tests and to the lack of clarity at the time of using diverse terms as specific cognitive alterations, mild cognitive impairment and dementia.

During the last years there is an increased interest in studying and describing cognitive deficit associated with PD (Aarsland et al., 2003; Giannaula, 2010; Locascio, Corkin & Growdon, 2003; Ostrosky-Solís, 2000; Perea-Bartolomé, 2001; Weintraub et al., 2004). This interest is justified if keeping numbers in mind. It is saying, the totality of PD patients show alterations from initial phases in tasks requiring attention, visuospatial, mnesic o executive functions. Also, about 20% to 30% of the patients with PD reach dementia along the evolution of the illness (Caixeta & Vieira, 2008; Halvorsen & Tynes, 2007; Hilker et al, 2005).

It has been emphasized in diverse studies that the diagnosis of dementia in PD is often underestimated (Caixeta & Vieira, 2008; Halvorsen & Tynes, 2007; Hobson & Meara, 2004). Therefore, long term studies to be carried out with such patients will be needed in order to evaluate the type and scope of cognitive deficit associated with the PD. Caviness et al. (2007) carried out a study among 86 patients, showing the presence of signs of cognitive deterioration. In particular, they found that 62% of the participants were cognitive intactly, 21% were fulfilling criteria of mild cognitive impairment and only 17% had symptoms compatible with dementia according to DSM IV. The study results also proved that patients with mild cognitive impairment were characterized for having, principally, executive deficit and alterations of memory, especially in tasks of free delayed memory and working memory. Therefore, the above mentioned study emphasizes the need to detect signs of cognitive deterioration in PD patients from the very beginning of the illness, that is to say, to detect the early neuropsychological deficits, and to supervise the evolution and course of these cognitive deficits.

In the same line, Taylor et al. (2008) carried out a longitudinal study in a sample of newly diagnosed patients of PD, analyzing the relation between the appearance of dementia depending on variables such as alterations to movement and attention related deficit. They found that patients suffering major postural instability since the beginning of the illness, and those with attention deficits, had a significant probability of developing dementia. All of these patients had deficits in tasks such simple reaction time tasks, tasks of election and of attention related control. In addition to the executive, attention related and mnesic deficit, as possible risk factors of the development of dementia in PD patients (Taylor et al., 2008). It has been proved that other factors exist, precipitating the development of dementia, such as: alteration of the visuospatial function, advanced age, increased development of movement related symptoms, presence of emotional alterations (depression and anxiety) and psychotic disorders (Halvorsen & Tynes, 2007).

It has been observed that the prevalence of dementia depended on the studied population, on the definition of dementia elected and on the methods used to diagnose it (Caviness et al., 2007). The dementia observed in PD patients usually appears approximately in 20-30% of them, being more frequent in those with major age, depressive symptoms, and in those with severe movement related deficit (Vera-Cuesta et al., 2006).

But it is important that various recent investigations on neuropsychological deficit in PD have verified that the most frequent cognitive alteration in the debut of the illness it is not the presence of a mild cognitive impairment, nor of dementia, but the presence of one or several cognitive deficits which do not affect the complex and instrumental activities in daily life (Elgh et al., 2009; Giannaula, 2010; Halvorsen y Tysnes, 2007; Verbaan et al, 2007; Zgaljardic et al. 2003). The above mentioned cognitive deficits without interference in the activities of the daily life have been found from initial phases in patients de novo, that is to say in those without pharmacological treatment. In particular, the studies emphasize on the presence of specific cognitive deficit of executive type (deficit in planning, sequence, abstract reasoning and verbal fluency), visuospatials deficits and, also, difficulties in the mnesic function have been found in the delayed recall of information and in certain aspects of the implicit memory (Higginson et al., 2005; Kemps et al., 2005; Locascio, Corkin & Growdon, 2003; Muslimovic et al., 2005).

On the other hand, through neuroimaging techniques such as positron emission tomography (PET) and functional magnetic resonance imaging (fRMI), it has been proved that the deficit in executive functions and in working memory observed in the initial phases would depend partly on the alteration of frontostriatal circuits that connect the basal ganglions with the prefrontal dorsolateral cortex (Bruck et al., 2005; Pillon et al, 2000). That is to say, in patients in initial phases a hypo-activation of prefrontal dorsolaterals areas have been found during execution of tasks of executive function (Caballol, Martí & Tolosa, 2007; Castiello et al., 2009). Recent studies have found that these executive deficit partially decline with restoring dopaminergic medication, which has led to suggest the importance of the dopaminergic system in the genesis of this deficit (Nobili et al, 2009). These finds suggest that the neuropsychological deficits observed in initial phases of the illness must be identified and treated as soon as possible, since these measures might help to delay the appearance and severity of cognitive deterioration and they would also improve the quality of life for patients (Halvorsen & Tynes, 2007; Mamikonian et al, 2009; Zgaljardic et al., 2003).

The study and management of cognitive alterations, with behavioral and emotional disturbances, is determinate because implies a serious limitation in the execution of daily activities for patients, as well as in their social and familiar relations (Dubois et al, 2007).

The aim of the present chapter is to describe the main neuropsychogical alterations from initial phases of the illness in PD patients. In particular, we will focus on the deficits produced in attention, visuospatial, executive and mnesic functions. We will comment on the results obtained in several studies based on neuropsychological tests, related to the fronto-subcortical cognitive impairment in patients in initial phases of the illness, according to the scale of Hoehn and Yahr (Fahn, 1967). Also, we will give a few small recommendations on how these deficits can be rehabilitated, that is to say, on how to carrying out the necessary neuropsychological intervention in order to postpone the appearance and severity of cognitive disorders and thus to improve the quality of life of patients.

2. Main neuropsychological deficits in initial Parkinson´s disease

2.1 Attention deficits

Attentional deficits in patients with PD are related from the initial stages of the disease, and affect tasks involving simple reaction times and those that require attentional control and, therefore, require a flexible distribution of attentional resources (Caviness et al, 2007). That means, in these patients there is an increase in reaction time and a general slowing of information processing, a typical phenomenon observed in the PD bradyphrenia. This slowness may be increased due to a consequence of any extra effort of the cognitive processes involved, and of the association of complex of motor and cognitive responses, and finally this slowness may be caused also by the process of selecting the appropriate response (Caviness et al, 2007, Nobili et al, 2009; Ostrosky-Solís, 2001).

It has been suggested that, through the connections between the basal ganglia and prefrontal cortex, basal ganglia will regulate the main functions of this part of the cerebral cortex, based on the anterior and posterior attentional systems (Posner & DiGirolamo, 1998). That means, the *posterior attentional network*, which depends on the posterior parietal cortex, superior colliculus, the pulvinar thalamic nuclei and inferior temporal lobes, control the focused attention, visual orientation and recognition of objects and attributes located in space. However, the *anterior attentional network*, which depends on the proper functioning of the frontal lobe and cingulate areas, would be responsible for selective attention, attentional control and the initiation and inhibition of responses (Posner & DiGirolamo, 1998). From early stages of the disease, there is a change in both attentional systems (Alonso et al., 2003), especially in the anterior attentional system (Lewis et al, 2003). Patients had deficits in shifting attention to different regions of visual space, difficulties in directing the attentional system into different areas of the environment and to manage these resources based on the objectives. Generally, we can say that patients, from initial stages, show alterations in shifting the focus of attention and in inhibition of both motor and cognitive programs in a short time interval (Alonso et al, 2003).

In our research with patients in early stages (Muñiz Casado & Rodriguez Fernández, 2007), we observe that attentional tasks are affected since the debut of the disease in line with the results obtained by Owen (2004), Owen et al. (1992) and Zgaljardic et al. (2006). More specifically, we found out that patients have a *general slowing of information processing* (Caviness et al., 2007, Nobili et al., 2009; Ostrosky-Solís, 2001) that, in our case, is evaluated through:

- increasing the time spent in the copy of the Rey-Osterrieth Complex Figure Test;

- more time than the controls participants in the TMT (Trail Making Test) performance, both Part A and Part B;
- less scores in the Digit Symbol subtest of the WAIS (Wechsler Adults Intelligence Scale), and
- decrease the speed of auditory information processing in the test PASAT (Paced Auditory Serial Addition Test).

All these changes indicate that since the onset of the disease, there is decrease in the speed of information processing.

On the other hand, if we look at the performance on the Digit Span subtest of the WAIS (Wechsler Adults Intelligence Scale), we found significant differences in the backward and the total score. That means that our patients have an attentional span similar to the one of the control group participants, but have more difficulties in the inverse series, which may point to a *deficit in the distribution of attentional resources*. Furthermore, using the Stroop test, patients with initial PD have a lower score than controls in reading words and reading the color film, probably because of the processing speed deficit, already discussed, but also because of a deficit in *attentional control to inhibition the incoming information that is not relevant to the task* and the resistance to a new task, since we found significant differences in the Stroop interference. These data are consistent with those of Owen (2004), who found in newly diagnosed patients the presence of attentional deficits in tasks involving selective control and inhibition of irrelevant information, such as in the Stroop test.

The deficits of attentional control in initial PD have been demonstrated using different tests. On one site, the *problems presented in the cognitive flexibility* to produce fewer scores than the controls on the PASAT (Paced Auditory Serial Addition Test). Through the PASAT we can appreciate a deficit in the flexible distribution of resources at the time to sustain attention throughout the test, which brings us to conclude that our patients have *difficulties in sustained attention tasks* that require a flexible distribution of attentional resources. On the other site, the mistakes made in Part B of TMT (Trail Making Test), show alterations in their ability to alternate between two sequences, a fact that does not happen in Part A of this test in which there is a simple sequence and patients do not make mistakes, having a similar performance to that of the controls. In addition, our patients had fewer scores than the controls in a cancellation task, which shows: a *deficit in changing the focus of attention* to different regions of visual space, alterations in directing the attentional system into different areas of the space and a *challenge to manage these resources* based on the demands required. On the other hand, the sustained attention task CPT (Continuous Performance Test), although without significant differences in the hits relative to controls, patients make more false positives, which suggests a difficulty of stopping and controling unsuitable responses and even some difficulty in keeping the attention on a monotonous task like this.

As a summary, as other authors have found (Caviness et al, 2007, Alonso et al, 2003; Fuiza & Mayán, 2005; Owen, 2004), from the initial stages, our patients show alterations in attentional focus change and inhibition of both cognitive and motor programs. If we focus on this last point, we have observed in the different sections of a test GO / NO GO, which are the change of hand position and point of opposing reactions, those are significant differences although are not statistically significant.

About cognitive **rehabilitation** of attention is important that the patient, firstly, choose the time and place to enable him to be concentrate and free from stimuli that may interfere, and create a daily routine of mental stimulation. To improve the processing speed issues it is recommended to monitor the execution time of the exercises of attention, so this will allow him to compare his own performance on different occasions (using the same exercises at first and then similar tasks but with different stimuli).

In order to improve *sustained attention*, the patient will increase the duration of the exercises, beginning with short exercises, and as he feels less fatigue and reduce mistakes at the end of the exercise, he will progress to longer duration exercises. That means, when the patient will reduce his mistakes, he can gradually increase the complexity of the task.

To improve his *control attentional* ability in tasks involving selective and divided attention it is recommended that he starts with exercises that involve the detection of a single stimulus and it is different from the distracting ones, this way he is working his *selective attention* at a simple level. Once dominated the ability to choose a stimulus among several, it will progressively increase the difficulty to find a stimulus among several ones so similar and even will increase the number of stimuli to be search and the number of distractors. At last, to improve the patient's *divided attention*, once able to concentrate in a relax environment (sustained attention), he needs to direct his attentional focus inhibiting other stimuli (selective attention), the next step is when the patient perform two simple similar tasks simultaneously but in different sensory modalities. For example, a visual cancellation task with an auditory selective attention task, and then little by little, it will increase the degree of difficulty.

2.2 Visuospatial and visuoperceptual deficits

From the beginning of the illness the patients present visuospatial deficits in tasks of spatial location, implying dimensional positioning of objects and integrating them coherently in the space (Galtier et al., 2009; Levin, Tomer & Rey, 1992; Owen, 2004; Sánchez-Rodríguez, 2002). Functional neuroimaging studies have found a metabolic reduction in the frontal and parieto-occipital cortex in initial PD patients, associated with the poor execution of visuospatial tasks (Kemps et al., 2005).

The same studies (Levin, Tomer & King, 1992; Kemps et al., 2005) show that the facial recognition is the visual perceptive function which is the earliest that became affected. Also, the studies emphasize on deficit in visuoconstructive tasks like the copy of the Rey-Osterrieth Complex Figure Test (Cooper et al., 1991; Owen, 2004). This alteration becomes clearer with the further illness evolution (Caixeta & Vieira, 2008). The patients showed deficit in some of the subtests of the manipulative scale according to WAIS (Wechsler Adults Intelligence Scale), such as: picture completion, blocks design and object assembly (Levin, Tomer & Rey, 1992; Dubois & Pillon, 1997).

Regarding the visuoperceptional and visuospatial deficits in their patients in diverse stages of the illness, Levin, Tomer and King (1992) came to the following conclusions:

- With regard to the control group initial patients were showing similar results in tasks evaluating the skills to carry out mental rotations of objects and reconstruction of pieces to form a meaningful object. Meanwhile PD patients in groups of moderate and advanced evolution of the disease were presenting deficits in these areas. Also an increase in the deterioration of the judgment of linear orientation was observed in patients with more years of PD evolution.
- Facial recognition and the constructive praxis of drawings and complex models were altered from the beginning of the illness and deteriorate as the illness develops.

- The patients of the initial group presented worse results in the face recognition with regard to the control group. Nevertheless, it is necessary to consider such a task, in addition to evaluating perceptive and facial components as they are discriminated by different characteristics of positioning and shades or the vision of dimensional contrast between different aspects, it also implies analytic skills, based on the reasoning and judgments of deduction, which may be depended on some executive aspects (Possin et al., 2008). Certain studies have found complex visuospatial alterations when executive aspects increase, such as planning, sequences and generation of a movement plan (Kemps et al., 2005; Possin et al., 2008; Rudkin, Pearson & Logie, 2007).

The studies that we are carrying out coincide in this sense with the majority of previous investigations, which have demonstrated that the facial recognition is the first visual perceptive function that is altered from the debut of the disease (Levin, Tomer & Rey, 1992; Kemps et al, 2005). In particular, our patients obtained worse results than the control group in all the components of Benton's facial recognition test, presenting a deficit in the specific skill to identify and discriminate unfamiliar human faces.

Also we have found difficulties in visual constructive tasks such the copy of the complex figure of Rey-Osterrieth, as well as other studies (Cooper et al., 1991; Owen, 2004). Nevertheless, these studies were including patients of initial and moderate stages, and our study was including only initial patients. We have found that they present alteration in the copy of the Rey-Osterrieth Complex Figure Test that, which implies visualperceptive and visualconstructive components in addition to executive elements.

Finally, in the picture completion of subtest of WAIS (Wechsler Adults Intelligence Scale) our patients present deficit in the perception of difference in relevant details from the irrelevant ones and in the visual organization, results that could stand in the same line as the found by other authors (Levin, Tomer & Rey, 1992; Dubois & Pillon, 1997; Owen, 2004).

To **rehability** visuoperceptual, spatial and constructive deficits of patients, we propose, first of all, to assure an improvement in their attention related functions. For the rehabilitation of the *visuoconstructive alterations*, the recommendation is to start fine motricity exercises, in which the patient with a colored pencil follows numerated points of a drawing until finally managing to complete all the points and to identify the drawing. The aim is to start with simple and two-dimensional drawings, getting to complex drawings and three-dimensional figures. Next, the patient will be proposed to reproduce drawings of different grade of difficulty, firstly with a patter and later without it. Finally, he will be asked to complete incomplete drawings or such containing perceptive intrusive elements.

To improve his *visuoperceptive capacity*, he will be shown incomplete drawings, and he will have to identify the lacking element. On the other hand, he will be shown fragments of drawings and before the drawing is completed, the patient will have to identify it from the incomplete degraded versions of it. He will be shown stimuli in different tonalities of color and grades of lighting, so that he could identify them correctly. To increase even further his dimensional skills, he will be presented tasks in which he will have to indicate the position of the object, or tests in which he would have to mentally rotate drawings to identify them perceptively.

2.3 Executive function deficits

In many cases the deficits found at the beginning of the PD in executive functions has explained the changes in other cognitive areas (Caviness et al, 2007, Halvorsen & Tynes, 2007, Lewis et al, 2003, Nobili et al, 2009; Poussin et al., 2008, Vera-Cuesta et al., 2006).

Executive functions have considered as those higher cognitive processes which associate ideas, movements and actions to execute complex behaviors and enable human adaptation to its environment (Fuster, 2007; Stuss & Alexander, 2000; Tirapu-Ustárroz, Muñoz-Céspedes & Pelegrin-Valero, 2002). From the neuroanatomical point of view, it have been associated mainly to the dorsolateral prefrontal cortex (Sawamoto et al., 2007; Tinaz, Schendan & Stern, 2008; Tirapu-Ustárroz & Muñoz-Céspedes, 2005). Therefore, the dorsolateral circuit is related to executive functions as planning, manipulation of information in working memory, concept formation and mental flexibility (Caviness et al, 2007). However, throughout the prefrontal cortex and its various cortical and subcortical connections (mainly with the basal ganglia) will influence the functioning of executive functions.

Using the Wisconsin Card Shorting Test (WCST) has been found a reduction in the number of categories produced by these patients from initial stages, and a high number of perseverative mistakes (Cooper, Sagar & Sullivan, 1993, Dubois et al, 2007; Lewis et al, 2003; Ostrosky-Solís, 2000, Vera-Cuesta et al., 2006). PD patients have difficulties with the organization, the management and the replacement of some concepts with others more innovative and adaptive, so that show *problems in guided tasks only with internal search key*, highlighting the *difficulties in developing their own strategies* which guide their own behavior, causing a deficit in the generation of new concepts or sets, in the change and planning for them and in the search for the rule involved in the solution of the task (Mckinlay et al, 2008).

On the other hand, we know that executive control is concerned with: planning, control of the plans involved in the task, monitoring the inhibition of irrelevant information and to manage mental flexibility to change the focus of attention. These cognitive functions are involved in tasks such as: the TMT (Trail Making Test), verbal fluency task, the Mental Control subtest of the WMS (Wechsler Memory Scales), the Stroop test and the PASAT (Paced Auditory Serial Addition Test). Patients with initial stages of PD show alterations in most of these tests (Bruck et al., 2005, Lewis et al 2003, Williams-Gray et al, 2007). Thus there have been found evidence of deficits in the maintenance of a sequence in a flexible way, as it happen in the Trail Making Test (Cools et al., 2001, Williams-Gray et al, 2007).

It has been also found that from early stages, PD patients often have difficulties in verbal fluency task, of both phonological and semantic nature, which means that their production of words, compared to controls, is fewer and they use less access strategies to the lexical and semantic stores, showing a lack of monitoring of information. These results suggest that the alteration of verbal fluency, found in patients with de novo, involves a dysexecutive impairment more than a problem of semantic memory (Henry & Crawford, 2004, Williams-Gray et al., 2007; Zec et al, 1999).

Our results have shown, once again, that patients from initial stages show difficulties in executive tasks. In brief, our patients have deficits in executive processes as following:

- Mental flexibility and capacity inhibition to the interference of other not relevant issues (statement based on the results of the Stroop test).
- Generation of new concepts, abstract reasoning and change of set (according to the results of the Wisconsin Card Shorting Test (WCST) and the Similarities subtest of the WAIS (Wechsler Adults Intelligence Scale)).
- Ability to initiate and maintain a verbal task, sequencing and planning the execution of it (according to the results of the verbal fluency task (semantic and phonetic)).

- Ability to plan strategies and to solve problems (evidence obtained from the results of the Hanoi Tower and in the copy of the Rey-Osterrieth Complex Figure Test).

To **rehabilitation** his executive functions, firstly it is recommended to improve the patient's ability to *initiate the execution of tasks by himself*. For this, it is proposed to improve the occurrence of new ideas or the skill to invent a short story, thinking of dishes that normally do not cook or drawing pictures without a model.

In order to stimulate the categorization and abstract reasoning is suggested to perform tasks involving sorting and classifying items into categories, such as classifying countries by continents, organizing the closet by clothes for different seasons or preparing shopping list according to different types of food. To stimulate the *mental flexibility* and the *regulation of behavior*, it can be proposed different table games like cards or dominoes. With these tasks, the patient not only has to implement his plans and sequence the steps to reach them, but also has to be flexible and able to adapt to other people and circumstances involved in the game, as well as stimulate social aspects such as empathy and other social skills.

Finally, to improve *planning* and *sequencing of steps* to take in a task, we ask him to write and list the necessary steps in order to paint a wall, to prepare a birthday party or a holiday.

2.4 Memory deficits

Often PD patients have memory deficits on tasks involving spatial working memory, implicit learning of sequences, learning pairs of related words and visuospatial learning (Brown et al., 2003, Galtier et al, 2009; Higginson et al., 2005; Verbaan et al, 2007; Zizak et al, 2005).

Regarding to declarative *long-term memory*, patients often reduce performance as the disease progresses, of both episodic and semantic memory (Aarsland, Zaccai & Brayne, 2005; Caballol, Marti & Tolosa, 2007, Lewis et al., 2005). The specific alterations of these patients, especially at early stages, of both verbal and visuospatial material, probably because of a deficit in attentional and organizational control (Pillon et al, 1998, Nobili et al, 2009). It has shown that patients keep their storage capacity but often they have problems with *encoding and recovering of information* due to executive alterations (Janvin et al., 2003).

Several studies show that some aspects of *working memory* are more impaired than others (Higginson et al., 2005, Moustafa, Sherman & Frank, 2008, Williams-Gray et al., 2007). There has been found that patients, in early and moderate stages without dementia, show deficits on tests of visuospatial working memory (Galtier et al, 2009; Poussin et al., 2008), while them performance in a similar test of verbal working memory was preserved (Galtier et al, 2009; Owen, 2004). Therefore, patients show a deficit in *spatial working memory*, and, in part, this alteration reflects an executive deficit rather than a pure memory deficit, since patients de novo and without medication can have difficulties in visuospatial tasks involving strategic processes, organization and active manipulation of information stored temporarily (Rudkin, Pearson & Logie, 2007; Sawamoto et al, 2007). However, the Lewis et al. (2003) working team found out deficits in *verbal working memory* task in their initial patients, which involved manipulation of information (to sort submitted letters by certain rules), although the same patients kept intact them execution when only they were asked to maintain and recover the letters.

Regarding to alterations in *implicit memory*, we know that patients can learn new concepts, cognitive and motor, but with remarkable slowness (Owen et al., 1998). Muslimovic and colleagues (2007) suggest that patients have a deficit in implicit tests, which involve a sequential component like the paradigm of serial reaction time, but are able to learn the skill, although with more difficulty than controls. However, the acquisition of more perceptive skills such as mirror reading or repetitive motor skills that require less planning and organization are usually preserved in patients (Ferraro, Ballot & Connor, 1993). That means that patients, from early stages, often keep preserved them performance over the control participants in the paradigm of priming or facilitation effect (Chenery, Angwin & Copland, 2008; Muslimovic et al., 2007).

According to our results, patients with initial PD have a reduced *short-term memory* compared with controls (evaluated by the Digit Span subtest of the WAIS (Wechsler Adults Intelligence Scale)). Regarding the declarative *long-term memory* (evaluated by TAVEC which is the Spanish version of the CVLT (California Verbal Learning Test), patients recover fewer words in free recall tasks, in both short and long term, and they benefit less from semantic clustering than the controls. They also have perseverations in the long-term free recall, which may indicate a lack of monitoring when information is recovered. Furthermore they show the phenomenon of interference, in both the free recall test of the intrusive list (proactive interference) and the short-term memory of the first list (retroactive interference), and recognize fewer words than controls. However, we observed no differences in discriminability index, in the response bias, or in the commission of false positives during recognition. Therefore, patients keep what they have learned when distractors appear, and also their hits in the recognition are independent of the chance and are related to what they learned and stored.

Generally, our patients are able to store information and keep it but in a disorganized way. We have noticed that they learn new information but slower and with lower performance level than the controls, that means, they have fewer scores in memory tests, with and without clues, and in the recognition test. Probably, as other authors have found (Stefanova et al., 2001; Weintraub et al, 2004; Verbaan et al, 2007; Zizak et al, 2005), this deficit is due to inefficient use of strategies during the encoding and the storage, which involves a lower recovery because of the inefficiency in the planning and the organization of information. Other studies have found that executive deficits in patients with early PD such as lack of planning, the use of strategies and the phenomenon of interference, together with working memory deficits (as found in test and subtest Letters and Numbers of the WAIS (Wechsler Adults Intelligence Scale), could be the main reason of some of the alterations seen in short term and long term memory, in verbal and visual modalities (Cooper et al., 1991; Muñiz Casado & Rodríguez Fernández, 2007; Pillon et al, 1998)).

We have found in our initial patients a deficit in verbal working memory, using the subtest Digit Span (in backward form), Letters and Numbers and Arithmetic of the WAIS (Wechsler Adults Intelligence Scale). These results are consistent with those obtained by other authors, testing the verbal working memory, even in patients with newly diagnosed disease (Higginson, 2001; Lewis et al, 2003).

For the **rehabilitation** of the memory functions in patients, and taking into account that many of their difficulties in this area are explain by attention and executive deficits, we propose the following strategies to:

- focus on relevant information.
- associate the information with already known material by the patient.
- organize information to remember through the use of categories at the time of encode and store the information.

- use two different ways, verbal and visual, to recover previously stored information.
- perform exercises in semantic verbal fluency: naming in particular tense examples of a certain category.

3. Conclusions

Cognitive impairment is considered a common feature of this disease. The majority of PD patients have developed some early mild cognitive deficits in the course of their disease. Several studies demonstrated that between 20% and 50% PD patients will develop Mild Cognitive Impairment (MCI), that means, many patients will have executive deficits, memory impairment, visuospatial deficits and other cognitive and emotional symptoms at lower level than it occurs in patients with dementia, but these deficits also damage their daily activities.

Factors such as the patient age at the beginning of the disease, the educational level, the occupation, the presence of emotional disorders, the asymmetry of the symptoms at the onset of illness, relevant motor symptoms, the appropriate response to drug therapy and other types of personal and family history, will influence the cognitive deficits presented by the patient. That is to say, cognitive alterations in these patients are a powerful predictor of their quality of life.

Along the chapter we explain and describe the cognitive deficits in initial stages of PD, and how those deficits should be assessed and treated in order to prevent the appearance of one probably MCI or dementia. Specifically, we describe attentional, visuospatial, executive and memory deficits in early PD. We consider necessary to asses and identify cognitive and emotional deficits in PD patients because those kinds of deficits may cause impairments in the social and daily activities of the patients. Besides, these neuropsychological deficits may be treated and prevented in order to improve the quality of life in those PD patients and, indirectly, the burden of their caregivers will diminish.

4. Acknowledgment

First of all, we wish to thank all the participants of our research and their families because they have been possible this work.

We deeply thank the medical staff of Neurology Service of the Hospital Clinic San Carlos of Madrid (Spain), especially to Dr. Vázquez.

5. References

Aarsland D, Andersen K, Larsen JP, Lolk A, & Kragh-Sørensen P. (2003). Prevalence and characteristics of dementia in Parkinson disease. An 8-year prospective study. *Arch Neurol, 60*: 387-92.

Alonso PE, Esteban E, Trujillo MC, Fernández GE, Roussó VT & Cordero EA. (2003). Alteraciones específicas de la atención en estadios tempranos de la Enfermedad de Parkinson. *Rev Neurol, 36*(11):1015 - 18.

Brown RG, Jahanshahi M, Limousin-Dowsey P, Thomas D, Quinn NP & Rothwell JC. (2003). Pallidotomy and incidental sequence learning in Parkinson's disease. *Neuro Report, 14*, 21–4.

Bruck A, Aalto S, Nurmi E, Bergman J & Rinne JO. (2005). Cortical 6-[18F]fluoro-L-dopa uptake and frontal cognitive functions in early Parkinson's disease. *Neurobiol Aging, 26*:891-898.

Butter T, Van den Hout A, Matthews F, Larsen J, Brayne C & Aarsland D. (2008). Dementia and survival in Parkinson disease. *Neurology, 70,* 1017-22.

Caballol N, Martí M & Tolosa E. (2007). Cognitive dysfunction and dementia in Parkinson disease. *Mov Disord, 22*(Suppl 17): 358-66.

Caixeta, L. & Vieira, R.T. (2008). Dementia in Parkinson´s disease. *Rev Bras Psiquiatr, 30*(4): 375-83.

Castiello U, Ansuini C, Bulgheroni M, Scaravilli T & Nicoletti R. (2009). Visuomotor priming effects in Parkinson´s diasease patients depend on the match between the observed and the executed action. *Neuropsychologia, 47*(3): 835-42.

Caviness JN, Driver-Dunckley E, Connor DJ, Sabbagh MN, Hentz JG, Noble B, Evidente VG, Shill HA & Adler CH. (2007). Defining mild cognitive impairment in Parkinson´s disease. *Mov Disord.22*(9):1272-7.

Chenery HJ, Angwin AJ & Copland DA. (2008). The basal ganglia circuits, dopamine, and ambiguous word processing: a neurobiological account of priming studies in Parkinson´s disease. *J Int Neuropsychol Soc., 14*(3):351-64.

Cools R, Barker RA, Sahakian BJ & Robbins TW. (2001). Mechanisms of cognitive set flexibility in Parkinson's disease. *Brain, 124,* 2503-2512.

Cooper JA, Sagar HJ, Jordan N, Harvey NS & Sullivan EV. (1991). Cognitive impairment in early, untreated Parkinson's disease and its relationship to motor disability. *Brain, 114,* 2095–122.

Cooper JA, Sagar HJ & Sullivan EV. (1993). Short-term memory and temporal ordering in early Parkinson's disease: effects of disease chronicity and medication. *Neuropsychologia, 31,* 933–49.

Dubois B, Burn D, Goetz C, Aarsland D, Brown R, Broe G, et al. (2007). Diagnostic procedures for Parkinson's disease dementia: recommendations from the Movement Disorders Society Task Force. *Mov Disord, 22*: 2314-24.

Dubois B, Pillon B (1997). Cognitive deficits in Parkinson´s disease. *J Neurol, 244,* 2-8.

Elgh H, Domellöf M, Linder J, Edström M, Stenlund H & Forsgren L. (2009). Cognitive function in early Parkinson's disease: a population-based study. *European Journal of Neurology, 16*(12) : 1278-1284.

Ferraro FR, Balota DA & Connor LT. (1993). Implicit memory and the formation of new associations in nondemented Parkinson's disease individuals and individuals with senile dementia of the Alzheimer type: a serial reaction time (SRT) investigation. *Brain Cogn, 21,* 163–80.

Fuiza, MJ & Mayán, JM. (2003). Características de la enfermedad de Parkinson. M.J. Fiuza & J.M. Mayán (eds). *¿Qué es el Parkinson? Guía de tratamiento para el lenguaje, el habla y la voz.* Pirámide, Madrid, 2005.

Fuster, J. M. (2007). Jackson and the frontal executive hierarchy. *International Journal of Psychophysiology, 64*(1), 106-107.

Galtier I, Nieto A, Barroso J & Lorenzo JN. (2009). Deterioro del aprendizaje visoespacial en la enfermedad de Parkinson. *Psicothema, 21*(1), 21-26.

Giannaula, R (2010). Alteraciones cognitivas y demencia en la enfermedad de Parkinson. *Revista Neurologia, 50*(1), 13-16.

Halvorsen, O & Tysnes, OB (2007). Dementia in Parkinson´s disease. *Tidssk Nor Laegeforen, 127*(22): 2973-4.

Henry JD & Crawford JR. (2004). Verbal fluency deficits in Parkinson's disease: a meta-analysis. *J Int Neuropsychol Soc, 10*, 608-622.

Higginson CI, Wheelock VL, Carroll KE & Sigvardt KA. (2005). Recognition memory in Parkinosn´s disease with and without dementia: evidence inconsistent with the retrieval deficit hypothesis. *J Clin Neuropsychol. 27*(4): 516-28.

Hilker R, Thomas A, Klein J, Weisenbach S, Kalbe E, Burghaus L, et al. (2005). Dementia in Parkinson disease. Functional Imaging of cholinergic and dopaminergic pathways. *Neurology, 65*: 1716-22.

Hobson, P. & Meara, J. (2004). Risk and incidence of dementia in a cohort of older subjects with Parkinson's disease in the United Kingdom. *Mov Disord, 19*:1043-1049.

Janvin C, Aarsland D, Larsen JP & Hugdahl K. (2003). Neuropsychological profile of patients with Parkinson's disease without dementia. *Dement Geriatr Cogn Disord, 15*, 126-131.

Kemps E, Szmalec A, Vandierendonck A & Crevits L. (2005). Visuo-spatial processing in Parkinson´s disease: evidence for diminished visuo-spatial sketch pad and central executive resources. *Parkinsonism Relat Disorders. 11*(3): 181-6.

Levin BE, Tomer R, Rey GJ. (1992). Cognitive impairments in Parkinson's disease. *Neurol Clin., 10*, 471–85.

Lewis SJ, Dove A, Robbins TW, Barker RA & Owen AM. (2003). Cognitive impairments in early Parkinson's disease are accompanied by reductions in activity in frontostriatal neural circuitry. *J Neurosci, 23*: 6351–6.

Lewis SJ, Slabosz A, Robbins TW, Barker RA & Owen AM. (2005). Dopaminergic basis for deficits in working memory but not attentional set-shifting in Parkinson´s disease. *Neuropsychologia, 43*(6), 823-32.

Locascio, JJ, Corkin, S & Growdon, JH (2003). Relation between characteristics of Parkinson´s disease and cognitive declive. *J Clin Exp Neuropsychol, 25*: 49-109.

Mamikonian E, Moberg P, Siderowf A, Duda J, Have T, Hurtig H, et al. (2009). Mild cognitive impairment is common in Parkinson's disease patients with normal Mini-Mental State examination (MMSE) scores. *Parkinsonism Relat Disord, 15*: 226-31.

Martínez-Martín P. (2006). Repercusiones sobre la calidad de vida del deterioro cognitivo en la enfermedad de Parkinson. *Revista de Neurología, 43*: 168-172.

McKinlay A, Kaller CP, Grace RC, Dalrymple-Alford JC, Anderson TJ, Fink J & Roger D. (2008). Planning in Parkinson´s disease: a matter of problem structure?. *Neuropsychologia, 46*(1): 384-9.

Moustafa AA, Sherman SJ & Frank MJ. (2008). A dopaminergic basis for working memory, learning and attentional shifting in Parkinsonism. *Neuropsychologia, 46*(13): 3144-56.

Muñiz Casado, J & Rodríguez Fernández, R. (2007). Déficit de memoria en pacientes con enfermedad de Parkinson inicial. *Mapfre Medicina, 18*(1), 39-45.

Muslimovic D, Post B, Speelman JD & Schmand B. (2005). Cognitive profile of patients with newly diagnosed Parkinson's disease. *Neurology, 65*: 1239–45.

Muslimovic D, Post B, Speelman JD & Schmand B. (2007). Motor procedural learning in Parkinson´s disease. *Brain, 130*(11), 2887-97.

Nobili F, Abbruzzese G, Morbelli S, Marchese R, Girtler N, Dessi B, Brugnolo A, Canepa C, Drosos GC, Sambuccti G & Rodríguez G. (2009). Amnestic mild cognitive impairment in Parkinson´s disease: a brain perfusion SPECT study. *Mov Disorders, 24*(3): 414-21.

Ostrosky-Solis, F. (2000). Características neuropsicológicas de la enfermedad de Parkinson. *Revista de Neurología, 30*(8): 788-796.

Owen, AM (2004). Cognitive dysfunction in Parkinson´s disease: the role of frontoestriatal circuitry. *Neuroscientist, 10*(6):525-37

Owen AM, Doyon J, Dagher A, Sadikot A & Evans AC. (1998). Abnormal basal ganglia outflow in Parkinson's disease identified with PET. Implications for higher cortical functions. *Brain, 121,* 949–65.

Owen AM, James M, Leigh PN, Summers BA, Marsden CD, Quinn NP, et al. (1992). Fronto-striatal cognitive deficits at different stages of Parkinson's disease. *Brain,* 115: 1727–51.

Perea-Bartolomé, M.V. (2001). Deterioro cognitivo en la enfermedad de Parkinson. *Revista de Neurología, 32*(12): 1182-1187.

Pillon, B., Ardouin, C., Damier, P., Krack, P. & Houeto, L. (2000). Neuropsychological changes between off and on STN or Gpi stimulation in Parkinson´s disease. *Neurology, 55*: 411-418.

Pillon, B., Bernard, D., Vidailhet, M., Bonnet, A.M., Hahn-Barma, V. & Dubois, B. (1998). Is impaired memory for spatial location in Parkinson´s disease domain specific or dependent on "strategic" processes?. *Neuropsychologia, 36*(1), 1-9.

Posner M.I. & Digirolamo, G.J. (1998). Executive attention: Conflict, target detection and cognitive control. En R. Parasuraman (Ed.), *The attentive brain* (pp. 401-423). Cambridge: MIT Press.

Possin KL, Filoteo JV, Song DD & Salmon DP. (2008). Spatial and object working memory deficits in Parkinson´s disease are due to impairment in different underlying processes. *Neuropsychology, 22*(5), 585-95.

Rudkin SJ, Pearson DG & Logie RG. (2007). Executive processes in visual and spatial working memory tasks. *Q J Exp Psychol, 60*(1), 79-100.

Sánchez-Rodríguez, J. L. (2002). Déficit neuropsicológicos en la enfermedad de Parkinson. *Revista de Neurología, 35*(4), 310-317.

Sawamoto N, Honda M, Hanakawa T, Aso T, Inoue M & Toyoda H. (2007). Cognitive slowing in Parkinson disease is accompanied by hypofunctioning of the striatum. Neurology, 68, 1062–8.

Stefanova, E.D., Kostie, V.S., Ziropadja, L.J., Ocic, G.G. & Markovic, M. (2001). Declarative memory in early Parkinson´s disease: Serial position learning effects. *Journal of Clinical and Experimental Neuropsychology, 23*(5), 581-591.

Stuss, D. T., & Alexander, M. P. (2000). Executive functions and the frontal lobes: A conceptual view. *Psychological Reseach, 63,* 289-298.

Taylor JP, Rowan EN, Lett D, O´Brien JT, Mckeith IG & Burn DJ. (2008). Poor atentional function predicts cognitive decline in patients with non-demented Parkinson´s disease independent of motor fhenotipe. *J Neurol Neurosurg Psychiatry, 79*(12): 1318-23.

Tinaz S, Schendan HE & Stern CE. (2008). Fronto-striatal deficit in Parkinson´s disease during semantic event sequencing. *Neurobiol aging, 29*(3), 397-407.

Tirapu-Ustárroz J, Muñoz-Céspedes JM. (2005). Memoria y funciones ejecutivas. *Rev Neurol, 41,* 475-484.

Tirapu-Ustárroz, J., Muñoz-Céspedes, J. M., & Pelegrín-Valero, C. (2002). Funciones ejecutivas: Necesidad de una integración conceptual. *Revista de Neurología, 34*(7), 673-685.

Vera-Cuesta, H. Vera-Acosta, H., Álvarez-González, Fernández-Maderos, I. & Casabona-Fernández, E. (2006). Disfunción frontal en la enfermedad de Parkinson idiopática. *Revista de Neurología,* 42(2): 76- 84.

Verbaan D, Marinus J, Visser M, Van Rooden SM, Stiggelbout AM, Middelkoop HA & Van Hillten JJ. (2007). Cognitive impairment in Parkinson´s disease. *J Neurol Neurosurg Psychiatry, 78* (11): 1182-7.

Weintraub D, Moberg PJ, Culbertson WC, Duda JE & Stern MB. (2004). Evidence for impaired encoding and retrieval memory profiles in Parkinson disease. *Cog Behav Neurol, 17*(4): 195-200.

Williams-Gray CH, Foltynie T, Brayne CE, Robbins TW & Barker RA. (2007). Evolution of cognitive dysfunction in an incident Parkinson´s disease cohort. *Brain, 130*(7), 1787-98.

Zec RF, Landreth ES, Fritz S, Grames E, Hasara A, Fraizer W, et al. (1999). A comparison of phonemic, semantic, and alternating word fluency in Parkinson's disease. *Arch Clin Neuropsychol, 14,* 255-264.

Zgaljardic DJ, Borod JC, Foldi NS & Mattis PJ. (2003). A review of the cognitive and behavioural sequelae of Parkinson´s disease: relationship to frontoestriatal circuitry. *Cogn Behav Neurol., 16*(4):193-21.

Zizak VS, Filoteo JV, Possin KL, Lucas JA, Rilling LM, Davis JD, Peavy G, Wong A & Salmon DP. (2005). The ubiquity of memory retrieval deficits in patients with frontal-striatal dysfunction. *Cogn Behav Neurol, 18*(4), 198-205.

5

Pathophysiology of Drug-Induced Dyskinesias

Christopher A. Lieu[1,2], Vikram Shivkumar[1], Timothy P. Gilmour[1,2], Kala Venkiteswaran[1,2], Mark J. Nolt[1,3], Milind Deogaonkar[4] and Thyagarajan Subramanian[1,2]

[1]*Department of Neurology, The Pennsylvania State University College of Medicine and M.S. Hershey Medical Center, Hershey, Pennsylvania*

[2]*Department of Neural & Behavioral Sciences, The Pennsylvania State University College of Medicine and M.S. Hershey Medical Center, Hershey, Pennsylvania*

[3]*Functional Neurosurgical Services, Sentient, Inc., Hunt Valley, Maryland*

[4]*Center for Neurological Restoration, The Cleveland Clinic Foundation, Cleveland, Ohio*

USA

1. Introduction

Parkinson's disease (PD) is a common neurological movement disorder that is characterized by bradykinesia, muscle rigidity and tremor due to progressive loss of dopaminergic nigrostriatal neurons. Currently, pharmacological treatment with levodopa (LD), the precursor of dopamine (DA), or other DA replacement therapies, such as synthetic DA agonists, are used to ameliorate parkinsonian symptoms. Although these treatments are effective at alleviating parkinsonism during the early stages of the disease, most advanced PD patients develop disabling, motor complications known as drug-induced dyskinesias. In this chapter, we define drug-induced dyskinesias as abnormal, excessive involuntary movements that occur with oral, pharmacological anti-parkinsonian medications for PD. One classic example is LD-induced dyskinesias. These disabling movements limit the effectiveness of pharmacological treatments.

The aim of this chapter is to introduce the phenomenology of drug-induced dyskinesias and evaluate the current theories for drug-induced dyskinesias, covering recent studies that identify the underlying pathophysiological changes on the biochemical/molecular (receptors, enzymes, and neurotransmitter systems), cellular (basal ganglia connections), electrophysiological (basal ganglia neuronal activity) and behavioral level that have been proposed to influence the development of drug-induced dyskinesias. We will also describe various treatment strategies currently utilized for drug-induced dyskinesias including adjunct pharmacological therapies and functional neurosurgery, most of which are currently limited in effectively diminishing drug-induced dyskinesias or unattainable for many patients. Because of the disabling nature of drug-induced dyskinesias, understanding the factors that contribute to the onset of drug-induced dyskinesias in PD will allow for the development of improved and novel treatment strategies that prevent or mitigate drug-induced dyskinesias without diminution of anti-parkinsonian effects.

2. Behavioral characteristics of drug-induced dyskinesias

2.1 Drug-induced dyskinesias in Parkinson's disease

Peak-dose dyskinesias are the most common form of dyskinesias and occur in 75% to 80% of the patients experiencing dyskinesias (Zesiewicz et al., 2007). The major risk factor has been considered to be severity of the disease. Peak-dose dyskinesias are due to a high dose of LD and represent an overdosed state. The plasma levels of LD are high and there is presumably excess striatal DA. Chorea is the most common form of involuntary movement in these cases. However, in later stages, dystonia can also occur. Chorea is more prominent in the head, trunk and upper limbs (Thanvi et al., 2007). Reducing the individual dose of anti-parkinsonian medication ameliorates the dyskinesias but can cause deterioration of parkinsonism. Hence these patients typically need more frequent dosing of anti-parkinsonian medication. Sustained-release LD formulations may prolong the duration of dyskinesia.

Diphasic dyskinesias develop when plasma levels are rising or falling but not with peak levels. These dyskinesias predominantly occur in the lower limbs and tend to be dystonic or choreiform. Treatment of diphasic dyskinesias is more difficult than peak-dose dyskinesias. Higher doses of LD can induce peak-dose dyskinesias and other adverse effects, while lower doses cause worsening of parkinsonism. The use of DA agonists with a longer duration of action and LD as supplementary drug is the most effective approach.

Off-period dystonia occurs when the plasma levels of DA are low, particularly in the early morning. It can be precipitated by anxiety or attempts to walk. It is characterized by painful spasms of the foot on the more affected side. It is treated by preventing the "offs". This can be achieved by use of DA agonists or sustained release LD formulations (Zesiewicz et al., 2007).

2.2 Preclinical animal models of drug-induced dyskinesias

2.2.1 Rodent models

Unilateral injection of the neurotoxin 6-hydroxydopamine (6-OHDA) into the medial forebrain bundle (MFB) induces selective loss of nigrostriatal neurons (Ungerstedt & Arbuthnott, 1970) in the rat. This causes extensive loss of nigrostriatal neurons unilaterally (>95% loss), and significant loss of DA. This leads to a hemiparkinsonian rat model of PD that exhibits motor deficits in the forelimb contralateral to lesion. Administration of pharmacological DA replacement therapies such as LD or DA agonists induces abnormal involuntary, dyskinetic movements and contralateral rotational behavior. These abnormal involuntary movements are separated into orolingual dyskinesias (rapid protrusion of the tongue and chewing movements), truncal and neck dystonic posturing in the direction contralateral to lesion and hyperkinetic/dystonic posturing of the forelimb contralateral to lesion (Cenci et al., 1998; Steece-Collier et al., 2003; Lieu et al., 2010). Similar to the hemiparkinsonian rat, 6-OHDA can be injected into the MFB or striatum to create hemiparkinsonian dyskinetic mice (Lundblad et al., 2004; Pavon et al., 2006). In mice, knockout of the PitX3 gene prevents the development of nigrostriatal neurons. LD exposure induces dyskinesias in these animals in the form of hyperkinetic movements of the forelimbs and hindlimbs (Ding et al., 2011).

2.2.2 Primate models

Primates have played an important role in understanding the pathophysiological basis of drug-induced dyskinesias and in preclinical experimental therapeutics targeted at diminishing or preventing drug-induced dyskinesias. Investigators have utilized various species to model drug-induced dyskinesias that include squirrel monkeys, common marmosets, macaques and vervet nonhuman primates (Boyce et al., 1990; Pearce et al., 1995; Heimer et al., 2006; Liang et al., 2008). Exposure to the neurotoxin 1-methyl-4-phenyl-1,2,3,6-tetrahydropyridine (MPTP) leads to selective loss of dopaminergic nigrostriatal neurons, and is used in primates to induce parkinsonism. LD and other pharmacological DA replacement therapy induces hyperkinetic, abnormal involuntary movements (choreoathetosis, violent jerks, flailing of the limbs), dystonic, abnormal posturing in the extremities and trunk, and orolingual dyskinesias (purposeless protrusion of the tongue). This animal model displays dyskinesias more clinically similar to drug-induced dyskinesias in PD when compared to the parkinsonian rodent.

The extent of nigrostriatal damage necessary to induce dyskinesias in animal models has demonstrated varying results. In rats and mice, development of dyskinesias is typically after extensive loss of nigrostriatal neurons via MFB lesion, typically upward to 95% loss of dopaminergic neurons when compared to the unlesioned side. Single striatal injection of 6-OHDA as described previously (Sauer & Oertel, 1994) induces a partial lesion with approximately 50% degeneration. These rats do not develop dyskinesias with LD exposure. However, higher doses of 6-OHDA and multiple striatal injection sites can lead to extensive degeneration where such animals develop dyskinesias similar to the MFB-lesioned rat (Winkler et al., 2002). In the primate, some have demonstrated that normal monkeys without MPTP exposure or monkeys with minor nigrostriatal degeneration develop dyskinesias, whereas other investigators argue the necessity that extensive nigrostriatal damage bilaterally is essential for the development of dyskinesias (Kurlan et al., 1991; Pearce et al., 2001; Togasaki et al., 2001; Heimer et al., 2006; Liang et al., 2008). We have recently shown that macaque rhesus monkeys that are clinically hemiparkinsonian by intracarotid MPTP do not develop dyskinesias with chronic LD treatment (Lieu et al., 2011), indicating that bilateral parkinsonian rhesus monkey is a more suitable model for drug-induced dyskinesias in this species. We hypothesize that one mechanism by which hemiparkinsonian rhesus monkeys do not develop dyskinesias is by interhemispheric inhibition. This may be through the small percentage of nigrostriatal neurons from the contralateral hemisphere innervating the denervated striatum. In the hemiparkinsonian rat, our group has shown that there is a loss of interhemispheric nigrostriatal neurons in the hemiparkinsonian dyskinetic rat. However, interhemispheric nigrostriatal neurons are retained in normal and partial-lesioned non-dyskinetic rats (Lieu et al., 2009). This suggests that loss of interhemispheric nigrostriatal neurons may play a role in the development of drug-induced dyskinesias.

3. Differential diagnosis of dyskinesias

Drug-induced dyskinesias need to be differentiated from other hyperkinetic disorders in patients. They are as follows:

3.1 Tremor

In contrast to drug-induced dyskinesias which are involuntary, continual, abrupt, brief and irregular, tremors are oscillatory, rhythmic and regular and tend to affect the more distal parts of the upper extremities. Peak-dose dyskinesias, by definition, will appear only after administration of anti-PD medications (typically 60-90 min) while tremor in PD will frequently mitigate upon administration of anti-PD medication. Rarely, diphasic dyskinesias may have to be distinguished from lower extremity tremor. Diphasic dyskinesias and tremor are both seen when anti-PD medication levels are low. However, on administration of anti-PD medications, diphasic dyskinesias tend to disappear sooner and abruptly as compared to parkinsonian tremor, which will mitigate slowly.

3.2 Huntington's disease

Chorea is a frequent manifestation of Huntington's disease. However, Huntington's chorea is easily distinguished by the family history, absence of temporal relation to dosing of anti-PD medications and by presence of several other typical findings in Huntington's disease that separates this entity from PD. This issue is more complicated in juvenile Huntington's disease. In this case, typically the patient is parkinsonian (Roos, 2010), does not exhibit chorea and is often treated with anti-PD medications. In this scenario, if the patient develops choreiform movements, they need to be distinguished from drug-induced dyskinesias as opposed to natural occurrence due to progression of Huntington's disease. Following points may be used to make this distinction:

a. Drug-induced dyskinesias have a temporal course to timing of anti-PD medications while chorea occurring in Huntington's disease is random and has no temporal course.
b. Juvenile Huntington's disease is a more severe form and invariably the patient will have more symptoms in other neurological domains beyond simple parkinsonism (dementia, ataxia, etc.)

A third scenario is when an adult Huntington's disease patient is treated with anti-dopaminergic medications (e.g. Haloperidol). This drug can produce tardive dyskinesias which need to be distinguished from drug-induced dyskinesias.

3.3 Tics and stereotypies

Tics are abrupt, brief, repetitive and stereotyped movements which vary in intensity and are repeated at irregular intervals (Jankovic, 2009). Patients usually have a generalized urge preceding the actual movement or local discomfort in the region of the body where the tic appears. Tics can be voluntarily suppressed but these result in mounting inner tension leading to a rebound of tics. Tics can also persist during sleep. Stereotypies are involuntary, patterned, repetitive, continuous, coordinated, ritualistic movements or utterances. Unlike tics, stereotypies are not preceded by an urge and usually occur during periods of stress, excitement or when engrossed. They can be ceased by distraction or initiation of a new activity.

Tics and stereotypies can be differentiated from dystonia by the absence of worsening on attempted movements. Tics and stereotypies can be differentiated from drug-induced dyskinesias which are choreiform. Also, drug-induced dyskinesias cannot be voluntarily suppressed.

3.4 Tardive dyskinesias

These are involuntary movements that are seen as a complication of long-term DA receptor antagonist therapy and present with rapid, repetitive, stereotypic movements involving oral, buccal and lingual areas. In cases where the patient is currently on DA receptor antagonists and exhibits signs of parkinsonism and oro-bucco-lingual involuntary movements, it is easy to make the distinction between tardive dyskinesias and drug-induced dyskinesias. However, in very rare cases where the patient has been previously treated with one or more DA receptor antagonists for a short period but such information is not available at the time of clinical presentation, it becomes essential to differentiate between drug-induced dyskinesias and tardive dyskinesias. In such cases, the predominant oro-bucco-lingual involvement, lack of limb and trunk involvement and the absence of improvement on withdrawal of drugs help to differentiate tardive dyskinesias from drug-induced dyskinesias.

3.5 Myoclonus

Myoclonus is a sequence of repeated, often nonrhythmic, brief shock-like jerks due to sudden involuntary contraction or relaxation of one or more muscles. Myoclonus can be differentiated from dystonia by the lack of distinctive postures. Rhythmic myoclonus can be distinguished from chorea occurring in drug-induced dyskinesias by the predictable timing of movements. Asynchronous multifocal myoclonus is more difficult to distinguish but can be done so due to the simpler, shock-like movements of myoclonus compared to the more complex, randomly distributed movements in chorea.

4. Physiology of drug-induced dyskinesias

4.1 Functional models of the basal ganglia

Our current understanding of the functional connectivity for PD is based on the classic rate model of the "direct" and "indirect" pathways of the basal ganglia motor loop (Albin et al., 1989; Alexander et al., 1990; DeLong, 1990). In this model, the dopaminergic nigrostriatal pathway modulates the activity of two separate pathways in the striatum (STR) (DA D1-receptor mediated "direct" and DA D2-receptor mediated "indirect" pathways). With subsequent loss of DA due to nigrostriatal degeneration (neurons originating from substantia nigra pars compacta (SNC) and terminating in the STR) (Fig. 1A), the activity of the motor loops is altered, leading to parkinsonism. In the parkinsonian "direct" pathway, γ-Aminobutyric acid (GABA)-ergic striatal input to the globus pallidus interna/substantia nigra reticulata (GPI/SNR) is reduced, leading to a disinhibition and overactivity of the GABAergic GPI and SNR. In the parkinsonian "indirect" pathway, there is an increase in GABAergic striatal neuron activity to the globus pallidus externa (GPE) leading to inhibition of the GABAergic GPE. This leads to disinhibition of the glutamatergic subthalamic nucleus (STN) and overactivity of this nucleus. This pathway also causes increased activity of the GPI and SNR. Taken together, in the parkinsonian state, both the "direct" and "indirect" pathways lead to an excessive inhibition of the motor thalamus (THAL) and subsequently the motor cortex (CTX).

Based on this model, DA replacement therapy should result in balanced activity of the "direct" and "indirect" pathways (Fig. 1B). However, our group as well as other investigators has demonstrated that with oral pharmacological DA replacement treatment, various basal ganglia nuclei activity do not become "balanced" as the classic rate model would suggest (Heimer et al., 2002; Heimer et al., 2006; Gilmour et al., 2011).

The classic model described above would also predict that drug-induced dyskinesias would be accompanied by increased thalamocortical activity, reduced inhibitory output from GPI/SNR to the THAL, and therefore reduced STN glutamatergic output in the "indirect" pathway and increased striatal output in the "direct" pathway (Fig. 1C). While some studies have supported this hypothesis, others have argued against it utilizing lesioning and electrophysiological studies of various basal ganglia nuclei (Bergman et al., 1990; Hamada & DeLong, 1992; Papa et al., 1999; Baron et al., 2000). Therefore, this model does not adequately explain the pathophysiology of drug-induced dyskinesias.

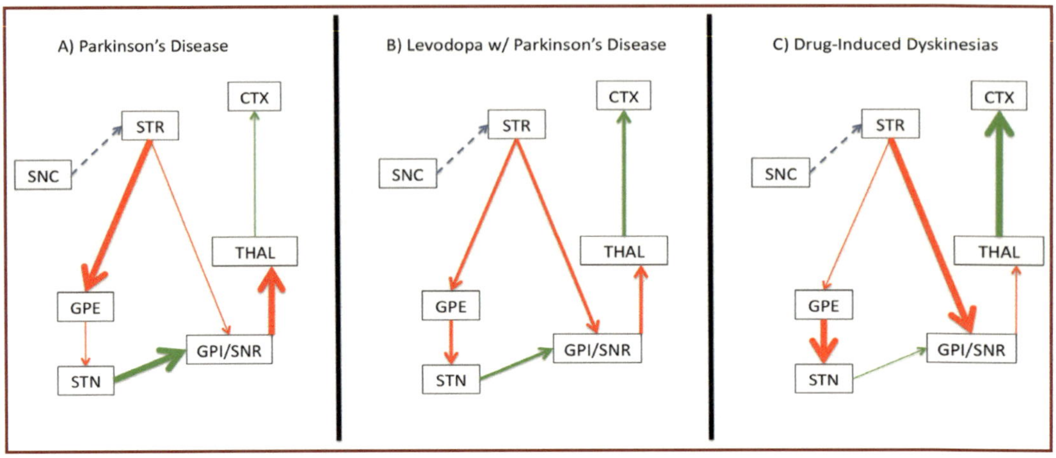

Fig. 1. Classic rate model of the basal ganglia. Red - GABA (Inhibitory); Green - Glutamate (Excitatory); Blue - Degenerated Dopaminergic Nigrostriatal Pathway. Size of arrows indicate extent of activity. In the normal state, the "direct" and "indirect" pathways would appear the same as Fig. 1B, except that SNC is intact.

4.2 Continuous versus pulsatile dopaminergic stimulation

DA is constitutively available in the brain, specifically via the nigrostriatal pathway in the normal state. With loss of DA in PD, the brain no longer has constitutive availability of DA, thus DA receptors are no longer tonically stimulated. It has been proposed that chronic intermittent, pulsatile treatment with pharmacological DA replacement therapies such as LD or DA agonists leads to supersensitivity of dopaminergic receptors (Chase et al., 1989). After oral administration of pharmacological anti-PD medications, plasma levels of these therapies will fluctuate throughout the day based on pharmacokinetics and half-life of the drug in PD patients, thus providing intermittent activation of DA receptors. Presence of intact nigrostriatal neurons allows the brain to store, release and re-uptake DA on demand. Since LD is a prodrug and has to be converted to DA, remaining intact nigrostriatal neurons are able to buffer, store, release on demand, and reuptake DA in early stages of PD. However, as the disease progresses to more advanced stages, there is extensive loss of nigrostriatal neurons and these mechanisms fail, leading to a more pulsatile activation of dopaminergic receptors. Drugs with longer half-lives, combinational pharmacological therapies and cell transplantation studies have provided evidence that continuous dopaminergic stimulation can both provide better symptomatic relief and mitigate/prevent drug-induced dyskinesias. Although there are groups working on biomarkers for drug-induced dyskinesias like positron emission tomography, there is no conclusive evidence that it can predict occurrence of dyskinesias (Feigin et al., 2001; Eidelberg, 2009).

5. Biochemical and molecular mechanisms of drug-induced dyskinesias

5.1 DA receptors

DA receptors are metabotropic G-protein-coupled receptors widely expressed throughout the basal ganglia but mainly in the striatum. The two main family subtypes of DA receptors are D1-like and D2-like receptors. The pathophysiological mechanisms of drug-induced dyskinesias have been attributed to striatal DA receptor supersensitivity. Earlier studies have shown that the presence of mRNA encoding for D1 receptors decreases and D2 receptors increases in response to dopaminergic denervation in earlier rodent studies (Gerfen et al., 1990), which is further confirmed in PD patients and MPTP-treated monkeys (Lee et al., 1978; Alexander et al., 1993; Morissette et al., 1996). More recently, Aubert et al. found differential changes of D1 and D2 receptor expression in dyskinetic monkeys, showing an increase in D2 mRNA and D2 ligand-binding compared to controls. D1 mRNA is also downregulated in MPTP monkeys but comparable to normal in LD treated parkinsonian monkeys. Further, they demonstrate that increased D1 receptor signaling is linearly related to dyskinesias (Aubert et al., 2005). It had been also been reported that there is an increase in both membrane and cytoplasmic striatal D1 receptor expression in MPTP-treated dyskinetic monkeys compared to normal monkeys, with only moderate changes in D2 receptor expression (Guigoni et al., 2007).

Therefore, previous studies demonstrate that plastic changes of DA receptors occur in response to DA denervation and pharmacological dopaminergic treatments. The notion of DA receptor supersensitivity is a combination of alterations to striatal DA receptor expression and subsequent G-protein second messenger signaling (see below). Although our understanding of DA receptor plasticity and supersensitivity has been studied mainly in the striatum for the underlying molecular changes associated with dyskinesias, future studies that examine alterations to the extrastriatal DA and receptor expression in the GPE, GPI, STN and SNR are warranted (Rommelfanger & Wichmann, 2010).

5.2 Second messenger signals

Neuronal second messenger signaling cascades are important for synaptic plasticity, modulation of downstream proteins and control of gene transcription factors (immediate early gene expression) which are modulated by DA receptors (Fig. 2). It has been reported that there is a significant increase of phosphorylation of ERK (P-ERK) in the DA denervated striatum in dyskinetic animals, and that blockade of ERK phosphorylation with the MEK1/2 inhibitor SL-327 or Ras inhibitor lovastatin significantly decreases dyskinesias (Pavon et al., 2006; Schuster et al., 2008; Ding et al., 2011). It has further been shown that phosphorylation of ERK increases in MSN after acute LD exposure but chronic LD exposure translates into a decrease in MSN ERK phosphorylation and reciprocal increases in cholinergic striatal interneurons. Similarly, another related second messenger signal, the DA- and cAMP-regulated phosphoprotein of 32 kDa (DARPP-32) has also been implicated in the onset of drug-induced dyskinesias (Santini et al., 2010). More specifically, increased phosphorylation on the Thr34 (P-Thr34) site of the protein seems to be associated with onset of drug-induced dyskinesias (Guan et al., 2007). We have shown that striatal DARPP-32 expression is selectively decreased in dyskinetic hemiparkinsonian rats compared to normal rats (Lieu et al., 2008). In the normal rat, we found relative uniformity of DARPP-32 immunohistochemical staining throughout the striatum bilaterally. However, in the LD-treated dyskinetic rat, we found decreased staining in dorsolateral areas of the striatum in the unlesioned hemisphere and an overall decrease in the density of staining in various regions of the lesioned hemisphere. Studies in dyskinetic rats and monkeys evaluating the transcription factors ΔFosB and ΔJunD within the striatum have also been implicated in the onset and maintenance of dyskinesias (Pavon et al., 2006; Berton et al., 2009; Cao et al., 2010). As mentioned previously, these maladaptive changes of second messenger signals are likely to be the direct result of DA receptor supersensitivity.

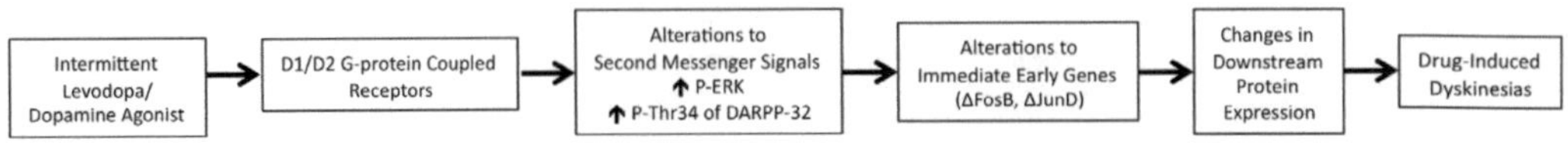

Fig. 2. Signal transduction in drug-induced dyskinesias in Parkinson's disease

5.3 GABA

GABA, being one of the major inhibitory neurotransmitters in the basal ganglia, is present in striatonigral and striatopallidal neurons. These 2 subsets of neurons express 2 isoforms of the GABA synthesizing enzymes, GAD65 and GAD67 (Mercugliano et al., 1992). Systematic administration of LD induces significant increases in GAD gene expression in striatonigral neurons (Soghomonian et al., 1996; Cenci et al., 1998; Carta et al., 2003; Nielsen & Soghomonian, 2004; Katz et al., 2005; Yamamoto & Soghomonian, 2009) and a small increase in GAD gene expression of striatopallidal neurons (Carta et al., 2003; Nielsen & Soghomonian, 2004; Carta et al., 2005). Although GABAergic striatal interneurons are not primarily affected in PD, as a result of progressive DA depletion, expression levels of GABA receptors change in the striatum. Subchronic administration of LD to 6-OHDA-lesioned rats induces marked increases in GABA release in the SNR (Yamamoto et al., 2006), and this increase was blocked by subchronic administration of an mGlutR5 agonist (Mela et al., 2007). This suggests that a GlutR5 agonist can efficiently decrease the severity of drug-induced dyskinesias in animal models of PD. Pulsatile dopaminergic stimulation can cause up-regulation of GABA receptors in GPI. GABA receptors were reported to be up-regulated in GPI of primates with drug-induced dyskinesias (Calon et al., 1999) and dyskinetic PD patients (Calon & Di Paolo, 2002). There have been reports on Modafinil preventing the MPTP-induced GABA-A receptor binding in the GPI of MPTP treated marmosets (Zeng et al., 2004). This study showed partial improvement in PD symptoms.

5.4 Glutamate

Glutamate is the main excitatory neurotransmitter in the basal ganglia. During the progression of PD, as a result of DA depletion in basal ganglia and treatment with LD or D1 receptor agonists, the glutamate levels are elevated, and have shown that increased expression of glutamate receptor resulted in dyskinetic behavior (Calon et al., 2002; Ouattara et al., 2010). Calon and colleagues (Calon et al., 2002; Calon et al., 2003) have shown an elevation of NMDA receptor binding in the putamen (53%) during motor fluctuation when compared to patients without motor fluctuation. Later in support of Calon's hypothesis, a number of ionotropic and metabotropic receptor antagonists have been shown to reduce drug-induced dyskinesias. A recent study showed a beneficial motor effect by AFQ056 (a metabotropic glutamate receptor type 5 antagonist) with LD in MPTP monkeys, supporting the therapeutic use of an mGluR5 antagonist to restore normal glutamatergic neurotransmission in PD and decrease dyskinesias (Gregoire et al., 2011).

5.5 Serotonin (5-HT)

Carta et al. (Carta et al., 2007) showed a prodyskinetic effect by the DA released by serotonergic neurons. When they transplanted fetal serotonergic neurons into the DA denervated striatum, the dyskinetic behaviors were induced by a single dose of LD itself in an already primed animal when compared to the pretransplantation score. When fetal dopaminergic neuronal grafts were introduced, this was able to reduce the abnormal involuntary movements significantly. It was previously reported that the partial 5-HT1A agonist buspirone reduced development and expression of drug-induced dyskinesias (Eskow et al., 2007). Recently Politis and colleagues (Politis et al., 2010) showed that dyskinesias were markedly attenuated by systemic administration of a serotonin receptor agonist (5HT1AR agonist) which dampened the transmitter release from serotonergic neurons indicating that the dyskinesias were caused by the serotonergic hyperinnervation. i.e, serotonergic neurons mediate dyskinetic side effects in PD patients with normal transplants. Recently Zeng et al. observed that striatal 5-HT hyperinnervation follows nigrostriatal pathway loss and provide the first evidence in primates that chronic LD treatment and the onset of dyskinesias are associated with a marked hypertrophy of striatal 5-HT axonal varicosities (Zeng et al., 2010).

5.6 Acetylcholine

Acetylcholine has been another neurotransmitter implicated in the modulation of drug-induced dyskinesias. A number of studies have demonstrated that in 6-OHDA lesioned rats and MPTP dyskinetic monkeys, long term exposure to nicotine, which acts on nicotinic acetylcholine receptors, can reduce drug-induced dyskinesias. Interestingly, the nicotinic receptor antagonist mecamylamine can also provide similar effects (Quik et al., 2007; Bordia et al., 2008; Bordia et al., 2010). It has been recently demonstrated that drug-induced dyskinesias can effectively be decreased by selective nicotinic receptor agonists in dyskinetic partially lesioned rats (Huang et al., 2011). The authors suggest that expression of nicotinic receptors on dopaminergic terminals may play a role in modulating dyskinesias. As mentioned previously, studies have also demonstrated an increase in striatal cholinergic interneuron activity in dyskinetic mice (Ding et al., 2011). Thus, although acetylcholine is not as widely expressed as other neurotransmitters (glutamate, GABA, and DA) within the basal ganglia, its role in dyskinesias warrants further research.

5.7 Adenosine

Adenosine A2A receptors are G-protein-coupled receptors that have been implicated in the pathophysiology of drug-induced dyskinesias. Adenosone A2A receptors are mainly present in GABAergic striatopallidal neurons, colocalized with enkephalin and D2 receptors. Adenosine A2A receptors mRNA levels in the putamen are known to be increased in PD patients with dyskinesias, when compared to normals or PD patients without dyskinesias. Furthermore, specific-binding to adenosine A2A receptors is elevated in dyskinetic PD patients compared to controls in the putamen, and elevated in PD patients when compared to normals in the GPE (Calon et al., 2004). These significant increases in A2A receptor mRNA have been further confirmed in the rat model of drug-induced dyskinesias when compared to sham-treated animals with LD treatment and 6-OHDA lesioned rats without LD (Tomiyama et al., 2004). Interestingly, increases in A2A receptor mRNA has been found in normal cynomolgus monkeys displaying dyskinesias with chronic

LD treatment (Zeng et al., 2000). Recently, it had been shown that genetic knock-out of forebrain A2A receptors in mice can attenuate dyskinesias after LD treatment (Xiao et al., 2006).

Adenosine A2A receptor antagonist administration in parkinsonism has been extensively examined, demonstrating that antagonism can increase anti-parkinsonian effects of pharmacological DA replacement therapies without exacerbating dyskinesias in preclinical models and in PD patients (Kanda et al., 1998; Lundblad et al., 2003; Xiao et al., 2006; LeWitt et al., 2008). Taken together, adenosine A2A receptor antagonists and pharmacological DA replacement treatment can be a useful combinational therapy to target dyskinesias.

5.8 Other chemical systems

Other chemical systems besides the traditional neurotransmitters are present throughout the basal ganglia and play an important role in dyskinesias. It has been shown that neuropeptide mRNA levels of striatal preproenkephalin (PPE) and preprodynorphin (PPD) are increased in dyskinetic MPTP-lesioned monkeys compared to control MPTP-lesioned monkeys, similar to previous reports in the 6-OHDA lesioned parkinsonian rat (Gerfen et al., 1990; Zeng et al., 2000; Morissette et al., 2006; Guan et al., 2007; Tamim et al., 2010).

Using opioid receptor-stimulated G-protein activation techniques, Chen and colleagues demonstrated that μ-opioid receptor-mediated G-protein activation is increased in the brain, specifically the cortex and basal ganglia in dyskinetic monkeys treated with LD. They also found binding changes in δ- and κ-opioid receptor in these animals (Chen et al., 2005). Furthermore, μ-opioid and δ-opioid stimulated binding in the striatum was positively correlated to dyskinesia severity. In a later study, it was shown that pre-treatment with the κ-opioid agonist U50,488 can reduce drug-induced dyskinesias in the parkinsonian rat and primate (Cox et al., 2007). However, U50,488 had the deleterious effects of reducing the anti-PD effects of LD.

Another system is the cannabinoid system which is also widely expressed in the basal ganglia, and modulates the activity of other neurotransmitter systems such as glutamate and DA. Cao and colleagues demonstrate the selective antagonism of cannabinoid type 1 receptor can increase the efficacy of LD without affecting the severity of dyskinesias in parkinsonian rhesus monkeys (Cao et al., 2007). Taken together, the biochemical and molecular mechanisms associated with dyskinesias are complex and still warrant further research.

6. Electrophysiological changes in drug-induced dyskinesias

6.1 Globus pallidus externa (GPE) and interna (GPI)

Most of the present electrophysiological studies of drug-induced dyskinesias are linked to an excessive decrease in activity in the GPI. In a study by Filion et al. (Filion et al., 1991), the mixed (D1 and D2) DA agonist apomorphine was injected in MPTP monkeys. They showed that all GPI neurons decreased their firing rate following apomorphine. The reverse was true of the predominant neuronal population in the GPE. A similar study by Boraud et al. (Boraud et al., 1998) supports the correlation between dyskinesias and an excessive decrease in the firing frequency of GPI neurons. A similar excessive decrease was reported by Papa and colleagues (Papa et al., 1999) in MPTP-treated monkeys treated with LD. This study showed that during dyskinesias, the firing rates declined profoundly in almost all cells of

GPI, with a decrease as low as 97% in individual cells. From recordings in parkinsonian patients treated with apomorphine, Lozano and colleagues suggested that dopaminergic agents act by decreasing GPI and STN activity, and increasing GPE activity (Lozano et al., 2000). They went on to suggest that drug-induced dyskinesias resulted from a large reduction in GPI firing.

The predominant electrophysiological signature of drug-induced dyskinesias at present is the excessive decrease in GPI activity. However, the idea that the hypoactivity in GPI is the primary mechanism by which drug-induced dyskinesias occurs is challenged by the fact that a pallidotomy, which abolishes activity in GPI, eliminates dyskinesias (Baron et al., 2000; Lozano et al., 2000). As a result, some have suggested that the pathophysiology of dyskinesias is not simply the result of the hypoactivity observed in GPI, but rather the result of a change in the firing pattern output of GPI. This would explain why a pallidotomy eliminates the drug-induced dyskinesias, as the abnormal firing pattern is removed (Obeso et al., 2002).

Other studies have examined the role of oscillatory activity in the basal ganglia with respect to drug-induced dyskinesias. In MPTP monkeys, Heimer and colleagues (Heimer et al., 2006) found increases in oscillatory activity and synchronization in GPI and GPE after induction of parkinsonism, and decreases in both following DA replacement therapy. Although DA replacement therapy had a reversal effect on the changes resulting from MPTP, they noted an imbalance in the oscillatory power and synchronization between GPI and GPE. Further studies on the electrophysiology of drug-induced dyskinesias must take into account the present results and explore the finer aspects of discharge characteristics like the firing patterns, multiple rhythms, oscillations, and synchronization in various regions of the basal ganglia circuitry.

6.2 Subthalamic nucleus (STN) and substantia nigra reticulata (SNR)

Since a change in the firing pattern of neurons from bursting to random pattern has also been implicated in the genesis of dyskinesias, recent work from our laboratory examined the effects of chronic LD treatments on the firing rate and firing pattern of STN and SNR neurons in the stable hemiparkinsonian monkey model of PD without dyskinesias (Gilmour et al., 2011). We also evaluated local field potentials (LFP) of both nuclei before and after LD treatments. We found that LD treatments did not significantly change the mean firing rate of STN neurons or bursting neuronal firing patterns. However, LD treatments induced a significant reduction of the mean firing rates of SNR neurons and a trend toward increased burstiness. The entropy of the spike sequences from STN and SNR was unchanged by LD treatment, but there was a shift of spectral power into higher frequency bands in LFP.

In a recent study that recorded LFP from STN using an externalized deep brain stimulator electrode, a desynchronizing effect of LD was noticed on two separate rhythms of STN (Priori et al., 2004). The oscillatory activity increased at low frequency (2–7 Hz range), while the beta oscillations significantly decreased in the low-beta range. Similar effects were observed with apomorphine. Others have shown that an increase in the theta/alpha band of the oscillatory activity can lead to drug-induced dyskinesias in the presence of excess DA in the SNR of the 6-OHDA-lesioned rat (Meissner et al., 2006). These studies add to the evidence that the imbalance of multiple rhythm systems may lead to drug-induced dyskinesias.

Another recent study examined the activity changes in the SNR of non-parkinsonian monkeys with apomorphine induced orofacial dyskinesias (Nevet et al., 2004). Recordings were performed before (no dyskinesias) and after (with dyskinesias) administration of apomorphine. They found that 96% of the cells recorded exhibited a change in firing rate after the dose of apomorphine, with 70% showing a reduction. As in our study with LD, they did not observe significant changes in firing pattern. As a result, the authors suggest that dyskinesias are more related to a decrease in neuronal firing rate in the SNR, rather than a change in the firing pattern. More work is needed to understand the role of basal ganglia neuronal firing patterns and its relationship to the long-term symptomatic effects of LD treatment.

6.3 Striatal medium-spiny neurons (MSN)

Striatal MSN respond to DA input to the striatum, mediated by D1 (excitatory) and D2 (inhibitory) DA receptors. The "direct" striatal output pathway largely consists of the D1 receptor type, whereas the "indirect" pathway consists of the D2 type. In a recent study, Liang and colleagues (Liang et al., 2008) recorded from MSN of severely parkinsonian monkeys during three periods: 1.) "OFF" states in which the monkeys exhibited parkinsonian disability; 2.) "ON" states in which the monkeys were treated with LD and regained motor control; and 3.) during high doses of LD which induced dyskinesias. During the OFF state, the authors found a significant increase in neuronal firing rate (2.7 – 52Hz), which is in contrast to what has been classically observed in the normal animal (0.5-2Hz). This increase in firing rate was observed in MSN from both the D1 and D2 pathway. In the ON state, an overall increase in activity was observed, although some neurons exhibited an increase in firing rate (63.6%) and some a decrease (33.6%). It is assumed that the increases and decreases corresponded to the excitatory and inhibitory pathways, respectively. In the dyskinetic state, the overall firing rate was similar to that observed in the ON state. However, some neurons showed an increase in firing rate from OFF to ON to ON with dyskinesias, and some neurons showed an increase from OFF to ON and then a decrease during ON with dyskinesias. The authors suggest that this combination of uni- and bidirectional changes with increases in DA leads to an imbalance of MSN activity. Interestingly, this result correlates with the suggestion by others that although enabling movement, this imbalance of striatal activity may result in dyskinesias (Wichmann & DeLong, 1996; Mink, 2003).

7. Graft-induced dyskinesias

Cell grafts have been increasingly researched over the past three decades as a method of endogenously resupplying DA to the depleted basal ganglia in a continuous fashion. The primary type of cells used in the early studies was fetal ventral mesencephalic cells, progenitors to the nigral cells which degenerate in PD. In the 1990s and early 2000s, after animal studies and open-label clinical trials had shown therapeutic benefits of cell transplants, two double-blind placebo-controlled multicenter studies were funded by the National Institutes of Health (NIH).

The results were disappointing; some patients received symptomatic benefits, but many patients did not (Freed et al., 2001; Olanow et al., 2003). Additionally, up to half of the patients developed dyskinetic movements that persisted even after multi-day withdrawal of dopaminergic medications. These symptoms have since been labeled graft-induced dyskinesias (GID) and look similar to diphasic dyskinesias. Several hypotheses have been proposed for the cause of these GID.

One of the first proposed causes of GID was that the grafts were producing "hotspots" of excessive DA in small, localized areas of the striatum. A related factor of dorsal versus ventral striatal placement was suspected. It was suggested that small DA-producing grafts might be reducing the striatal DA supersensitivity only in a small area around each graft, and this imbalanced and patchy reinnervation produced GID. In support of this hypothesis, Ma and colleagues (Ma et al., 2002) saw significantly increased uptake of ^{18}F-dopa in five patients with GID, with the increase localized to small focal areas in the grafted putamen. This hypothesis was also supported by a study by Carlsson and colleagues in a rat model of PD showing differential effects on drug-induced dyskinesias due to rostral versus caudal striatal grafts (Carlsson et al., 2006). However, Piccini and colleagues showed using another ^{18}F-dopa experiment that patients with GID did not show abnormal DA release from graft areas (Piccini et al., 2005), and subsequent post-hoc analysis of larger numbers of grafted patients showed no correlation between striatal reinnervation and GID (Hagell et al., 2002; Olanow et al., 2003).

Another hypothesis was that GID were caused by immune system rejection of the grafts. Early analyses showed that some patients with GID showed low-level inflammation around their grafts (Hagell et al., 2002), and GID worsened in some patients after immunosuppression was stopped (Piccini et al., 2005). However, a recent experiment which induced graft rejection in a rat model did not show an increase in abnormal involuntary movements, suggesting that inflammation and rejection alone may not be the primary cause of GID (Lane et al., 2008).

Because the risk of developing GID has been shown to vary depending on the patient, another hypothesis for the origin of GID is that it stems from the same pathophysiology as drug-induced dyskinesias. All of the original patients in the Freed and Olanow NIH studies who developed GID had previously been exposed to many years of intermittent LD therapy, suggesting possible priming and hypersensitization of the striatum. Pre-transplant drug-induced dyskinesias has been implicated in the development of GID and is increasingly seen as a counterindication for transplant (Lane et al., 2010). Experiments in rodent PD models have similarly shown correlations between pre-transplant drug-induced dyskinesias and post-transplant amphetamine-induced dyskinesias (Lane et al., 2006; Lane et al., 2009; Lane et al., 2009).

Another hypothesis is that GID is the result of aberrant synaptic graft-host connectivity. Studies have previously shown degeneration of dendrites and dendritic spines on the striatal MSN in advanced PD (Stephens et al., 2005). Soderstrom and colleagues recently looked at synaptic connections to dendrites near graft sites, showing that decreases in tyrosine hydroxylase-positive synapses onto striatal dendritic spines and increases in asymmetric excitatory synapses correlate with GID in rat models (Soderstrom et al., 2008). Further studies showed that chronic administration of nimodipine, a calcium channel blocker which had been shown to preserve striatal dendritic spines, reduced GID (Soderstrom et al., 2010). Another approach to avoiding aberrant graft synaptic connectivity has been the use of retinal pigment epithelial (RPE) cells, which produce LD and possibly DA but do not form axons or synaptic connections (Subramanian et al., 2002; Bakay et al., 2004). These RPE cells have been shown to provide symptomatic benefit in both animal trials and open-label clinical studies. Promising recent research with new inducible pluripotent stem cells and inducible neuron-like cells shows progress toward dopaminergic therapeutic grafts developed from patients' own donor cells (Wernig et al., 2008; Vierbuchen et al., 2010).

A final hypothesis for the cause of GID is the accidental inclusion of serotonergic cells in the dopaminergic graft. Serotonergic neurons are known to be able to convert, store, and release DA under certain conditions (Tanaka et al., 1999). The patients in the Freed NIH study who developed GID had been transplanted with neurons which had been cultured for several days, a technique which is known to increase the proportion of serotonergic neurons compared to dopaminergic neurons. It was recently shown in a rat PD model that serotonergic striatal grafts increased drug-induced dyskinesia activity (Carta et al., 2007; Carlsson et al., 2009). Drug-induced dyskinesias is not identical to GID, as drug-induced dyskinesias is seen during and after the surge in DA which follows LD ingestion (de la Fuente-Fernandez et al., 2004), and some studies show no relationship between GID and serotonergic innervation in the rat model (Lane et al., 2009). However, recent studies in human patients continue to support the serotonergic cograft hypothesis for GID. Politis and colleagues used ^{11}C-DASB PET to show that two grafted patients with GID showed much higher levels of striatal serotonin receptor expression than other grafted patients without GID (Politis et al., 2010). Furthermore, GID was significantly reduced by systemic administration of buspirone, a 5-hydroxytryptamine agonist which reduces serotonin release.

In summary, the exact cause of GID still remains to be clarified, and several factors may well be involved. Promising hypotheses for reducing GID are garnering increasing experimental support, including selection of patients without severe drug-induced dyskinesias, optimization of novel cell sources and transplant techniques to reduce immune reaction and decrease serotonergic progenitor cells, and pharmacological methods of preserving striatal spines and increasing striatal dopaminergic reinnervation.

8. Adjunct drugs to reduce drug-induced dyskinesias

8.1 Amantadine

Amantadine is a NMDA receptor antagonist and has been found to be efficacious in the treatment of drug-induced dyskinesias without reducing antiparkinsonian benefits. Its antidyskinetic effect gives support to the glutamatergic theory as a pathophysiological mechanism. Double-blind placebo-controlled studies have demonstrated 45% to 60% reductions in dyskinesia. Benefits are typically seen in 3 weeks following initiation of treatment. The benefits of Amantadine have been shown to last for only 8 months to 1 year in some studies (Sawada et al., 2010). A more recent study has shown that the antidyskinetic effects last longer than 1 year and has advocated the continued use of Amantadine for the treatment of dyskinesias (Wolf et al., 2010). Also, discontinuation of Amantadine has been shown to worsen dyskinesias. Amantadine is initiated at a dose of 100 mg/day and can be increased up to 300 mg/day. Potential side effects are confusion, hallucination, edema of feet and livedo reticularis.

8.2 Sarizotan

Sarizotan is a 5-HT1A receptor agonist and is a high affinity antagonist for D3 and D4 receptors. The beneficial effects of Sarizotan are probably due to its 5-HT1A agonist properties. It has been found to reduce dyskinesia in 6-OHDA lesioned rats and in MPTP-lesioned monkeys (Bibbiani et al., 2001). In open label studies, Sarizotan in a dose range of 4 to 20 mg/day showed promising results in decreasing dyskinesias (Olanow et al., 2004). A double-blinded placebo-controlled study demonstrated significant decrease in the duration and severity of dyskinesias on the Unified Parkinson's Disease Rating Scale (UPDRS) with 2 mg/day Sarizotan compared to placebo. UPDRS is a standard rating tool used in clinical research. Other clinical tools to measure dyskinesias (patients' home diary and abnormal involuntary movements scale score) did not show any changes while on this dose. Higher doses were associated with worsening of parkinsonism with no additional anti-dyskinetic benefits (Goetz et al., 2007). Sarizotan is well-tolerated and studies have not shown any adverse effect compared to placebo.

8.3 Levetiracetam

Levetiracetam is an anti-epileptic drug. It has been found to reduce dyskinesias in MPTP lesioned primates. We were the first to report improvement in drug-induced dyskinesias upon treatment with low doses of Levetiracetam in an open label study (Tousi & Subramanian, 2005). Other open label studies provided mixed efficacy results and poor tolerability due to somnolence. More recently, two double-blinded placebo-controlled studies have evaluated the efficacy and safety of Levetiracetam in the treatment of dyskinesias (Stathis et al., 2010; Wolz et al., 2010). In one study (Wolz et al., 2010), patients received 250 mg/day titrated gradually to a dose of 2000 mg/day over 7 weeks followed by a 4-week maintenance phase. There was a significant difference in UPDRS dyskinesia ratings (duration and severity) between the two groups. There was no significant change in abnormal involuntary movements scale score. In the other study (Stathis et al., 2010), patients received 500 mg/day and 1000 mg/day each for 2 weeks. 'On with dyskinesia' time decreased and 'On without dyskinesia' time increased significantly in the treatment group. Duration of dyskinesias decreased significantly while, severity decreased but the change was not significant. Both studies did not demonstrate worsening of parkinsonian symptoms. The most common side effects are somnolence and dizziness. However, in contrast to the open label studies that reported intolerable side effects leading to high dropout rates, the double-blinded placebo-controlled studies did not report severe adverse effects. The mechanisms of the antidyskinetic effects of Levetiracetam are unknown. It has been hypothesized that it could be due to modulation of the pathological synchronization and desynchronization of neuronal circuits of the basal ganglia and maladaptive DA release and reuptake at the presynaptic level. The recent trials provide promising data that Levetiracetam might be useful for treatment of drug-induced dyskinesias without reducing the efficacy of antiparkinsonian therapy.

8.4 DA agonists

DA agonists are often used as adjuncts to LD in advanced PD. DA agonists exert their pharmacological effect by directly activating the DA receptors bypassing the presynaptic synthesis of DA. These include non-ergot compounds, such as Ropinirole and Pramipexole, and apomorphine. DA agonists when used as the initial form of therapy can help to delay onset of LD-induced complications. In patients who have already developed dyskinesias, addition of a DA agonist may permit a reduction in LD dose without worsening of parkinsonism. The addition of a DA agonist might result in worsening of dyskinesias but this can be corrected by lowering the dose of LD. If lowering the dose of LD results in increased "off" states, then the agonist dose needs to be increased. However, patients experiencing severe dyskinesias are rarely controlled with this regimen in the long term. Apomorphine being water-soluble can be injected subcutaneously or applied intranasally. The use of continuous subcutaneous apomorphine infusion has been found to abort "off" periods, reduce dyskinesias, and improve PD motor scores, with the added benefit of an LD-sparing effect (Deleu et al., 2004). Apomorphine can cause severe nausea and vomiting due to its fast onset of action. Hence the patient should be pretreated to prevent nausea. Ropinirole and Pramipexole are initiated at a dose of 0.25 mg and 0.125 mg three times a day respectively and titrated to effect (Hinson, 2010). In contrast to the traditional ergot agonists, the non-ergots have a lower risk of complications such as peptic ulcer disease, vasoconstrictive effects, erythromelalgia and valvular heart disease. Other common adverse effects include drowsiness, sleep attacks, confusion, orthostatic hypotension, nausea and leg/ankle edema. Ropinirole has a higher incidence of hypotension and somnolence while Pramipexole is associated with a higher risk of hallucinations (Jankovic & Aguilar, 2008).

9. Surgical management of drug-induced dyskinesias

Drug-induced dyskinesias have a treatment limiting effect on pharmacological approaches in the treatment of PD. In these patients, surgical intervention becomes necessary. Ablative surgeries in the past had a relatively limited role due to the nature of the procedure, irreversibility and the inability to modulate the therapy according to the need of the patient. Since the advent of deep brain stimulation (DBS), surgical options have become more accepted in these patients (Rezai et al., 2008). Both ablative and DBS procedures are effective in the treatment of LD-induced motor complications, such as drug-induced dyskinesias, that cannot be satisfactorily controlled with medical therapies (Guridi et al., 2008). The modalities by which surgical interventions reduce dyskinesias are multifold: 1) Reduction in daily DA intake; 2) Increasing on-time and thus reducing the repetitive LD dosing schedules; 3) Direct anti-dyskinesia effect.

9.1 Ablative procedures

Ablative procedures effective in controlling drug-induced dyskinesias include:

9.1.1 Thalamotomy

The anti-dyskinesia effect of thalamotomy has been variable. Ventral intermedius nucleus (VIM) of thalamus is not a part of the pallidal receiving area and hence does not have an anti-dyskinesia effect (Tasker et al., 1997). A lesion in the pallidal receiving area of thalamus (nucleus ventralis oralis and ventralis posterior VoA and VoP) has been shown to have profound anti-dyskinesia effects (Narabayashi et al., 1984). In a study of thalamotomy in MPTP monkeys, Page et al. found that a lesion of the pallidal outflow receiving areas of the thalamus had a significant anti-dyskinesia effect but similar lesions in cerebellar or nigral outflow receiving areas (VIM) had no anti-dyskinesia effect (Page, 1992; Page et al., 1993).

9.1.2 Pallidotomy

Posteroventral pallidotomy has been shown to have a significant and sustained anti-dyskinesia effect (Lozano et al., 1995; Baron et al., 1996). A randomized, controlled trial by

Vitek et al. (Vitek et al., 2003) comparing unilateral pallidotomy with medical therapy showed improvement in contralateral dyskinesias in all patients with a significant reduction in ipsilateral dyskinesias. Several other studies have confirmed the significant and sustained anti-dyskinesia effect of pallidotomy (de Bie et al., 1999; Merello et al., 1999). The mechanism of action of pallidotomy in reducing drug-induced dyskinesias is more complex. Pallidotomy improves PD symptoms by reducing pallidal neuronal activity, which in turn restores thalamocortical excitability. This should theoretically worsen the drug-induced dyskinesias. The anti-dyskinetic effect of pallidotomy is considered the function of normalizing the pattern of firing of GPI (Guridi et al., 2008). The optimal lesion location within the GPI has been variously argued to be anteromedial (Gross et al., 1999) and posteroventral (Krauss et al., 1997).

9.1.3 Subthalamotomy

Subthalamotomy is performed in a small number of patients due to the risk involved in the procedure. Alvarez et al. (Alvarez et al., 2001) reported no anti-dyskinesia effect of unilateral subthalamotomy in the short-term or long-term (Alvarez et al., 2009) follow-up. Around 15% of patients (14 patients) with unilateral subthalamotomy in this study developed postoperative hemichorea-ballism which required an additional pallidotomy in eight patients (Alvarez et al., 2009). On the other hand, Su et al. (Su et al., 2003) reported a significant reduction (75%) in dyskinesias after unilateral subthalamotomy in their study. They also state that the lesions in patients with anti-dyskinesia effect were larger and probably affected the pallidofugal fibers. With a significant risk of developing postoperative hemichorea-ballism and variable anti-dyskinetic response, subthalamotomy is probably the least useful procedure for treating dyskinesias.

All of these ablative procedures are associated with an increased risk of hemorrhage and bilateral ablative procedures are associated with further risks, including speech, swallowing, and cognitive problems. With the advent of DBS, ablative lesions are now rarely performed.

9.2 Deep Brain Stimulation

DBS for PD is routinely performed on patients with medically intractable PD. The targets for DBS in PD have included a number of nodal points in the basal ganglia thalamocortical circuit. These include the VIM of the thalamus, the GPI and the STN (Rezai et al., 2008). VIM DBS predominately improves tremor; GPI and STN have been the primary targets for the treatment of the motor symptoms associated with PD. Though GPI and STN DBS both improve PD symptoms (e.g., tremor, rigidity and bradykinesia), there is a continued debate over which site is more effective in improving motor symptoms, reducing PD medications and controlling medication associated side effects such as drug-induced dyskinesias and motor fluctuations (Krack et al., 1998; Burchiel et al., 1999; Limousin-Dowsey et al., 1999; Allert et al., 2001; Krause et al., 2001; Volkmann, 2004; Anderson et al., 2005). Another area of interest is stimulation of the pedunculopontine nucleus (PPN) for PD.

9.2.1 VIM DBS

VIM DBS provides excellent tremor relief, but does not have anti-dyskinesia effect, as shown in various studies (Benabid et al., 1996; Tasker et al., 1996; Limousin-Dowsey et al., 1999). However, some anti-dyskinesia effect is observed in VIM DBS when the electrode is more posterior, medial, and deeper, probably modulating the centromedian and parafascicular complex (Caparros-Lefebvre et al., 1993).

9.2.2 GPI DBS

Most major studies have reported that GPI DBS is effective in reducing all the cardinal motor signs of PD as well as improving motor fluctuations, reducing dyskinesias and increasing on time (The Deep-Brain Stimulation for Parkinson's Disease Study Group, 2001). Ghika et al. (Ghika et al., 1998) reported that the mean off time decreased from 40% to 10%, and the mean dyskinesia scores were reduced to one-third. Burchiel et al. reported a significant reduction in dyskinesias (Burchiel et al., 1999), while Kumar et al. reported that the reduction in the total "on" dyskinesias score was 66% (Kumar et al., 2000). Volkmann et al. reported a sustained reduction in dyskinesias at 5 years follow up of 64% (Volkmann et al., 2004). Rodrigues et al. reported a reduction in dyskinesia scores by 76% (Rodrigues et al., 2007) out 4 years. Several such studies have confirmed that pallidal stimulation is associated with a marked reduction in contralateral drug-induced dyskinesias in addition to improvements in "off"-period. The duration of benefit on motor complications following DBS-GPI is sustained. The location of the DBS lead has an effect on the anti-dyskinetic effect of GPI DBS. Bejjani et al. (Bejjani et al., 1997; Bejjani et al., 1998) have demonstrated different clinical effects after stimulation of the dorsal and the posteroventral part of the GP. With stimulation in the more dorsal portions of the pallidum, they reported improvement in akinesia and rigidity, but an exacerbation of dyskinesias. Stimulation in the posteroventral portion of the GP had a pronounced anti-dyskinetic effect, but worsened bradykinesia.

9.2.3 STN DBS

STN DBS has been the established modality of therapy for advanced PD patients since the initial studies by the group of Dr. Benabid in Grenoble. STN DBS has shown a dramatic and sustained anti-dyskinesia effect in various major studies (Limousin et al., 1995; Krack et al., 1997; Limousin et al., 1998; Benabid et al., 2000). The effect of STN DBS on drug-induced dyskinesias is homogeneous and well accepted. Patients undergoing STN DBS have a significant antidyskinetic effect that can be closely correlated with a reduction in LD dose (Guridi et al., 2008). STN DBS improves peak-dose as well as biphasic dyskinesia (Krack et al., 1997). It also results in significant reduction (47%) in LD dose (Krack et al., 1997). The reduction in dose and drug-induced dyskinesias is sustained over a long period. In a survey published by Hamani et al. of multiple studies involving 737 patients in 34 neurosurgery units, STN DBS improved drug-induced dyskinesias by 73% at 6 months and 94% at 12 months in the on-stimulation on-medication state in comparison to the preoperative on-medication scores (Hamani et al., 2005). Long-term studies of bilateral DBS-STN in patients with advanced PD demonstrate the stability of this therapeutic efficacy.

9.2.4 PPN DBS

PPN DBS has been used in a number of PD patients for gait and postural impairment (Tsang et al., 2010). Early studies suggested that PPN DBS could be utilized in patients who respond poorly to anti-PD medications or other neurosurgical treatments (Plaha & Gill, 2005). This was later confirmed in patients receiving both PPN and STN DBS (Stefani et al., 2007). Although the authors suggest that this procedure is appropriate for treating parkinsonian symptoms, they indicate that PPN DBS is not suitable in targeting drug-induced dyskinesias. In 2010, Ferraye and colleagues found that PPN DBS only provided modest amelioration of parkinsonian symptoms. According to their findings, dyskinesias were not alleviated with PPN stimulation (Ferraye et al., 2010).

9.2.5 DBS Conclusion

It is evident that DBS is an effective therapy for PD patients with motor complications like drug-induced dyskinesias. The primary benefit of DBS is on dyskinesia and "off" time. Stimulation of both the GPI and the STN are effective in treating the motor features of PD and LD related motor complications like drug-induced dyskinesias, but the preferable target remains a controversial topic. It is possible that stimulation of the GPI has a more direct effect in blocking dyskinesias, while reduction in dyskinesias with STN DBS may primarily relate to a reduction in LD dose. A recent study compared the effects of STN DBS and GPI DBS (Follett et al., 2010). Subthalamic and pallidal DBS resulted in improvement in motor function, reduction in dyskinesias and reduction in dose of dopaminergic medications. Effects on motor function and dyskinesias did not differ significantly between the two groups. Patients undergoing subthalamic stimulation required a significantly lower dose of dopaminergic agents than did those undergoing pallidal stimulation. The difference may be an important consideration in patients having side effects, as a reduction in medications may lead to a better quality of life.

10. Key points for the pathophysiology of drug-induced dyskinesias

- The classic rate model of the basal ganglia does not completely explain drug-induced dyskinesias.
- Despite numerous advances in understanding the changes to neurochemical sub-systems in the striatum and downstream nuclei in the basal ganglia in dyskinesias, the prevailing hypothesis of D1 and D2 receptor supersensitivity due to loss of continuous dopaminergic stimulation is still the unifying conceptual idea for drug-induced dyskinesias. However, this idea still does not entirely explain the phenomenology of drug-induced dyskinesias.
- Alternate theories for drug-induced dyskinesias include: basal ganglia neuronal firing pattern abnormalities, interhemispheric inhibition, and alterations to second messenger systems as complementary pathophysiological mechanisms.
- Despite significant advances in the field, treatment for drug-induced dyskinesias in PD is largely unsatisfactory for many patients.
- We have made excellent advances in clinical distinction of drug-induced dyskinesias from other syndromes.
- Many new treatments are currently being examined, and understanding the pathophysiological basis of drug-induced dyskinesias will allow for better development of these novel therapies.

11. References

The Deep-Brain Stimulation for Parkinson's Disease Study Group. (2001). Deep-brain stimulation of the subthalamic nucleus or the pars interna of the globus pallidus in Parkinson's disease. *N Engl J Med,* Vol. 345, No. 13, pp. 956-963

Albin, R. L.; Young, A. B. & Penney, J. B. (1989). The functional anatomy of basal ganglia disorders. *Trends Neurosci,* Vol. 12, No. 10, pp. 366-375

Alexander, G. E.; Crutcher, M. D. & DeLong, M. R. (1990). Basal ganglia-thalamocortical circuits: parallel substrates for motor, oculomotor, "prefrontal" and "limbic" functions. *Prog Brain Res,* Vol. 85, No., pp. 119-146

Alexander, G. M.; Schwartzman, R. J.; Grothusen, J. R.; Brainard, L. & Gordon, S. W. (1993). Changes in brain dopamine receptors in MPTP parkinsonian monkeys following L-dopa treatment. *Brain Res,* Vol. 625, No. 2, pp. 276-282

Allert, N.; Volkmann, J.; Dotse, S.; Hefter, H.; Sturm, V. & Freund, H. J. (2001). Effects of bilateral pallidal or subthalamic stimulation on gait in advanced Parkinson's disease. *Mov Disord,* Vol. 16, No. 6, pp. 1076-1085

Alvarez, L.; Macias, R.; Guridi, J.; Lopez, G.; Alvarez, E.; Maragoto, C.; Teijeiro, J.; Torres, A.; Pavon, N.; Rodriguez-Oroz, M. C.; Ochoa, L.; Hetherington, H.; Juncos, J.; DeLong, M. R. & Obeso, J. A. (2001). Dorsal subthalamotomy for Parkinson's disease. *Mov Disord,* Vol. 16, No. 1, pp. 72-78

Alvarez, L.; Macias, R.; Pavon, N.; Lopez, G.; Rodriguez-Oroz, M. C.; Rodriguez, R.; Alvarez, M.; Pedroso, I.; Teijeiro, J.; Fernandez, R.; Casabona, E.; Salazar, S.; Maragoto, C.; Carballo, M.; Garcia, I.; Guridi, J.; Juncos, J. L.; DeLong, M. R. & Obeso, J. A. (2009). Therapeutic efficacy of unilateral subthalamotomy in Parkinson's disease: results in 89 patients followed for up to 36 months. *J Neurol Neurosurg Psychiatry,* Vol. 80, No. 9, pp. 979-985

Anderson, V. C.; Burchiel, K. J.; Hogarth, P.; Favre, J. & Hammerstad, J. P. (2005). Pallidal vs subthalamic nucleus deep brain stimulation in Parkinson disease. *Arch Neurol,* Vol. 62, No. 4, pp. 554-560

Aubert, I.; Guigoni, C.; Hakansson, K.; Li, Q.; Dovero, S.; Barthe, N.; Bioulac, B. H.; Gross, C. E.; Fisone, G.; Bloch, B. & Bezard, E. (2005). Increased D1 dopamine receptor signaling in levodopa-induced dyskinesia. *Ann Neurol,* Vol. 57, No. 1, pp. 17-26

Bakay, R. A.; Raiser, C. D.; Stover, N. P.; Subramanian, T.; Cornfeldt, M. L.; Schweikert, A. W.; Allen, R. C. & Watts, R. (2004). Implantation of Spheramine in advanced Parkinson's disease (PD). *Front Biosci,* Vol. 9, No., pp. 592-602

Baron, M. S.; Vitek, J. L.; Bakay, R. A.; Green, J.; Kaneoke, Y.; Hashimoto, T.; Turner, R. S.; Woodard, J. L.; Cole, S. A.; McDonald, W. M. & DeLong, M. R. (1996). Treatment of advanced Parkinson's disease by posterior GPi pallidotomy: 1-year results of a pilot study. *Ann Neurol,* Vol. 40, No. 3, pp. 355-366

Baron, M. S.; Vitek, J. L.; Bakay, R. A.; Green, J.; McDonald, W. M.; Cole, S. A. & DeLong, M. R. (2000). Treatment of advanced Parkinson's disease by unilateral posterior GPi pallidotomy: 4-year results of a pilot study. *Mov Disord,* Vol. 15, No. 2, pp. 230-237

Bejjani, B.; Damier, P.; Arnulf, I.; Bonnet, A. M.; Vidailhet, M.; Dormont, D.; Pidoux, B.; Cornu, P.; Marsault, C. & Agid, Y. (1997). Pallidal stimulation for Parkinson's disease. Two targets? *Neurology,* Vol. 49, No. 6, pp. 1564-1569

Bejjani, B. P.; Damier, P.; Arnulf, I.; Papadopoulos, S.; Bonnet, A. M.; Vidailhet, M.; Agid, Y.; Pidoux, B.; Cornu, P.; Dormont, D. & Marsault, C. (1998). Deep brain stimulation in Parkinson's disease: opposite effects of stimulation in the pallidum. *Mov Disord,* Vol. 13, No. 6, pp. 969-970

Benabid, A. L.; Benazzouz, A.; Limousin, P.; Koudsie, A.; Krack, P.; Piallat, B. & Pollak, P. (2000). Dyskinesias and the subthalamic nucleus. *Ann Neurol,* Vol. 47, No. 4 Suppl 1, pp. S189-192

Benabid, A. L.; Pollak, P.; Gao, D.; Hoffmann, D.; Limousin, P.; Gay, E.; Payen, I. & Benazzouz, A. (1996). Chronic electrical stimulation of the ventralis intermedius nucleus of the thalamus as a treatment of movement disorders. *J Neurosurg,* Vol. 84, No. 2, pp. 203-214

Bergman, H.; Wichmann, T. & DeLong, M. R. (1990). Reversal of experimental parkinsonism by lesions of the subthalamic nucleus. *Science,* Vol. 249, No. 4975, pp. 1436-1438

Berton, O.; Guigoni, C.; Li, Q.; Bioulac, B. H.; Aubert, I.; Gross, C. E.; Dileone, R. J.; Nestler, E. J. & Bezard, E. (2009). Striatal overexpression of DeltaJunD resets L-DOPA-induced dyskinesia in a primate model of Parkinson disease. *Biol Psychiatry,* Vol. 66, No. 6, pp. 554-561

Bibbiani, F.; Oh, J. D. & Chase, T. N. (2001). Serotonin 5-HT1A agonist improves motor complications in rodent and primate parkinsonian models. *Neurology,* Vol. 57, No. 10, pp. 1829-1834

Boraud, T.; Bezard, E.; Guehl, D.; Bioulac, B. & Gross, C. (1998). Effects of L-DOPA on neuronal activity of the globus pallidus externalis (GPe) and globus pallidus internalis (GPi) in the MPTP-treated monkey. *Brain Res,* Vol. 787, No. 1, pp. 157-160

Bordia, T.; Campos, C.; Huang, L. & Quik, M. (2008). Continuous and intermittent nicotine treatment reduces L-3,4-dihydroxyphenylalanine (L-DOPA)-induced dyskinesias in a rat model of Parkinson's disease. *J Pharmacol Exp Ther,* Vol. 327, No. 1, pp. 239-247

Bordia, T.; Campos, C.; McIntosh, J. M. & Quik, M. (2010). Nicotinic receptor-mediated reduction in L-DOPA-induced dyskinesias may occur via desensitization. *J Pharmacol Exp Ther,* Vol. 333, No. 3, pp. 929-938

Boyce, S.; Rupniak, N. M.; Steventon, M. J. & Iversen, S. D. (1990). Characterisation of dyskinesias induced by L-dopa in MPTP-treated squirrel monkeys. *Psychopharmacology (Berl),* Vol. 102, No. 1, pp. 21-27

Burchiel, K. J.; Anderson, V. C.; Favre, J. & Hammerstad, J. P. (1999). Comparison of pallidal and subthalamic nucleus deep brain stimulation for advanced Parkinson's disease: results of a randomized, blinded pilot study. *Neurosurgery,* Vol. 45, No. 6, pp. 1375-1382; discussion 1382-1374

Calon, F. & Di Paolo, T. (2002). Levodopa response motor complications--GABA receptors and preproenkephalin expression in human brain. *Parkinsonism Relat Disord,* Vol. 8, No. 6, pp. 449-454

Calon, F.; Dridi, M.; Hornykiewicz, O.; Bedard, P. J.; Rajput, A. H. & Di Paolo, T. (2004). Increased adenosine A2A receptors in the brain of Parkinson's disease patients with dyskinesias. *Brain,* Vol. 127, No. Pt 5, pp. 1075-1084

Calon, F.; Morissette, M.; Ghribi, O.; Goulet, M.; Grondin, R.; Blanchet, P. J.; Bedard, P. J. & Di Paolo, T. (2002). Alteration of glutamate receptors in the striatum of dyskinetic 1-methyl-4-phenyl-1,2,3,6-tetrahydropyridine-treated monkeys following dopamine agonist treatment. *Prog Neuropsychopharmacol Biol Psychiatry,* Vol. 26, No. 1, pp. 127-138

Calon, F.; Morissette, M.; Goulet, M.; Grondin, R.; Blanchet, P. J.; Bedard, P. J. & Di Paolo, T. (1999). Chronic D1 and D2 dopaminomimetic treatment of MPTP-denervated monkeys: effects on basal ganglia GABA(A)/benzodiazepine receptor complex and GABA content. *Neurochem Int*, Vol. 35, No. 1, pp. 81-91

Calon, F.; Rajput, A. H.; Hornykiewicz, O.; Bedard, P. J. & Di Paolo, T. (2003). Levodopa-induced motor complications are associated with alterations of glutamate receptors in Parkinson's disease. *Neurobiol Dis*, Vol. 14, No. 3, pp. 404-416

Cao, X.; Liang, L.; Hadcock, J. R.; Iredale, P. A.; Griffith, D. A.; Menniti, F. S.; Factor, S.; Greenamyre, J. T. & Papa, S. M. (2007). Blockade of cannabinoid type 1 receptors augments the antiparkinsonian action of levodopa without affecting dyskinesias in 1-methyl-4-phenyl-1,2,3,6-tetrahydropyridine-treated rhesus monkeys. *J Pharmacol Exp Ther*, Vol. 323, No. 1, pp. 318-326

Cao, X.; Yasuda, T.; Uthayathas, S.; Watts, R. L.; Mouradian, M. M.; Mochizuki, H. & Papa, S. M. (2010). Striatal overexpression of DeltaFosB reproduces chronic levodopa-induced involuntary movements. *J Neurosci*, Vol. 30, No. 21, pp. 7335-7343

Caparros-Lefebvre, D.; Blond, S.; Vermersch, P.; Pecheux, N.; Guieu, J. D. & Petit, H. (1993). Chronic thalamic stimulation improves tremor and levodopa induced dyskinesias in Parkinson's disease. *J Neurol Neurosurg Psychiatry*, Vol. 56, No. 3, pp. 268-273

Carlsson, T.; Carta, M.; Munoz, A.; Mattsson, B.; Winkler, C.; Kirik, D. & Bjorklund, A. (2009). Impact of grafted serotonin and dopamine neurons on development of L-DOPA-induced dyskinesias in parkinsonian rats is determined by the extent of dopamine neuron degeneration. *Brain*, Vol. 132, No. Pt 2, pp. 319-335

Carlsson, T.; Winkler, C.; Lundblad, M.; Cenci, M. A.; Bjorklund, A. & Kirik, D. (2006). Graft placement and uneven pattern of reinnervation in the striatum is important for development of graft-induced dyskinesia. *Neurobiol Dis*, Vol. 21, No. 3, pp. 657-668

Carta, A. R.; Fenu, S.; Pala, P.; Tronci, E. & Morelli, M. (2003). Selective modifications in GAD67 mRNA levels in striatonigral and striatopallidal pathways correlate to dopamine agonist priming in 6-hydroxydopamine-lesioned rats. *Eur J Neurosci*, Vol. 18, No. 9, pp. 2563-2572

Carta, A. R.; Tronci, E.; Pinna, A. & Morelli, M. (2005). Different responsiveness of striatonigral and striatopallidal neurons to L-DOPA after a subchronic intermittent L-DOPA treatment. *Eur J Neurosci*, Vol. 21, No. 5, pp. 1196-1204

Carta, M.; Carlsson, T.; Kirik, D. & Bjorklund, A. (2007). Dopamine released from 5-HT terminals is the cause of L-DOPA-induced dyskinesia in parkinsonian rats. *Brain*, Vol. 130, No. Pt 7, pp. 1819-1833

Cenci, M. A.; Lee, C. S. & Bjorklund, A. (1998). L-DOPA-induced dyskinesia in the rat is associated with striatal overexpression of prodynorphin- and glutamic acid decarboxylase mRNA. *Eur J Neurosci*, Vol. 10, No. 8, pp. 2694-2706

Chase, T. N.; Baronti, F.; Fabbrini, G.; Heuser, I. J.; Juncos, J. L. & Mouradian, M. M. (1989). Rationale for continuous dopaminomimetic therapy of Parkinson's disease. *Neurology*, Vol. 39, No. 11 Suppl 2, pp. 7-10; discussion 19

Chen, L.; Togasaki, D. M.; Langston, J. W.; Di Monte, D. A. & Quik, M. (2005). Enhanced striatal opioid receptor-mediated G-protein activation in L-DOPA-treated dyskinetic monkeys. *Neuroscience*, Vol. 132, No. 2, pp. 409-420

Cox, H.; Togasaki, D. M.; Chen, L.; Langston, J. W.; Di Monte, D. A. & Quik, M. (2007). The selective kappa-opioid receptor agonist U50,488 reduces L-dopa-induced dyskinesias but worsens parkinsonism in MPTP-treated primates. *Exp Neurol*, Vol. 205, No. 1, pp. 101-107 de Bie, R. M.; de Haan, R. J.; Nijssen, P. C.; Rutgers, A. W.; Beute, G. N.; Bosch, D. A.; Haaxma, R.; Schmand, B.; Schuurman, P. R.; Staal, M. J. & Speelman, J. D. (1999). Unilateral pallidotomy in Parkinson's disease: a randomised, single-blind, multicentre trial. *Lancet*, Vol. 354, No. 9191, pp. 1665-1669

de la Fuente-Fernandez, R.; Sossi, V.; Huang, Z.; Furtado, S.; Lu, J. Q.; Calne, D. B.; Ruth, T. J. & Stoessl, A. J. (2004). Levodopa-induced changes in synaptic dopamine levels increase with progression of Parkinson's disease: implications for dyskinesias. *Brain*, Vol. 127, No. Pt 12, pp. 2747-2754

Deleu, D.; Hanssens, Y. & Northway, M. G. (2004). Subcutaneous apomorphine : an evidence-based review of its use in Parkinson's disease. *Drugs Aging*, Vol. 21, No. 11, pp. 687-709

DeLong, M. R. (1990). Primate models of movement disorders of basal ganglia origin. *Trends Neurosci*, Vol. 13, No. 7, pp. 281-285

Ding, Y.; Won, L.; Britt, J. P.; Lim, S. A.; McGehee, D. S. & Kang, U. J. (2011). Enhanced striatal cholinergic neuronal activity mediates L-DOPA-induced dyskinesia in parkinsonian mice. *Proc Natl Acad Sci U S A*, Vol. 108, No. 2, pp. 840-845

Eidelberg, D. (2009). Metabolic brain networks in neurodegenerative disorders: a functional imaging approach. *Trends Neurosci*, Vol. 32, No. 10, pp. 548-557

Eskow, K. L.; Gupta, V.; Alam, S.; Park, J. Y. & Bishop, C. (2007). The partial 5-HT(1A) agonist buspirone reduces the expression and development of l-DOPA-induced dyskinesia in rats and improves l-DOPA efficacy. *Pharmacol Biochem Behav*, Vol. 87, No. 3, pp. 306-314

Feigin, A.; Fukuda, M.; Dhawan, V.; Przedborski, S.; Jackson-Lewis, V.; Mentis, M. J.; Moeller, J. R. & Eidelberg, D. (2001). Metabolic correlates of levodopa response in Parkinson's disease. *Neurology*, Vol. 57, No. 11, pp. 2083-2088

Ferraye, M. U.; Debu, B.; Fraix, V.; Goetz, L.; Ardouin, C.; Yelnik, J.; Henry-Lagrange, C.; Seigneuret, E.; Piallat, B.; Krack, P.; Le Bas, J. F.; Benabid, A. L.; Chabardes, S. & Pollak, P. (2010). Effects of pedunculopontine nucleus area stimulation on gait disorders in Parkinson's disease. *Brain*, Vol. 133, No. Pt 1, pp. 205-214

Filion, M.; Tremblay, L. & Bedard, P. J. (1991). Effects of dopamine agonists on the spontaneous activity of globus pallidus neurons in monkeys with MPTP-induced parkinsonism. *Brain Res*, Vol. 547, No. 1, pp. 152-161

Follett, K. A.; Weaver, F. M.; Stern, M.; Hur, K.; Harris, C. L.; Luo, P.; Marks, W. J., Jr.; Rothlind, J.; Sagher, O.; Moy, C.; Pahwa, R.; Burchiel, K.; Hogarth, P.; Lai, E. C.; Duda, J. E.; Holloway, K.; Samii, A.; Horn, S.; Bronstein, J. M.; Stoner, G.; Starr, P. A.; Simpson, R.; Baltuch, G.; De Salles, A.; Huang, G. D. & Reda, D. J. (2010). Pallidal versus subthalamic deep-brain stimulation for Parkinson's disease. *N Engl J Med*, Vol. 362, No. 22, pp. 2077-2091

Freed, C. R.; Greene, P. E.; Breeze, R. E.; Tsai, W. Y.; DuMouchel, W.; Kao, R.; Dillon, S.; Winfield, H.; Culver, S.; Trojanowski, J. Q.; Eidelberg, D. & Fahn, S. (2001). Transplantation of embryonic dopamine neurons for severe Parkinson's disease. *N Engl J Med*, Vol. 344, No. 10, pp. 710-719

Gerfen, C. R.; Engber, T. M.; Mahan, L. C.; Susel, Z.; Chase, T. N.; Monsma, F. J., Jr. & Sibley, D. R. (1990). D1 and D2 dopamine receptor-regulated gene expression of striatonigral and striatopallidal neurons. *Science*, Vol. 250, No. 4986, pp. 1429-1432

Ghika, J.; Villemure, J. G.; Fankhauser, H.; Favre, J.; Assal, G. & Ghika-Schmid, F. (1998). Efficiency and safety of bilateral contemporaneous pallidal stimulation (deep brain stimulation) in levodopa-responsive patients with Parkinson's disease with severe motor fluctuations: a 2-year follow-up review. *J Neurosurg,* Vol. 89, No. 5, pp. 713-718

Gilmour, T. P.; Lieu, C. A.; Nolt, M. J.; Piallat, B.; Deogaonkar, M. & Subramanian, T. (2011). The effects of chronic levodopa treatments on the neuronal firing properties of the subthalamic nucleus and substantia nigra reticulata in hemiparkinsonian rhesus monkeys. *Exp Neurol,* Vol. 228, No. 1, pp. 53-58

Goetz, C. G.; Damier, P.; Hicking, C.; Laska, E.; Muller, T.; Olanow, C. W.; Rascol, O. & Russ, H. (2007). Sarizotan as a treatment for dyskinesias in Parkinson's disease: a double-blind placebo-controlled trial. *Mov Disord,* Vol. 22, No. 2, pp. 179-186

Gregoire, L.; Morin, N.; Ouattara, B.; Gasparini, F.; Bilbe, G.; Johns, D.; Vranesic, I.; Sahasranaman, S.; Gomez-Mancilla, B. & Di Paolo, T. (2011). The acute antiparkinsonian and antidyskinetic effect of AFQ056, a novel metabotropic glutamate receptor type 5 antagonist, in l-Dopa-treated parkinsonian monkeys. *Parkinsonism Relat Disord,* doi: 10.1016/j.parkreldis.2011.01.008

Gross, R. E.; Lombardi, W. J.; Lang, A. E.; Duff, J.; Hutchison, W. D.; Saint-Cyr, J. A.; Tasker, R. R. & Lozano, A. M. (1999). Relationship of lesion location to clinical outcome following microelectrode-guided pallidotomy for Parkinson's disease. *Brain,* Vol. 122 (Pt 3), No., pp. 405-416

Guan, Q.; Zhan, Q.; He, Y. & Tan, L. (2007). Changes in the prodynorphin gene and DARPP-32 state in 6-OHDA-lesioned rats following long-term treatment with l-dopa. *Neurosci Lett,* Vol. 426, No. 1, pp. 64-68

Guigoni, C.; Doudnikoff, E.; Li, Q.; Bloch, B. & Bezard, E. (2007). Altered D(1) dopamine receptor trafficking in parkinsonian and dyskinetic non-human primates. *Neurobiol Dis,* Vol. 26, No. 2, pp. 452-463

Guridi, J.; Obeso, J. A.; Rodriguez-Oroz, M. C.; Lozano, A. A. & Manrique, M. (2008). L-dopa-induced dyskinesia and stereotactic surgery for Parkinson's disease. *Neurosurgery,* Vol. 62, No. 2, pp. 311-323; discussion 323-315

Hagell, P.; Piccini, P.; Bjorklund, A.; Brundin, P.; Rehncrona, S.; Widner, H.; Crabb, L.; Pavese, N.; Oertel, W. H.; Quinn, N.; Brooks, D. J. & Lindvall, O. (2002). Dyskinesias following neural transplantation in Parkinson's disease. *Nat Neurosci,* Vol. 5, No. 7, pp. 627-628

Hamada, I. & DeLong, M. R. (1992). Excitotoxic acid lesions of the primate subthalamic nucleus result in transient dyskinesias of the contralateral limbs. *J Neurophysiol,* Vol. 68, No. 5, pp. 1850-1858

Hamani, C.; Richter, E.; Schwalb, J. M. & Lozano, A. M. (2005). Bilateral subthalamic nucleus stimulation for Parkinson's disease: a systematic review of the clinical literature. *Neurosurgery,* Vol. 56, No. 6, pp. 1313-1321; discussion 1321-1314

Heimer, G.; Bar-Gad, I.; Goldberg, J. A. & Bergman, H. (2002). Dopamine replacement therapy reverses abnormal synchronization of pallidal neurons in the 1-methyl-4-phenyl-1,2,3,6-tetrahydropyridine primate model of parkinsonism. *J Neurosci,* Vol. 22, No. 18, pp. 7850-7855

Heimer, G.; Rivlin-Etzion, M.; Bar-Gad, I.; Goldberg, J. A.; Haber, S. N. & Bergman, H. (2006). Dopamine replacement therapy does not restore the full spectrum of normal pallidal activity in the 1-methyl-4-phenyl-1,2,3,6-tetra-hydropyridine primate model of Parkinsonism. *J Neurosci,* Vol. 26, No. 31, pp. 8101-8114

Hinson, V. K. (2010). Parkinson's disease and motor fluctuations. *Curr Treat Options Neurol,* Vol. 12, No. 3, pp. 186-199

Huang, L. Z.; Campos, C.; Ly, J.; Ivy Carroll, F. & Quik, M. (2011). Nicotinic receptor agonists decrease L-dopa-induced dyskinesias most effectively in partially lesioned parkinsonian rats. *Neuropharmacology,* Vol. 60, No. 6, pp. 861-868

Jankovic, J. (2009). Treatment of hyperkinetic movement disorders. *Lancet Neurol,* Vol. 8, No. 9, pp. 844-856

Jankovic, J. & Aguilar, L. G. (2008). Current approaches to the treatment of Parkinson's disease. *Neuropsychiatr Dis Treat,* Vol. 4, No. 4, pp. 743-757

Kanda, T.; Jackson, M. J.; Smith, L. A.; Pearce, R. K.; Nakamura, J.; Kase, H.; Kuwana, Y. & Jenner, P. (1998). Adenosine A2A antagonist: a novel antiparkinsonian agent that does not provoke dyskinesia in parkinsonian monkeys. *Ann Neurol,* Vol. 43, No. 4, pp. 507-513

Katz, J.; Nielsen, K. M. & Soghomonian, J. J. (2005). Comparative effects of acute or chronic administration of levodopa to 6-hydroxydopamine-lesioned rats on the expression of glutamic acid decarboxylase in the neostriatum and GABAA receptors subunits in the substantia nigra, pars reticulata. *Neuroscience,* Vol. 132, No. 3, pp. 833-842

Krack, P.; Limousin, P.; Benabid, A. L. & Pollak, P. (1997). Chronic stimulation of subthalamic nucleus improves levodopa-induced dyskinesias in Parkinson's disease. *Lancet,* Vol. 350, No. 9092, pp. 1676

Krack, P.; Pollak, P.; Limousin, P.; Hoffmann, D.; Xie, J.; Benazzouz, A. & Benabid, A. L. (1998). Subthalamic nucleus or internal pallidal stimulation in young onset Parkinson's disease. *Brain,* Vol. 121 (Pt 3), No., pp. 451-457

Krause, M.; Fogel, W.; Heck, A.; Hacke, W.; Bonsanto, M.; Trenkwalder, C. & Tronnier, V. (2001). Deep brain stimulation for the treatment of Parkinson's disease: subthalamic nucleus versus globus pallidus internus. *J Neurol Neurosurg Psychiatry,* Vol. 70, No. 4, pp. 464-470

Krauss, J. K.; Desaloms, J. M.; Lai, E. C.; King, D. E.; Jankovic, J. & Grossman, R. G. (1997). Microelectrode-guided posteroventral pallidotomy for treatment of Parkinson's disease: postoperative magnetic resonance imaging analysis. *J Neurosurg,* Vol. 87, No. 3, pp. 358-367

Kumar, R.; Lang, A. E.; Rodriguez-Oroz, M. C.; Lozano, A. M.; Limousin, P.; Pollak, P.; Benabid, A. L.; Guridi, J.; Ramos, E.; van der Linden, C.; Vandewalle, A.; Caemaert, J.; Lannoo, E.; van den Abbeele, D.; Vingerhoets, G.; Wolters, M. & Obeso, J. A. (2000). Deep brain stimulation of the globus pallidus pars interna in advanced Parkinson's disease. *Neurology,* Vol. 55, No. 12 Suppl 6, pp. S34-39

Kurlan, R.; Kim, M. H. & Gash, D. M. (1991). Oral levodopa dose-response study in MPTP-induced hemiparkinsonian monkeys: assessment with a new rating scale for monkey parkinsonism. *Mov Disord,* Vol. 6, No. 2, pp. 111-118

Lane, E. L.; Bjorklund, A.; Dunnett, S. B. & Winkler, C. (2010). Neural grafting in Parkinson's disease unraveling the mechanisms underlying graft-induced dyskinesia. *Prog Brain Res,* Vol. 184, No., pp. 295-309

Lane, E. L.; Brundin, P. & Cenci, M. A. (2009). Amphetamine-induced abnormal movements occur independently of both transplant- and host-derived serotonin innervation following neural grafting in a rat model of Parkinson's disease. *Neurobiol Dis,* Vol. 35, No. 1, pp. 42-51

Lane, E. L.; Soulet, D.; Vercammen, L.; Cenci, M. A. & Brundin, P. (2008). Neuroinflammation in the generation of post-transplantation dyskinesia in Parkinson's disease. *Neurobiol Dis,* Vol. 32, No. 2, pp. 220-228

Lane, E. L.; Vercammen, L.; Cenci, M. A. & Brundin, P. (2009). Priming for L-DOPA-induced abnormal involuntary movements increases the severity of amphetamine-induced dyskinesia in grafted rats. *Exp Neurol,* Vol. 219, No. 1, pp. 355-358

Lane, E. L.; Winkler, C.; Brundin, P. & Cenci, M. A. (2006). The impact of graft size on the development of dyskinesia following intrastriatal grafting of embryonic dopamine neurons in the rat. *Neurobiol Dis,* Vol. 22, No. 2, pp. 334-345

Lee, T.; Seeman, P.; Rajput, A.; Farley, I. J. & Hornykiewicz, O. (1978). Receptor basis for dopaminergic supersensitivity in Parkinson's disease. *Nature,* Vol. 273, No. 5657, pp. 59-61

LeWitt, P. A.; Guttman, M.; Tetrud, J. W.; Tuite, P. J.; Mori, A.; Chaikin, P. & Sussman, N. M. (2008). Adenosine A2A receptor antagonist istradefylline (KW-6002) reduces "off" time in Parkinson's disease: a double-blind, randomized, multicenter clinical trial (6002-US-005). *Ann Neurol,* Vol. 63, No. 3, pp. 295-302

Liang, L.; DeLong, M. R. & Papa, S. M. (2008). Inversion of dopamine responses in striatal medium spiny neurons and involuntary movements. *J Neurosci,* Vol. 28, No. 30, pp. 7537-7547

Lieu, C. A.; Deogaonkar, M.; Bakay, R. A. & Subramanian, T. (2011). Dyskinesias do not develop after chronic intermittent levodopa therapy in clinically hemiparkinsonian rhesus monkeys. *Parkinsonism Relat Disord,* Vol. 17, No. 1, pp. 34-39

Lieu, C. A.; Kunselman, A. R.; Manyam, B. V.; Venkiteswaran, K. & Subramanian, T. (2010). A water extract of Mucuna pruriens provides long-term amelioration of parkinsonism with reduced risk for dyskinesias. *Parkinsonism Relat Disord,* Vol. 16, No. 7, pp. 458-465

Lieu, C. A.; Marupudi, N. I.; Berk, M. A.; Ramachandra, R. & Subramanian, T. (2009). Interhemisphric nigrostriatal connections and their potential role in the genesis of drug-induced dyskinesias in Parkinson's disease. *Cell Transplantation,* Vol. 18, No. 2, pp. 19

Lieu, C. A.; Stull, A. M.; Petticoffer, A. C.; Manyam, B. V. & Subramanian, T. (2008). Drug-induced dyskinesias and the involvement of DARPP-32 in the hemiparkinsonian rat. *Cell Transplantation,* Vol. 17, No. 4, pp. 471-472

Limousin, P.; Krack, P.; Pollak, P.; Benazzouz, A.; Ardouin, C.; Hoffmann, D. & Benabid, A. L. (1998). Electrical stimulation of the subthalamic nucleus in advanced Parkinson's disease. *N Engl J Med,* Vol. 339, No. 16, pp. 1105-1111

Limousin, P.; Pollak, P.; Benazzouz, A.; Hoffmann, D.; Broussolle, E.; Perret, J. E. & Benabid, A. L. (1995). Bilateral subthalamic nucleus stimulation for severe Parkinson's disease. *Mov Disord,* Vol. 10, No. 5, pp. 672-674

Limousin-Dowsey, P.; Pollak, P.; Van Blercom, N.; Krack, P.; Benazzouz, A. & Benabid, A. (1999). Thalamic, subthalamic nucleus and internal pallidum stimulation in Parkinson's disease. *J Neurol,* Vol. 246 Suppl 2, No., pp. II42-45

Lozano, A. M.; Lang, A. E.; Galvez-Jimenez, N.; Miyasaki, J.; Duff, J.; Hutchinson, W. D. & Dostrovsky, J. O. (1995). Effect of GPi pallidotomy on motor function in Parkinson's disease. *Lancet*, Vol. 346, No. 8987, pp. 1383-1387

Lozano, A. M.; Lang, A. E.; Levy, R.; Hutchison, W. & Dostrovsky, J. (2000). Neuronal recordings in Parkinson's disease patients with dyskinesias induced by apomorphine. *Ann Neurol*, Vol. 47, No. 4 Suppl 1, pp. S141-146

Lundblad, M.; Picconi, B.; Lindgren, H. & Cenci, M. A. (2004). A model of L-DOPA-induced dyskinesia in 6-hydroxydopamine lesioned mice: relation to motor and cellular parameters of nigrostriatal function. *Neurobiol Dis*, Vol. 16, No. 1, pp. 110-123

Lundblad, M.; Vaudano, E. & Cenci, M. A. (2003). Cellular and behavioural effects of the adenosine A2a receptor antagonist KW-6002 in a rat model of l-DOPA-induced dyskinesia. *J Neurochem*, Vol. 84, No. 6, pp. 1398-1410

Ma, Y.; Feigin, A.; Dhawan, V.; Fukuda, M.; Shi, Q.; Greene, P.; Breeze, R.; Fahn, S.; Freed, C. & Eidelberg, D. (2002). Dyskinesia after fetal cell transplantation for parkinsonism: a PET study. *Ann Neurol*, Vol. 52, No. 5, pp. 628-634

Meissner, W.; Ravenscroft, P.; Reese, R.; Harnack, D.; Morgenstern, R.; Kupsch, A.; Klitgaard, H.; Bioulac, B.; Gross, C. E.; Bezard, E. & Boraud, T. (2006). Increased slow oscillatory activity in substantia nigra pars reticulata triggers abnormal involuntary movements in the 6-OHDA-lesioned rat in the presence of excessive extracellular striatal dopamine. *Neurobiol Dis*, Vol. 22, No. 3, pp. 586-598

Mela, F.; Marti, M.; Dekundy, A.; Danysz, W.; Morari, M. & Cenci, M. A. (2007). Antagonism of metabotropic glutamate receptor type 5 attenuates l-DOPA-induced dyskinesia and its molecular and neurochemical correlates in a rat model of Parkinson's disease. *J Neurochem*, Vol. 101, No. 2, pp. 483-497

Mercugliano, M.; Soghomonian, J. J.; Qin, Y.; Nguyen, H. Q.; Feldblum, S.; Erlander, M. G.; Tobin, A. J. & Chesselet, M. F. (1992). Comparative distribution of messenger RNAs encoding glutamic acid decarboxylases (Mr 65,000 and Mr 67,000) in the basal ganglia of the rat. *J Comp Neurol*, Vol. 318, No. 3, pp. 245-254

Merello, M.; Nouzeilles, M. I.; Kuzis, G.; Cammarota, A.; Sabe, L.; Betti, O.; Starkstein, S. & Leiguarda, R. (1999). Unilateral radiofrequency lesion versus electrostimulation of posteroventral pallidum: a prospective randomized comparison. *Mov Disord*, Vol. 14, No. 1, pp. 50-56

Mink, J. W. (2003). The Basal Ganglia and involuntary movements: impaired inhibition of competing motor patterns. *Arch Neurol*, Vol. 60, No. 10, pp. 1365-1368

Morissette, M.; Dridi, M.; Calon, F.; Hadj Tahar, A.; Meltzer, L. T.; Bedard, P. J. & Di Paolo, T. (2006). Prevention of levodopa-induced dyskinesias by a selective NR1A/2B N-methyl-D-aspartate receptor antagonist in parkinsonian monkeys: implication of preproenkephalin. *Mov Disord*, Vol. 21, No. 1, pp. 9-17

Morissette, M.; Goulet, M.; Calon, F.; Falardeau, P.; Blanchet, P. J.; Bedard, P. J. & Di Paolo, T. (1996). Changes of D1 and D2 dopamine receptor mRNA in the brains of monkeys lesioned with 1-methyl-4-phenyl-1,2,3,6-tetrahydropyridine: correction with chronic administration of L-3,4-dihydroxyphenylalanine. *Mol Pharmacol*, Vol. 50, No. 5, pp. 1073-1079

Narabayashi, H.; Yokochi, F. & Nakajima, Y. (1984). Levodopa-induced dyskinesia and thalamotomy. *J Neurol Neurosurg Psychiatry*, Vol. 47, No. 8, pp. 831-839

Nevet, A.; Morris, G.; Saban, G.; Fainstein, N. & Bergman, H. (2004). Discharge rate of substantia nigra pars reticulata neurons is reduced in non-parkinsonian monkeys with apomorphine-induced orofacial dyskinesia. *J Neurophysiol,* Vol. 92, No. 4, pp. 1973-1981

Nielsen, K. M. & Soghomonian, J. J. (2004). Normalization of glutamate decarboxylase gene expression in the entopeduncular nucleus of rats with a unilateral 6-hydroxydopamine lesion correlates with increased GABAergic input following intermittent but not continuous levodopa. *Neuroscience,* Vol. 123, No. 1, pp. 31-42

Obeso, J. A.; Rodriguez-Oroz, M. C.; Rodriguez, M.; Arbizu, J. & Gimenez-Amaya, J. M. (2002). The basal ganglia and disorders of movement: pathophysiological mechanisms. *News Physiol Sci,* Vol. 17, No., pp. 51-55

Olanow, C. W.; Damier, P.; Goetz, C. G.; Mueller, T.; Nutt, J.; Rascol, O.; Serbanescu, A.; Deckers, F. & Russ, H. (2004). Multicenter, open-label, trial of sarizotan in Parkinson disease patients with levodopa-induced dyskinesias (the SPLENDID Study). *Clin Neuropharmacol,* Vol. 27, No. 2, pp. 58-62

Olanow, C. W.; Goetz, C. G.; Kordower, J. H.; Stoessl, A. J.; Sossi, V.; Brin, M. F.; Shannon, K. M.; Nauert, G. M.; Perl, D. P.; Godbold, J. & Freeman, T. B. (2003). A double-blind controlled trial of bilateral fetal nigral transplantation in Parkinson's disease. *Ann Neurol,* Vol. 54, No. 3, pp. 403-414

Ouattara, B.; Hoyer, D.; Gregoire, L.; Morissette, M.; Gasparini, F.; Gomez-Mancilla, B. & Di Paolo, T. (2010). Changes of AMPA receptors in MPTP monkeys with levodopa-induced dyskinesias. *Neuroscience,* Vol. 167, No. 4, pp. 1160-1167

Page, R. D. (1992). The use of thalamotomy in the treatment of levodopa-induced dyskinesia. *Acta Neurochir (Wien),* Vol. 114, No. 3-4, pp. 77-117

Page, R. D.; Sambrook, M. A. & Crossman, A. R. (1993). Thalamotomy for the alleviation of levodopa-induced dyskinesia: experimental studies in the 1-methyl-4-phenyl-1,2,3,6-tetrahydropyridine-treated parkinsonian monkey. *Neuroscience,* Vol. 55, No. 1, pp. 147-165

Papa, S. M.; Desimone, R.; Fiorani, M. & Oldfield, E. H. (1999). Internal globus pallidus discharge is nearly suppressed during levodopa-induced dyskinesias. *Ann Neurol,* Vol. 46, No. 5, pp. 732-738

Pavon, N.; Martin, A. B.; Mendialdua, A. & Moratalla, R. (2006). ERK phosphorylation and FosB expression are associated with L-DOPA-induced dyskinesia in hemiparkinsonian mice. *Biol Psychiatry,* Vol. 59, No. 1, pp. 64-74

Pearce, R. K.; Heikkila, M.; Linden, I. B. & Jenner, P. (2001). L-dopa induces dyskinesia in normal monkeys: behavioural and pharmacokinetic observations. *Psychopharmacology (Berl),* Vol. 156, No. 4, pp. 402-409

Pearce, R. K.; Jackson, M.; Smith, L.; Jenner, P. & Marsden, C. D. (1995). Chronic L-DOPA administration induces dyskinesias in the 1-methyl-4- phenyl-1,2,3,6-tetrahydropyridine-treated common marmoset (Callithrix Jacchus). *Mov Disord,* Vol. 10, No. 6, pp. 731-740

Piccini, P.; Pavese, N.; Hagell, P.; Reimer, J.; Bjorklund, A.; Oertel, W. H.; Quinn, N. P.; Brooks, D. J. & Lindvall, O. (2005). Factors affecting the clinical outcome after neural transplantation in Parkinson's disease. *Brain,* Vol. 128, No. Pt 12, pp. 2977-2986

Plaha, P. & Gill, S. S. (2005). Bilateral deep brain stimulation of the pedunculopontine nucleus for Parkinson's disease. *Neuroreport,* Vol. 16, No. 17, pp. 1883-1887

Politis, M.; Wu, K.; Loane, C.; Quinn, N. P.; Brooks, D. J.; Rehncrona, S.; Bjorklund, A.; Lindvall, O. & Piccini, P. (2010). Serotonergic neurons mediate dyskinesia side effects in Parkinson's patients with neural transplants. *Sci Transl Med,* Vol. 2, No. 38, pp. 38ra46

Priori, A.; Foffani, G.; Pesenti, A.; Tamma, F.; Bianchi, A. M.; Pellegrini, M.; Locatelli, M.; Moxon, K. A. & Villani, R. M. (2004). Rhythm-specific pharmacological modulation of subthalamic activity in Parkinson's disease. *Exp Neurol,* Vol. 189, No. 2, pp. 369-379

Quik, M.; Cox, H.; Parameswaran, N.; O'Leary, K.; Langston, J. W. & Di Monte, D. (2007). Nicotine reduces levodopa-induced dyskinesias in lesioned monkeys. *Ann Neurol,* Vol. 62, No. 6, pp. 588-596

Rezai, A. R.; Machado, A. G.; Deogaonkar, M.; Azmi, H.; Kubu, C. & Boulis, N. M. (2008). Surgery for movement disorders. *Neurosurgery,* Vol. 62 Suppl 2, No., pp. 809-838; discussion 838-809

Rodrigues, J. P.; Walters, S. E.; Watson, P.; Stell, R. & Mastaglia, F. L. (2007). Globus pallidus stimulation in advanced Parkinson's disease. *J Clin Neurosci,* Vol. 14, No. 3, pp. 208-215

Rommelfanger, K. S. & Wichmann, T. (2010). Extrastriatal dopaminergic circuits of the Basal Ganglia. *Front Neuroanat,* Vol. 4, No., pp. 139

Roos, R. A. (2010). Huntington's disease: a clinical review. *Orphanet J Rare Dis,* Vol. 5, No. 1, pp. 40

Santini, E.; Sgambato-Faure, V.; Li, Q.; Savasta, M.; Dovero, S.; Fisone, G. & Bezard, E. (2010). Distinct changes in cAMP and extracellular signal-regulated protein kinase signalling in L-DOPA-induced dyskinesia. *PLoS One,* Vol. 5, No. 8, pp. e12322

Sauer, H. & Oertel, W. H. (1994). Progressive degeneration of nigrostriatal dopamine neurons following intrastriatal terminal lesions with 6-hydroxydopamine: a combined retrograde tracing and immunocytochemical study in the rat. *Neuroscience,* Vol. 59, No. 2, pp. 401-415

Sawada, H.; Oeda, T.; Kuno, S.; Nomoto, M.; Yamamoto, K.; Yamamoto, M.; Hisanaga, K. & Kawamura, T. (2010). Amantadine for dyskinesias in Parkinson's disease: a randomized controlled trial. *PLoS One,* Vol. 5, No. 12, pp. e15298

Schuster, S.; Nadjar, A.; Guo, J. T.; Li, Q.; Ittrich, C.; Hengerer, B. & Bezard, E. (2008). The 3-hydroxy-3-methylglutaryl-CoA reductase inhibitor lovastatin reduces severity of L-DOPA-induced abnormal involuntary movements in experimental Parkinson's disease. *J Neurosci,* Vol. 28, No. 17, pp. 4311-4316

Soderstrom, K. E.; Meredith, G.; Freeman, T. B.; McGuire, S. O.; Collier, T. J.; Sortwell, C. E.; Wu, Q. & Steece-Collier, K. (2008). The synaptic impact of the host immune response in a parkinsonian allograft rat model: Influence on graft-derived aberrant behaviors. *Neurobiol Dis,* Vol. 32, No. 2, pp. 229-242

Soderstrom, K. E.; O'Malley, J. A.; Levine, N. D.; Sortwell, C. E.; Collier, T. J. & Steece-Collier, K. (2010). Impact of dendritic spine preservation in medium spiny neurons on dopamine graft efficacy and the expression of dyskinesias in parkinsonian rats. *Eur J Neurosci,* Vol. 31, No. 3, pp. 478-490

Soghomonian, J. J.; Pedneault, S.; Blanchet, P. J.; Goulet, M.; Di Paolo, T. & Bedard, P. J. (1996). L-DOPA regulates glutamate decarboxylases mRNA levels in MPTP-treated monkeys. *Brain Res Mol Brain Res,* Vol. 39, No. 1-2, pp. 237-240

Stathis, P.; Konitsiotis, S.; Tagaris, G. & Peterson, D. (2010). Levetiracetam for the management of levodopa-induced dyskinesias in Parkinson's disease. *Mov Disord,* doi: 10.1002/mds.23355

Steece-Collier, K.; Collier, T. J.; Danielson, P. D.; Kurlan, R.; Yurek, D. M. & Sladek, J. R., Jr. (2003). Embryonic mesencephalic grafts increase levodopa-induced forelimb hyperkinesia in parkinsonian rats. *Mov Disord,* Vol. 18, No. 12, pp. 1442-1454

Stefani, A.; Lozano, A. M.; Peppe, A.; Stanzione, P.; Galati, S.; Tropepi, D.; Pierantozzi, M.; Brusa, L.; Scarnati, E. & Mazzone, P. (2007). Bilateral deep brain stimulation of the pedunculopontine and subthalamic nuclei in severe Parkinson's disease. *Brain,* Vol. 130, No. Pt 6, pp. 1596-1607

Stephens, B.; Mueller, A. J.; Shering, A. F.; Hood, S. H.; Taggart, P.; Arbuthnott, G. W.; Bell, J. E.; Kilford, L.; Kingsbury, A. E.; Daniel, S. E. & Ingham, C. A. (2005). Evidence of a breakdown of corticostriatal connections in Parkinson's disease. *Neuroscience,* Vol. 132, No. 3, pp. 741-754

Su, P. C.; Tseng, H. M.; Liu, H. M.; Yen, R. F. & Liou, H. H. (2003). Treatment of advanced Parkinson's disease by subthalamotomy: one-year results. *Mov Disord,* Vol. 18, No. 5, pp. 531-538

Subramanian, T.; Marchionini, D.; Potter, E. M. & Cornfeldt, M. L. (2002). Striatal xenotransplantation of human retinal pigment epithelial cells attached to microcarriers in hemiparkinsonian rats ameliorates behavioral deficits without provoking a host immune response. *Cell Transplant,* Vol. 11, No. 3, pp. 207-214

Tamim, M. K.; Samadi, P.; Morissette, M.; Gregoire, L.; Ouattara, B.; Levesque, D.; Rouillard, C. & Di Paolo, T. (2010). Effect of non-dopaminergic drug treatment on Levodopa induced dyskinesias in MPTP monkeys: common implication of striatal neuropeptides. *Neuropharmacology,* Vol. 58, No. 1, pp. 286-296

Tanaka, H.; Kannari, K.; Maeda, T.; Tomiyama, M.; Suda, T. & Matsunaga, M. (1999). Role of serotonergic neurons in L-DOPA-derived extracellular dopamine in the striatum of 6-OHDA-lesioned rats. *Neuroreport,* Vol. 10, No. 3, pp. 631-634

Tasker, R. R.; DeCarvalho, G. C.; Li, C. S. & Kestle, J. R. (1996). Does thalamotomy alter the course of Parkinson's disease? *Adv Neurol,* Vol. 69, No., pp. 563-583

Tasker, R. R.; Munz, M.; Junn, F. S.; Kiss, Z. H.; Davis, K.; Dostrovsky, J. O. & Lozano, A. M. (1997). Deep brain stimulation and thalamotomy for tremor compared. *Acta Neurochir Suppl,* Vol. 68, No., pp. 49-53

Thanvi, B.; Lo, N. & Robinson, T. (2007). Levodopa-induced dyskinesia in Parkinson's disease: clinical features, pathogenesis, prevention and treatment. *Postgrad Med J,* Vol. 83, No. 980, pp. 384-388

Togasaki, D. M.; Tan, L.; Protell, P.; Di Monte, D. A.; Quik, M. & Langston, J. W. (2001). Levodopa induces dyskinesias in normal squirrel monkeys. *Ann Neurol,* Vol. 50, No. 2, pp. 254-257

Tomiyama, M.; Kimura, T.; Maeda, T.; Tanaka, H.; Kannari, K. & Baba, M. (2004). Upregulation of striatal adenosine A2A receptor mRNA in 6-hydroxydopamine-lesioned rats intermittently treated with L-DOPA. *Synapse,* Vol. 52, No. 3, pp. 218-222

Tousi, B. & Subramanian, T. (2005). The effect of levetiracetam on levodopa induced dyskinesia in patients with Parkinson's disease. *Parkinsonism Relat Disord,* Vol. 11, No. 5, pp. 333-334

Tsang, E. W.; Hamani, C.; Moro, E.; Mazzella, F.; Poon, Y. Y.; Lozano, A. M. & Chen, R. (2010). Involvement of the human pedunculopontine nucleus region in voluntary movements. *Neurology,* Vol. 75, No. 11, pp. 950-959

Ungerstedt, U. & Arbuthnott, G. W. (1970). Quantitative recording of rotational behavior in rats after 6-hydroxy-dopamine lesions of the nigrostriatal dopamine system. *Brain Res,* Vol. 24, No. 3, pp. 485-493

Vierbuchen, T.; Ostermeier, A.; Pang, Z. P.; Kokubu, Y.; Sudhof, T. C. & Wernig, M. (2010). Direct conversion of fibroblasts to functional neurons by defined factors. *Nature,* Vol. 463, No. 7284, pp. 1035-1041

Vitek, J. L.; Bakay, R. A.; Freeman, A.; Evatt, M.; Green, J.; McDonald, W.; Haber, M.; Barnhart, H.; Wahlay, N.; Triche, S.; Mewes, K.; Chockkan, V.; Zhang, J. Y. & DeLong, M. R. (2003). Randomized trial of pallidotomy versus medical therapy for Parkinson's disease. *Ann Neurol,* Vol. 53, No. 5, pp. 558-569

Volkmann, J. (2004). Deep brain stimulation for the treatment of Parkinson's disease. *J Clin Neurophysiol,* Vol. 21, No. 1, pp. 6-17

Volkmann, J.; Allert, N.; Voges, J.; Sturm, V.; Schnitzler, A. & Freund, H. J. (2004). Long-term results of bilateral pallidal stimulation in Parkinson's disease. *Ann Neurol,* Vol. 55, No. 6, pp. 871-875

Wernig, M.; Zhao, J. P.; Pruszak, J.; Hedlund, E.; Fu, D.; Soldner, F.; Broccoli, V.; Constantine-Paton, M.; Isacson, O. & Jaenisch, R. (2008). Neurons derived from reprogrammed fibroblasts functionally integrate into the fetal brain and improve symptoms of rats with Parkinson's disease. *Proc Natl Acad Sci U S A,* Vol. 105, No. 15, pp. 5856-5861

Wichmann, T. & DeLong, M. R. (1996). Functional and pathophysiological models of the basal ganglia. *Curr Opin Neurobiol,* Vol. 6, No. 6, pp. 751-758

Winkler, C.; Kirik, D.; Bjorklund, A. & Cenci, M. A. (2002). L-DOPA-induced dyskinesia in the intrastriatal 6-hydroxydopamine model of parkinson's disease: relation to motor and cellular parameters of nigrostriatal function. *Neurobiol Dis,* Vol. 10, No. 2, pp. 165-186

Wolf, E.; Seppi, K.; Katzenschlager, R.; Hochschorner, G.; Ransmayr, G.; Schwingenschuh, P.; Ott, E.; Kloiber, I.; Haubenberger, D.; Auff, E. & Poewe, W. (2010). Long-term antidyskinetic efficacy of amantadine in Parkinson's disease. *Mov Disord,* Vol. 25, No. 10, pp. 1357-1363

Wolz, M.; Lohle, M.; Strecker, K.; Schwanebeck, U.; Schneider, C.; Reichmann, H.; Grahlert, X.; Schwarz, J. & Storch, A. (2010). Levetiracetam for levodopa-induced dyskinesia in Parkinson's disease: a randomized, double-blind, placebo-controlled trial. *J Neural Transm,* Vol. 117, No. 11, pp. 1279-1286

Xiao, D.; Bastia, E.; Xu, Y. H.; Benn, C. L.; Cha, J. H.; Peterson, T. S.; Chen, J. F. & Schwarzschild, M. A. (2006). Forebrain adenosine A2A receptors contribute to L-3,4-dihydroxyphenylalanine-induced dyskinesia in hemiparkinsonian mice. *J Neurosci,* Vol. 26, No. 52, pp. 13548-13555

Yamamoto, N.; Pierce, R. C. & Soghomonian, J. J. (2006). Subchronic administration of L-DOPA to adult rats with a unilateral 6-hydroxydopamine lesion of dopamine neurons results in a sensitization of enhanced GABA release in the substantia nigra, pars reticulata. *Brain Res*, Vol. 1123, No. 1, pp. 196-200

Yamamoto, N. & Soghomonian, J. J. (2009). Metabotropic glutamate mGluR5 receptor blockade opposes abnormal involuntary movements and the increases in glutamic acid decarboxylase mRNA levels induced by l-DOPA in striatal neurons of 6-hydroxydopamine-lesioned rats. *Neuroscience*, Vol. 163, No. 4, pp. 1171-1180

Zeng, B. Y.; Iravani, M. M.; Jackson, M. J.; Rose, S.; Parent, A. & Jenner, P. (2010). Morphological changes in serotoninergic neurites in the striatum and globus pallidus in levodopa primed MPTP treated common marmosets with dyskinesia. *Neurobiol Dis*, Vol. 40, No. 3, pp. 599-607

Zeng, B. Y.; Pearce, R. K.; MacKenzie, G. M. & Jenner, P. (2000). Alterations in preproenkephalin and adenosine-2a receptor mRNA, but not preprotachykinin mRNA correlate with occurrence of dyskinesia in normal monkeys chronically treated with L-DOPA. *Eur J Neurosci*, Vol. 12, No. 3, pp. 1096-1104

Zeng, B. Y.; Smith, L. A.; Pearce, R. K.; Tel, B.; Chancharme, L.; Moachon, G. & Jenner, P. (2004). Modafinil prevents the MPTP-induced increase in GABAA receptor binding in the internal globus pallidus of MPTP-treated common marmosets. *Neurosci Lett*, Vol. 354, No. 1, pp. 6-9

Zesiewicz, T. A.; Sullivan, K. L. & Hauser, R. A. (2007). Levodopa-induced dyskinesia in Parkinson's disease: epidemiology, etiology, and treatment. *Curr Neurol Neurosci Rep*, Vol. 7, No. 4, pp. 302-310

6

Preclinical Solutions for Insight in Premotor Parkinson

Ingrid H.C.H.M. Philippens and Peternella S. Verhave
Biomedical Primate Research Centre (BPRC), The Netherlands

1. Introduction

Parkinson's disease is second only to Alzheimer's disease, among the main chronic and progressive neurodegenerative disorders. Although neurodegenerative disease may appear at any age, the risk increases with ageing. Therefore, the increasing prevalence of neurodegenerative diseases is an increasing concern for ageing western societies. The problem has been well-recognized and triggered research efforts to develop strategies to limit the progression of neurodegenerative diseases, such as Parkinson's disease.

The clinical features of Parkinson's disease were first described by the English surgeon James Parkinson in his "Essay on the shaking palsy" in 1817. Notably, it took another hundred years after Parkinson's publication before the first Parkinson's disease brain pathology was described. The great breakthrough in Parkinson's disease started in the 1950s by the Swedish scientist Carlsson (Fahn, 2008) who recognized dopamine as the neurotransmitter involved in the pathological process. This subsequently led to research into parkinsonian brains by the Austrian scientists Ehringer and Hornykiewicz. They demonstrated that the level of the neurotransmitter dopamine in parkinsonian brains was dramatically reduced (Ehringer & Hornykiewicz, 1960). This reduction was caused by the degeneration of dopamine neurons in the *substantia nigra*. Only one year later the first patients were treated with the dopamine replacement drug L-dihydroxy-phenylalanine (L-DOPA) (Birkmayer & Hornykiewicz, 1961). L-DOPA therapy for Parkinson's disease was designed and described by the English physician Cotzias (Fahn, 2008).

Nowadays, treatment is still heavily dependent on dopamine replacement therapy, which is primarily aimed at symptom control and can be associated with severe side effects. Furthermore, with this treatment approach there is no prevention or retardation of dopaminergic neuron degeneration. Therefore, it would be a better approach to focus on a medical intervention in the cell death processes to stop or slow down progression in order to increase the quality of life of these patients. This strategy has been well-recognized (Jankovic, 2005; Philippens et al., 2010; Tolosa et al., 2009) and research efforts to develop neuroprotective treatment strategies is the current focus of both clinicians and basic scientists. To achieve this strategy, early identification of individuals at risk and an early start of neuroprotective treatment to prevent the progressive loss of neurons are important. Once it is established that a person is at risk of developing Parkinson's disease, progressive loss of neurons must be prevented.

Generally, patients enter the clinic with motor-related problems regardless of the fact that they have been suffering from non-motor problems, such as olfactory dysfunction, mood changes and sleep problems for years before the actual diagnosis. Since there are no specific early diagnostic biological markers for Parkinson's disease, the clinical diagnosis is still entirely based on the presence of the characteristic motor features that start after the time when more than 50 % of the dopaminergic neurons have already been lost. At this stage neuroprotective strategies can only have a limited effect. Therefore, it is essential to establish markers to identify subjects at risk before motor manifestation. James Parkinson already described the difficulty of the awareness of this slow progressive neurodegenerative process in the early stages of the disease. He wrote: "*So slight and nearly imperceptible are the first inroads of this malady, and so extremely slow its progress, that it rarely happens, that the patient can form any recollection of the precise period of its commencement*". This formulates well the obstacles in the investigation of the early stages of Parkinson's disease and prompts us to find markers for the early stage of Parkinson's disease in humans and in animal models. In particular, animal models offer an opportunity to link low-level neurodegeneration to disease manifestation and a possibility to investigate strategies for intervention therapy. Despite all the research performed during the last five decades, neither the cause of sporadic Parkinson's disease, nor a preventive method and an acceptable symptom treatment have been found. We emphasize that a shift should be made from a diagnosis that is based on motor complications towards early recognition of premotor symptoms supported by the first indications of Parkinson's disease pathology. The ultimate goal will be treatment of individuals at risk with a neuroprotective therapy, thereby significantly prolonging their normal life style.

2. Parkinson's disease

Normal control of movement is a result of the complex interplay of various groups of nerve cells in the central nervous system. Neurons in the basal ganglia (*striatum, pallidum, subthalamic nucleus* and *substantia nigra*) are the key players in motor function and are responsible for the fine-tuning of movements. They are regarded as components of several largely segregated basal ganglia-thalamocortical circuits serving cognitive, oculomotor and motor functions (Joshua et al., 2009). Most important to the motor disorder, Parkinson's disease, are a group of neurons located in the *substantia nigra,* situated in the ventral midbrain. Neurons of the *substantia nigra* communicate with other neurons in the basal ganglia through dopamine neurotransmission. At the time of Parkinson's disease diagnosis, based on typical motor symptoms, patients have already lost at least 50% of the dopamine neurons in the *substantia nigra* (Jellinger, 2008). Together with the loss of these neurons, dopamine synthesis and dopamine release are drastically reduced. Owing to the disturbances in the striatal-thalamocortical circuit as a result of the decline of dopamine, the reinforcing influence of the motor circuitry upon cortically initiated movements is reduced (Alexander & Crutcher, 1990; Wichmann & DeLong, 2003). Indeed, in non-human primate models of Parkinson's disease, the reduction of *substantia nigra pars compacta* output leads to decreased facilitation of cortical motor areas and subsequent development of akinesia and bradykinesia (Wichmann & DeLong, 2003). Together with this neurodegeneration in the *substantia nigra,* intraneural protein inclusions are found in the *substantia nigra* and other brain regions (Braak et al., 2003). The marked neurodegeneration in the *substantia nigra* together with the occurrence of protein inclusions called Lewy bodies form the post-mortem confirmation of Parkinson's disease diagnosis.

2.1 Etiology of Parkinson's disease

Although Parkinson's disease has been studied for almost 200 years, the precise mechanisms leading to progressive cell death still need to be resolved; the actual cause and the mechanism(s) associated with the pathogenesis of Parkinson's disease are still unknown. However, it has been proposed that several factors including oxidative stress, excitotoxicity, mitochondrial dysfunction, environmental toxins, proteasome dysfunction, inflammatory aspects and genetic defects may contribute to the neurodegenerative process causing Parkinson's disease. Whatever the cause is, it is clear that Parkinson's disease is a multi-factorial disorder resulting from the combined effect of age, environmental factors, genetic susceptibility and complex genetic-environmental interactions (Fig. 1) (Chan et al., 1998; Le Couteur et al., 2002; Migliore & Coppede, 2009; Schapira, 2009). Many epidemiological studies support the role of pesticide exposure in Parkinson's disease. For example, rural living (Chen et al., 2009), drinking well-water (Gatto et al., 2009) and occupation-based exposure (Goldman et al., 2005) are potential risk factors that support the above possibility.

Independent of the actual cause, neurodegeneration in Parkinson's disease is based on an endogenous excitotoxicity, i.e. a Parkinson's disease patient basically destroys, and has destroyed, his or her own *substantia nigra* neurons by endogenously generated activity, combined with disturbed homeostatic control of the neurons. There is an obvious inbalance between energy supply and demand in neurons occurring during activation, but this may be the consequence of over-excitation. An alternative explanation is that the problem is related to neuronal homeostatic maintenance processes. Since Parkinson's disease is a slowly progressing disease, it is likely that the excitotoxic state is not always present, and only occasionally induces neuronal death. An excitotoxic state may be directly based on over-excitation, or due to suppression of neuronal maintenance processes; or (more likely) both. Alternatively, factors related to neuronal maintenance processes may be of great importance for understanding slow gradual neurodegeneration. In neurodegenerative disorders, already weakened neurons may not survive glutamate concentrations that would not normally be lethal. These weakening factors may represent susceptibility processes, which are perhaps more easily influenced and would require pharmacological interventions which are less invasive than those currently in use.

2.2 Molecular and cellular mechanisms of Parkinson's disease

Recently, at least eight defined genetic loci have been associated with autosomal dominant or recessive familial Parkinson's disease, wherein thus far five causative mutations have been identified (Nuytemans et al., 2010). Mutations in the following genes have been reported to cause familial Parkinson's disease: alpha-synuclein (SNCA), leucine-rich repeat kinase (LRRK2), parkin (PARK2), PINK1 (PARK6) and DJ-1 (PARK7). Although these familial forms of Parkinson's disease are rare compared with the frequency of sporadic cases, they are very important for understanding the molecular basis or cause of disease pathology. The cellular processes involved are thought to be related with age, environment, genes or a combination of these. They are: mitochondrial dysfunction, glutamate excitotoxicity, oxidative stress, inflammatory responses and proteasome dysfunction (Alexi et al., 2000; Betarbet et al., 2000; Dauer & Przedborski, 2003; Jenner, 2003a; Philippens et al, 2010). In this regard, neurons may die by necrosis, caused by changes in ion dynamics, cellular swelling resulting in the disintegration of the cell and its organelles and removal of cell debris by phagocytosis. Neurons can also go into apoptosis initiated by exogenous toxins, which are mediated by e.g. oxidative stress and the release of cytochrome c by mitochondria.

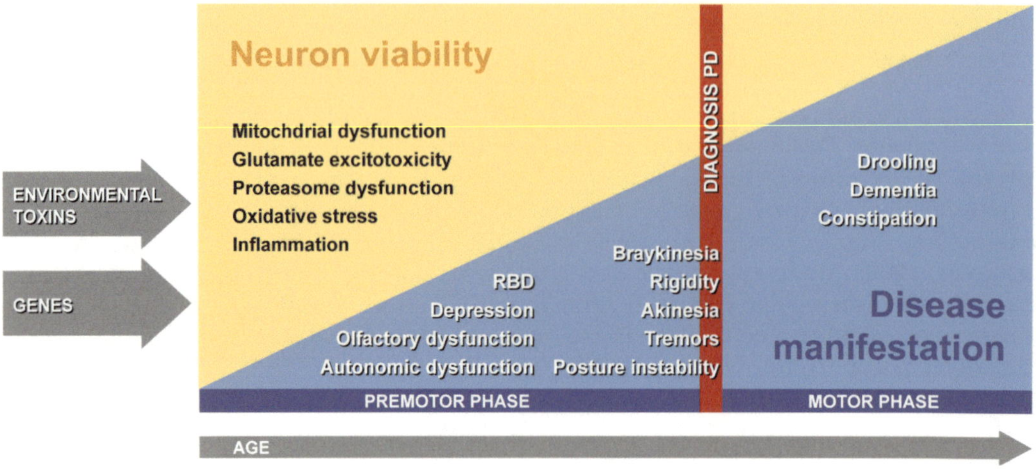

Fig. 1. Schematic diagram depicting the pathology and symptomatology of Parkinson's disease.

The disease manifestation is divided into the premotor phase, before Parkinson's disease diagnosis and the motor phase starting around the time of diagnosis. The multi-factorial nature of the disease is depicted by the possible causes of Parkinson's disease: environmental toxins, genes and age that are depicted by the grey arrows. Neuron viability is reduced over time as shown in the yellow triangle with the proposed features that cause the degeneration of neurons in random order. The occurrence of symptoms increases over time as shown in the blue triangle with the different symptoms that occur at each phase of the disease. PD: Parkinson's disease; RBD: rapid eye movement sleep behavior disorder.

2.3 Parkinson's disease manifestation

Parkinson's disease is strongly progressive, meaning that the symptoms worsen with time. Even under currently available medication, motor incapacitation appears five to ten years after onset of the disease. The progressive neurodegeneration in Parkinson's disease results in a wide range of disabling motor and non-motor symptoms (Fig. 1). Generally, patients enter the clinic with motor-related problems when they are in their fifties. At the time of diagnosis they are suffering from bradykinesia (slowness of movements) and one or more of the other classic motor-related problems: tremor at rest (typically in the hands), rigidity of movements, akinesia (impaired movements) and/or postural instability (balance problems). Besides motor problems, patients may suffer from disturbing non-motor problems like depression, constipation and dementia. Since there are no early diagnostic biological markers for Parkinson's disease, clinical diagnosis is currently entirely based on the presence of the characteristic motor features. However, diagnostics based on live imaging of the dopamine transporter in brain scans and non-motor symptoms like olfactory dysfunction are under current investigation (Deeb et al., 2010). Many patients report having suffered from abnormal olfaction, mood disorders, autonomic dysfunction and sleep problems years before the motor symptoms-based diagnosis (Berg, 2008; Tolosa et al., 2009). Of these non-motor symptoms, sleep problems are reported in around 80% of all Parkinson's disease patients (Tandberg et al., 1998; Garcia-Borreguero et al., 2003; Oerlemans & de Weerd, 2002). Sleep problems can range from reduced sleep efficiency, difficulty in turning in bed, to motor problems during rapid eye movement (REM) sleep, diagnosed as REM Sleep Behavior Disorder (RBD). The latter observation has been proposed as a useful preclinical biomarker for Parkinson's disease (Iranzo et al., 2006; Postuma et al., 2006). Together with the classic motor symptoms, these sleep problems are very disturbing for patients and their (bed) partners. All together, with or without medication, patients are heavily disabled by a wide range of problems, which invariably increase over time.

2.4 Neuroprotective treatment

Recently, deep brain stimulation (DBS) has gained popularity as a treatment for tremors in advanced Parkinson's disease (Sydow, 2008) by suppressing the neuronal firing pattern in the target area (*subtalamic nucleus*) either directly or by inducing the release of inhibitory transmitters (Hilker et al., 2008). Thousands of patients worldwide have undergone DBS treatment. Although temporarily effective, these Parkinson's disease therapies do not stop or reduce the neurodegenerative state and therefore do not actually cure the disease. The current priority in Parkinson's disease research is, therefore, to move beyond symptom control and to develop neuroprotective treatments.

Several strategies have been proposed which can protect the brain from neurodegeneration. One of these strategies is the neurorestorative cell therapy treatment, which is still under investigation. However, major ethical and practical issues need to be resolved before they can be tested in the clinic (Xi & Zhang, 2008). Therefore, we still rely on pharmacological approaches. Most of the neuroprotective compounds either act as anti-oxidants or as anti-apoptotic agents. Some of the anti-oxidants have already been tested in the clinic such as tocopherol, the monoamine oxidase B (MAO-B) inhibitor l-deprenyl, the mitochondrial stabilizer coenzyme Q10. The anti-apoptotic compound rasagiline has also been investigated (ParkinsonStudyGroup, 1993; Shults et al., 2002). Anti-apoptotic compounds such as neuro-immunophilin, pramipexole and ropinirole have also been tested for their neuroprotective efficacy in Parkinson's disease patients (Gold & Nutt, 2002; ParkinsonStudyGroup, 2002; Sethi et al., 1998).

Besides these drugs, some treatments are directed against inflammation, glutamate release or excitotoxicity, or addressing the disturbed mitochondrial energy supply or neuronal maintenance, thereby ultimately aiming at reducing apoptosis and necrosis of the dopamine neuron. Examples are riluzole, a versatile anti-excitotoxic compound and a possible candidate for neuroprotection in Parkinson's disease (Bensimon et al., 2009), and trophic factors like glial cell-derived neurotrophic factor (GDNF) (Nutt et al., 2003) and the dopamine replacement L-DOPA (Fahn, 2005). Some of the above mentioned compounds have shown promising neuroprotective effects in the clinic, whereas others have not fared well. The neuroprotective efficacy is generally measured by the delay in time before starting L-DOPA therapy, changes in Parkinson's disease symptoms, or imaging of dopamine markers. The following factors may lead to difficulties in assessing the effectiveness of a neuroprotective compound (Olanow et al., 2008; Ravina et al., 2003):

1. None of the outcome measures used in clinical trials directly reflect neurodegeneration;
2. The outcome measures were confounded with the symptomatic or pharmacological effects of the intervention;
3. Dosing to achieve neuroprotective action of a compound is often a guess, based on parameters which have been identified in animal studies, but may not be relevant in humans;
4. Diagnosis can be mistaken for other related parkinsonian disorders;
5. And patients included in the trials have already been diagnosed with Parkinson's disease and are thus in a progressive state of neurodegeneration.

Especially the fifth factor may be an important reason for the lack of neuroprotective effect, because the neurodegenerative process has already proceeded substantially before the first motor symptoms allowed the clinical diagnosis of Parkinson's disease in these patients.
Although several neuroprotective compounds are good candidates and have been tested in both animal models and patients, none have led to a neuroprotective treatment for Parkinson's disease approved by the Food and Drug Administration (FDA). Neuroprotection in patients remains the ultimate goal. However, it has to be combined with extensive preclinical screening, early diagnosis and exclusive neuroprotection markers.

3. Modeling Parkinson's disease

Studying Parkinson's disease neurobiology in combination with disease manifestation in humans is limited to clinical trials and post-mortem material. Therefore, in order to find new targets for neuroprotective therapies, the availability of adequate animal models would be an excellent asset in current Parkinson's disease research. Cell cultures or invertebrate models are useful (Botella et al., 2009; Schule et al., 2009) but they can only model Parkinson's disease to a certain extent.
Animal models should ideally mimic the main features of the disease pathology and additionally show the typical parkinsonian syndrome. In this regard, four scientific criteria have been proposed (van der Staay et al., 2009) to judge the validity of a model: face, predictive, construct and external validity. The dopamine deficiency observed in Parkinson's disease is the main cause underlying the pathophysiology of the motor symptomatology.
Animal models can feature the typical –preferably progressive- loss of dopamine neurons in the *substantia nigra* in combination with the associated dopamine reduction in the *striatum.* This is called face validity or the degree of descriptive similarity between the symptoms in the animal model and in humans affected by Parkinson's disease. Often the presence of the typical Parkinson's disease behaviors or the Parkinson's disease specific Lewy body formation can be an important addition to answer the research question addressed in an animal model. In the pharmacological context, predictive validity refers to the ability of a model to correctly identify the efficacy of a therapeutic strategy. Therefore L-DOPA-induced improvement of motor behavior is a key issue in animal models for Parkinson's disease.
Because of the multi-factorial nature of Parkinson's disease, construct validity is the most difficult scientific criterion in modeling idiopathic Parkinson's disease. Construct validity is the degree of similarity between the mechanisms underlying behavior in the model and those in the condition being modeled. Animal models can mimic the pathology and the symptomatology of the disease but not easily the etiology. However, factors like genes, environment and age can be altered separately or in combination in animal models thereby

ensuring construct validity to a certain extent. External validity represents the way results obtained using a particular model can be generalized or applied to and across populations. The ultimate Parkinson's disease model has not yet been described. However, there are several experimental models that meet the above criteria. Some Parkinson's disease models rely on selective neurotoxins to chemically destroy dopamine neurons or on precise targeting of the specific brain regions using stereotactic surgery. Others are focused on genetic defects.

Having a relatively short lifespan, mice are of interest for disease models owing to their rapid progression through the disease stages and their consistent neurological defect. Mutant mice are valuable models for investigating various pathological conditions that modify brain function either during development or in adulthood. There are also several pharmacologically induced Parkinson's disease models available, such as the 1-methyl-4-phenyl-1,2,3,6-tetrahydropyridine (MPTP) mouse model (Schmidt & Ferger, 2001). However, unlike humans and monkeys, mice need a relatively high systemic dose of MPTP to induce dopamine neurodegeneration (Jackson-Lewis et al., 1995) and they show a relatively restricted Parkinson's disease-like symptomatology. Therefore, face validity is not optimal (Luchtman et al., 2009). Furthermore, the behavioral changes due to Parkinson's disease induction recover very fast after the MPTP challenge (Schmidt & Ferger, 2001). Thus, mice are mainly of interest for neuropathology and molecular changes after neurodegeneration of dopamine neurons and not suited for extensive research into clinically based symptomatology.

While, physiological and pharmacological questions can often be studied well in rodent models, issues concerning complex behavior can be addressed more accurately in primates. Therefore, non-human primate models are preferred in clinically focused behavioral studies because their disease manifestation can be translated directly to the human situation (Annett et al., 1994; Di Monte et al., 2000; Eslamboli, 2005).

In this regard, the common marmoset (*Callithrix jacchus*) is an established model in neuroscience. Compared to humans, these monkeys have a similar *striatum* structure, hand-foot use and motor behavioral reaction (construct validity), and for example a similar response to dopamine replacement therapy (predictive validity) (Blanchet et al., 2004; Eslamboli, 2005; Hardman et al., 2002; Jenner, 2003b). Additionally, non-human primates are genetically closer to humans than rodents and react similarly to pharmacological interventions (face validity) (Smith et al., 2001). The small and easy to handle marmoset is thus of major importance as a model in behavioral studies (Willner, 1986).

Non-human primates are generally appreciated as model species because of their great validity for simulating conditions in humans. Monkeys are, like humans, very sensitive to MPTP (Burns et al., 1983; Jenner et al., 1984) and after this treatment they express many features of clinical Parkinson's disease which might reflect their genetic, physiological and behavioral proximity to humans. They have a similar *striatum* structure, similar hand-foot use and comparable responsiveness to all dopaminergic medications known to be effective in Parkinson's disease (Eslamboli, 2005); this makes them a valuable addition to the range of available Parkinson's disease models. They also have optimal face validity and predictive validity. Old-world monkeys with high cognitive abilities, such as macaque monkeys (Burns et al., 1983) and baboons (Hantraye et al., 1993) are interesting because they can handle complex behavioral tasks enabling testing of cognitive deficits in the late stage of Parkinsonism. New-world monkeys, such as squirrel monkeys, capuchin monkeys and common marmoset monkeys are, although somewhat less sensitive to MPTP, especially useful because of the aforementioned abilities, but also for their size and are consequently easy to handle in the laboratory. The popular marmoset MPTP model offers several advantages in studying disease therapies and neuroprotective methods (Philippens, 2009). Unlike rodent models (Jackson-Lewis et al., 1995; Mandel et al., 2003; Meredith et al., 2008), MPTP-treated marmoset monkeys show optimal face validity with a wide range of parkinsonian behaviors (Jenner et al 1984; van Vliet et al., 2006) including the L-DOPA-induced dyskinesia (Visanji et al., 2006) and hallucinations (Fox et al., 2006). The "clinical" condition of the parkinsonian state in this MPTP monkey model is generally focused on the motor symptoms. Motor symptoms reported in marmosets use extensive rating scales (Iravani et al., 2003; Jenner, 2003b; Pearce et al., 1996; van Vliet et al., 2006) and tests towards locomotor activity (Obinu et al., 2002; van Vliet et al., 2006), hand-eye coordination (Annett et al., 1994; van Vliet et al., 2006) and akinesia and jumping behavior (Verhave et al., 2009). Non-motor symptoms are apathy (van Vliet et al., 2006) and bladder problems (Albanese et al., 1988). More recently, we can also add sleep related symptoms to this list (Verhave et al., 2011). Because of the striking similarity in sleep macrostructure between marmoset monkeys and humans, changes in sleep due to MPTP treatment can be used as a premotor sign in early stage of Parkinson's disease. A more in-depth insight of the non-motor symptoms would be a valuable addition to this model in order to investigate the effect of dopaminergic drugs as reviewed by Jenner (Jenner, 2009).

3.1 Chemically induced Parkinson's disease

The most potent toxin to induce Parkinson-like dopamine neurodegeneration is 1-methyl-4-phenyl-1,2,3,6-tetrahydropyridine (MPTP). MPTP is a neurotoxin that easily crosses the blood-brain barrier and is specific for dopamine neurons. The MPTP model induces face validity through a specific lesion in the *substantia nigra* and it shows predictive validity with the use of L-DOPA. The MPTP model is actually environmentally induced parkinsonism, and therefore has construct validity to a certain extent. Since MPTP induces reproducible Parkinson's disease in mice, monkeys and humans it offers appropriate external validity.

Other useful toxins are the non-specific 6-hydroxidopamine (6-OHDA), rotenone and paraquat. 6-OHDA is recognized by *substantia nigra* neurons as dopamine and is taken up by the cell where it then exerts its toxic properties. As 6-OHDA does not cross the blood-brain barrier it needs to be locally administered, which is not a trivial procedure. As a result of this local administration, the severity of the lesion depends on the separation of the point of application from the region of interest, which makes this model less suitable for studying the molecular mechanisms of neurodegeneration (Bove et al., 2005). An advantage of this model is that unilateral 6-OHDA lesions, generally used in rats, have proven to be very reproducible over time, in which the non-infused hemisphere can serve as intra-animal control (Blandini et al., 2007). Unlike paraquat which offers contradictory results in mice, repeated systemic administration of rotenone, which easily penetrates the blood-brain barrier, is another potential alternative for inducing Parkinson's disease in experimental animals (Sherer et al., 2003; Schmidt & Alam, 2006). Both paraquat and rotenone affect neurons by disturbing processes such as the glutamate balance, increasing reactive oxygen species (ROS) production, the mitochondrial respiration or misfolding of proteins as reviewed by Bove et al. 2005.

3.1.1 MPTP

Since the serendipitous discovery of the neurotoxic effects of 1-methyl-4-phenyl-1,2,3,6-tetrahydropyridine (MPTP) in young Calnifornian drug users in the 1980s (Langston et al.,

1983), it has become the preferred agent to induce parkinsonism in laboratory animals. This drug represents the most important and most frequently used neurotoxin in animal models. MPTP selectively damages dopaminergic neurons (Javitch et al., 1985), which invariably leads to impaired dopamine neurotransmission.

After entering the brain, glia cells facilitate the conversion of MPTP into 1-methyl-2,3-dihydropyridinium ($MPDP^+$) by the enzyme MAO-B. Thereafter, the actual toxic metabolite, 1-methyl-4-phenylpyridinium (MPP^+), is formed by oxidation. MPP^+ leaves the glia cells and enters the dopamine cells via the dopamine transporter. Once inside the neuron MPP^+ is taken up in vesicles by the vesicular monoamine transporter and then into mitochondria using an energy demanding process (Del Zompo et al., 1993). In mitochondria, MPP^+ blocks the electron transport enzyme ubiquinone oxidoreductase (complex I) (Nicklas et al., 1985) and leads to a reduction in cellular ATP.

4. Markers for the early phase of Parkinson's disease

A maximally beneficial effect of neuroprotective therapies in the treatment of Parkinson's disease can only be achieved with early diagnosis and an early intervention. But unfortunately, early diagnosis of Parkinson's disease may be difficult. Nowadays the clinical diagnosis of Parkinson's disease is still primarily based on overt clinical motor symptoms, such as unilateral rest tremor, reduced arm swing, and slowed hand movement. These symptoms emerge relatively late in the course of the underlying neurodegenerative process when more than 50 % of the dopamine neurons are already lost.

Therefore, the identification and validation of biomarkers, such as premotor symptoms, are critical to facilitate the early diagnosis of Parkinson's disease. Examples of premotor symptoms of early Parkison's disease are olfactory decline, alterations in mood and autonomic function, and most notably disturbed sleep (Berg, 2008; Tolosa et al., 2009). For instance, complaints of insomnia are reported in approximately 80% of all Parkinson's disease patients (Oerlemans & de Weerd, 2002; Tandberg et al., 1998), and excessive movement during sleep frequently occur in Parkinson's disease patients (van Hilten et al., 1994).

But the slow onset of the clinical impairments in relation to the progression of neurodegeneration makes studies correlating neuropathology to symptom manifestation in human subjects difficult. Therefore, research efforts should be focused on the identification of biomarkers for early diagnosis and neuroprotective treatment in relevant animal models of the disease with an emphasis on human validity. The non-motor symptoms of Parkinson's disease have only recently started to become of interest to the scientific community (Park & Stacy, 2009). In animal models this is a very new field so that non-motor parameters are generally not yet part of the symptom description. However, there are reports on olfaction problems in the MPTP-treated marmoset (Miwa et al., 2004), and several studies on sleep problems in non-human primates (Almirall et al., 1999; Barraud et al., 2009), as well as on constipation (Anderson et al., 2007).

Hence, the MPTP treated marmoset monkey may fill this gap and provide insights into the course of non-motor effects in relation to the underlying neurodegeneration of the brain. Since the focus in Parkinson's disease research has recently shifted from the motor phase to the premotor phase of the disease (Berg, 2008; Marek & Jennings, 2009; Philippens et al., 2010; Stephenson et al., 2009; Tolosa et al., 2009; Tolosa & Poewe, 2009), it is of particular interest to investigate further the validity of the classic MPTP model of Parkinson's disease for the study of premotor symptoms. The stages in which premotor symptoms are apparent and precede the motor phase of Parkinson's disease need to be identified, in order to investigate early pathological processes of the disease and to develop early treatment approaches. In addition, as there are currently still no blood or cerebrospinal fluid biomarkers of Parkinson's disease, we rely completely on non-invasive markers based on the early premotor symptoms.

4.1 Brain imaging

Post-mortem pathological changes in the brain can be used as a definitive diagnostic marker for Parkinson's disease. However, for the living patient during the early stage of the disease this diagnostic tool is of no use in the clinic. For animal research post-mortem necropsy studies can be very useful for measuring the efficacy of a neuroprotective treatment at selected time points. MPTP induces selective lesions in the dopaminergic neurons of the *substantia nigra pars compacta.* The damage to the dopaminergic neurons can be identified with tyrosine hydroxylase (TH) staining, which is the first and rate-limiting enzyme in the synthesis of the catecholamines, and is often used as a quick and sensitive method to visualize surviving dopaminergic neurons (Pearson et al., 1983; Waters et al., 1987). Beside the immunohistochemistry, neurochemical changes in the striatum, such as the level of dopamine and its metabolites 3,4-dihydroxyphenylacetic acid (DOPAC) and homovanillic acid (HVA), but also other monoamines, such as noradrenaline and serotonin, can be used to quantify the severity of neurodegeneration (Gerlach et al., 1991). Important in the interpretation of these data is the possible discrepancy between the TH-positive neurons and surviving dopamine neurons as it has been suggested that MPTP can reduce TH activity without cell loss (Tatton et al., 1990).

Nevertheless, these neuropathological measures are invasive and static read-out values. Dynamic changes in the brain due to cell death, recovery and compensation mechanisms cannot be explored with these techniques. Brain imaging techniques, such as positron emission tomography (PET) using radioactive [^{18}F]6-fluoro-DOPA (F-DOPA), single proton emission computed tomography (SPECT) using the dopamine uptake ligand [^{123}I]beta-CIT, and magnetic resonance imaging (MRI) can cover this lacuna as these techniques are non-invasive and can be repeated over time. The PET scan quantifies the reduction of dopamine metabolism caused by dopaminergic neuronal death. The SPECT scan targets the dopamine transporter on the dopamine neuronal terminals indicating the loss of these axons. Dopamine transporter imaging using SPECT (DatSPECT), a technique that has been approved for use in Europe, offers one way of improving diagnosis of Parkinson's disease. There is a high density of dopamine transporter target sites in the striatum, the region of the brain that is primarily affected by Parkinson's disease. Continued neuronal degeneration with Parkinson's disease progression shows up as diminished uptake of the radiotracer on the dopamine transporter imaging. In clinical studies, MRI and magnetic resonance spectroscopy (MRS) are very versatile techniques that examine structural and physiological processes in living organism and are widely used in clinical and experimental research (Dijkhuizen & Nicolay, 2003). These neuronal imaging techniques may be useful for the early detection of Parkinson's disease. Therefore, investigational imaging techniques could soon provide earlier and more definitive diagnosis of Parkinson's disease.

In animal studies, these techniques can also have scientific and ethical benefit as the animal acts as its own control thereby reducing animal usage for research. The advantage is that these non-invasive techniques can be applied repeatedly over a prolonged period with the opportunity of following the progress of the disease over time.

4.1.1 Magnetic resonance imaging and spectroscopy (MRI and MRS)

A typical **MRI** technique used for Parkinson's disease research is T2-weighted imaging in which changes in signal intensities are partly due to an altered water content of a tissue, mostly caused by the presence of extracellular edema (Dijkhuizen & Nicolay, 2003). Earlier examinations with T2-weighted imaging on the effect of MPTP intoxication in animals showed changes in relevant brain areas like the *substantia nigra pars compacta, caudate nucleus* and *putamen* (Miletich et al., 1994; Podell et al., 2003; Zhang et al., 1999).

MRS, on the other hand, visualizes signals from carbon-bound protons from various metabolites (Kauppinen & Williams, 1994). But with MRS only few metabolites can be examined. The most frequently used neuronal marker with MRS is N-acetyl aspartate (NAA) (Gujar et al., 2005; Castillo et al., 1996). Reductions of NAA levels have been observed in the striatum and *substantia pars compacta* in parkinsonian mice, cats, cynomolgus monkeys and marmoset monkeys (Boska et al., 2005; Brownell et al., 1998; Podell et al., 2003; van Vliet et al., 2008). An example of brain imaging of a marmoset brain slice from a region of interest for MRS analysis is given in figure 2.

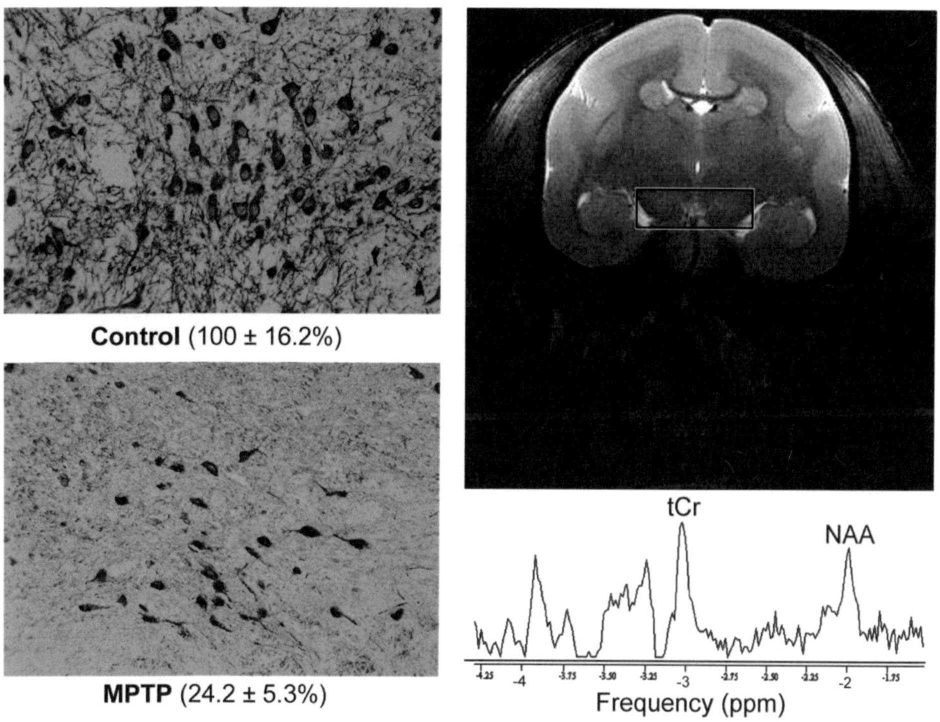

Fig. 2. Examples of neuronal brain imagings of marmoset monkey brain.

Left: An example of post-mortem immunochemistry imaging TH staining of neurons in the *substantia nigra pars compacta* in a healthy contol marmoset monkey (100 % TH-positive neurons) and of a monkey treated with a total dose of 6 mg/kg MPTP (24 % TH-positive neurons). Right side: A magnitic resonance brain image of a marmoset brain slice (Bregma - 0.6 mm) with an outlined region for single voxel spectroscopy (squared box) in which the *substantia nigra* is located for the MRS analyses. Below is an example of an original MRS spectrum, which is used for data analyses of proton emission. NAA: N-acetyl aspartate; tCr: total (phospho) creatine.

In the MPTP treated marmoset monkey Parkinson's disease model magnetic resonance techniques were validated as a supplement for Parkinson's research towards neuroprotection (van Vliet et al., 2008). Both MRI and MRS were applied to investigate the neuroprotective effects of the vigilance-stimulating compound modafinil (Modiodal®) using a 4.7 T NMR spectrometer (Varian, Palo Alto, California). Modafinil was chosen because of its neuroprotective effects on dopamine neurons in the *substantia nigra pars compacta* in the marmoset MPTP model (Jenner et al., 2000; van Vliet et al., 2006).
In this particular study the MPTP intoxication resulted in a significant reduction of about 75 % of TH positive dopaminergic neurons as shown in figure 2, whereas this neurodegeneration level was significantly reduced to only 39 % in the modafinil treated parkinsonian monkeys.
In the MRI scan, MPTP intoxication resulted in a tendency for reduced T2 relaxation times in the *substantia nigra*: we found a tendency to decreased relative relaxation times in the placebo treated parkinsonian monkeys, which was not observed following modafinil treatment (van Vliet et al., 2008). This was in contrast with earlier reports in which an increase of T2-weighted signal intensities was described in the *substantia nigra* and dopaminergic projection areas (Miletich et al., 1994; Podell et al., 2003; Zhang et al., 1999). The differences between these and our studies were the extended time between MPTP treatment and the execution of the brain-imaging scan in our study compared to the other studies, in which the interval was several hours to several days. Also, we used a lower dose of MPTP in our study, which was only 6 mg/kg. This approach prevented extracellular edema, which generally results in an increase in T2 relaxation time (Dijkhuizen & Nicolay, 2003). Indeed, in contrast to the other studies, we found a similar reduction of the T2 relaxation time in the *substantia nigra* as has also been reported in Parkinson's disease patients (Kosta et al., 2006).
In the MRS scan MPTP intoxication resulted in a reduction of the NAA/total creatine (tCr) ratio: we found a significant reduction of the NAA/tCr ratio in the placebo treated parkinsonian monkeys. On the other hand, the NAA/tCR ratio after modafinil treatment was significantly increased following MPTP-intoxication compared to baseline values (van Vliet et al., 2008). The decrease in the NAA/tCr ratios has also been seen in other MPTP studies. Mice also show a clear decrease in the absolute NAA concentration in the *substantia nigra* both at 2 and 6 days after MPTP intoxication (Boska et al., 2005). Cats show decreased NAA/tCr ratios in the striatum 12 hours after MPTP intoxication (Podell et al., 2003). Furthermore, chronic MPTP intoxicated cynomolgus monkeys show a persistent reduction in NAA/tCr ratio in the caudate and putamen (Brownell et al., 1998).
The neuroprotective action of modafinil, measured in the brain by immunohistochemistry TH staining and brain imaging using MRI and MRS shows a clear correlation with the observed clinical parkinsonian symptoms, which indicates the value of both markers in neuroprotection research (van Vliet et al., 2008). It can be concluded that MRS (NAA/tCR ratio) is a valuable tool for neuroprotective research in the MPTP intoxicated marmoset as correlations indicate a clear relationship between motor functional deficits and measurements of brain damage.

4.2 Sleep

Unlike the nocturnal preference and fragmented pattern of sleep in mice and rats, the architecture of marmosets' sleep resembles that of humans (Philippens et al., 2004; Verhave et al., 2011). Marmosets are diurnal and, as in humans, their night sleep architecture consists of a recurring pattern of cycles with light, deep and REM sleep. Further, quantifying the different stages in marmoset monkeys can be performed with the classical sleep scoring system directly adapted from human scoring (Rechtschaffen & Kales, 1968). Because of the striking similarity in sleep macrostructure between marmoset monkeys and humans, a demonstration of early abnormalities during sleep in the marmoset MPTP model would be of significant value as potential biomarkers for the early stage of idiopathic Parkinson's disease.

Although rodent studies are frequently used for Parkinson's disease research, the nocturnal nature of these animals' behavior and the short sleep bouts (Monaca et al., 2004; Yi et al., 2007) make them less suitable as models for sleep in Parkinson's disease. Nevertheless, sleep changes have been reported in the rat (Lima et al., 2007). In rats, MPTP induces a temporary reduction of REM sleep and increases sleep efficiency (Lima et al., 2007). However, possible changes in muscle tone during REM sleep were not addressed in this study. In the marmoset MPTP model, with a mild parkinsonian state, resembling an early phase of Parkinson's disease in humans, selective abnormalities in muscle tone during REM sleep phases were found (Verhave et al., 2011). In figure 3 an example is shown of electroencephalogram (EEG) traces during REM sleep combined with the electromyogram (EMG) indicating complete atonia during the normal healthy situation and with severe muscle tone indicating the presence of RBD.

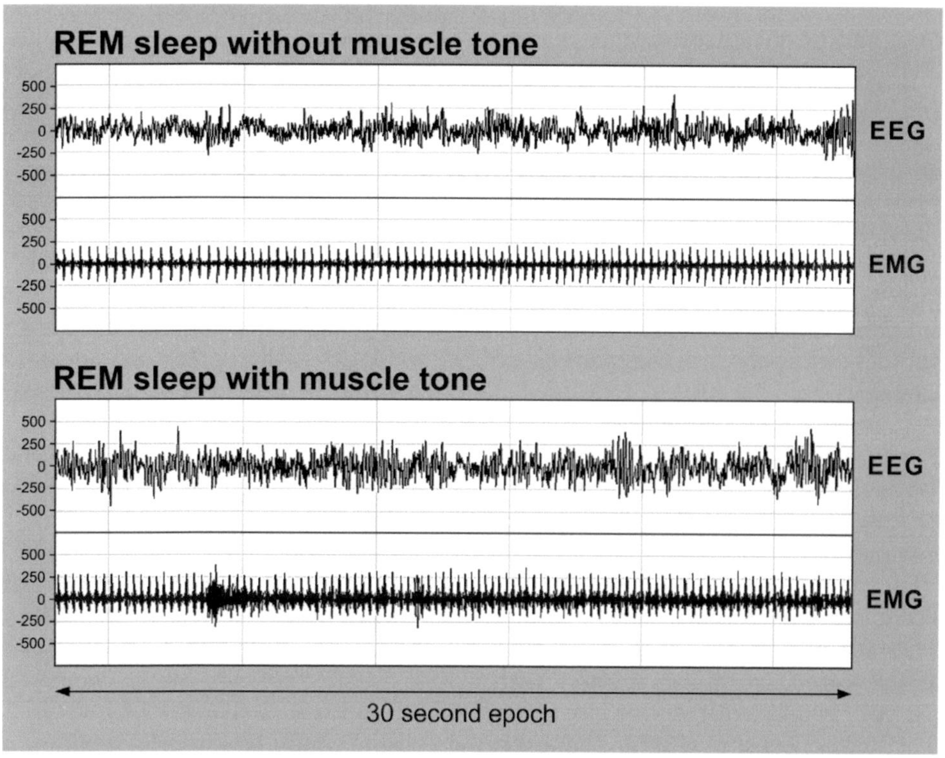

Fig. 3. Example of EEG and EMG epoch during REM sleep with and without RBD.

A 30-second epoch of an electroencephalogram (EEG) for measuring the sleep stage and electromyogram (EMG) for measuring the muscle tone during REM sleep of a normal

healthy marmoset monkey (upper level): the 30-second trace consists of random fast EEG while the EMG showed no muscle activity, and of a marmoset monkey suffering from RBD (bottom level): the trace consists of random fast EEG in the presence of 50-100% muscle tension in the EMG (Verhave et al., 2011).
The regular spikes are artefacts of the heart rate.

4.2.1 Rapid eye movement behavior disorder as a sleep marker for early Parkinson's disease

Rapid eye movement sleep behavior disorder (RBD) is characterized by increased muscle activity during rapid eye movement (REM) sleep, which can lead to injury either to oneself or to a bed partner. The core symptom of RBD, namely the lack of normal muscle atonia during REM sleep (Comella et al., 1993; Ondo et al., 2001), can emerge in two ways: (1) tonic muscle activity characterized by at least 50% of the time muscle activity in a 30-second REM sleep epoch or (2) phasic muscle activity and twitches within 30-second epochs (Lapierre & Montplaisir, 1992). RBD is a disorder of considerable interest for understanding early pathological processes in Parkinson's disease. At least one-third of Parkinson's disease patients have increased and irregular chin muscle tone during REM sleep (Comella et al., 1993; Gagnon et al., 2002) and many meet the criteria for RBD. More importantly, disturbances in sleep usually begin years before Parkinson's disease is diagnosed (Iranzo et al., 2005; Postuma et al., 2006; Tolosa et al., 2009). RBD is a key symptom during the early phases of Parkinson's disease, since one-third of all patients initially diagnosed with RBD are later diagnosed with Parkinson's disease within 3 to 13 years after the initial RBD diagnosis (Gagnon et al., 2002; Iranzo et al., 2006; Schenck et al., 1996). Moreover, 40% of all RBD cases reported eventually go on to develop a neurological disorder, most notably Parkinson's disease (Ferini-Strambi & Zucconi, 2000).
We investigated the effects of MPTP treatment on sleep architecture in marmoset monkeys, with special attention to RBD-like changes in muscle tone during REM sleep (Verhave et al., 2011). Because of the direct link between RBD and Parkinson's disease (Gagnon et al., 2002; Iranzo et al., 2005; Iranzo et al., 2006; Postuma et al., 2006; Schenck et al., 1996; Stiasny-Kolster et al., 2005), we evaluated different sleep components, particularly the REM sleep chin muscle disturbances in the marmoset MPTP model. To achieve this, the general sleep characteristics and the muscle tone (EMG) changes during REM sleep in the marmoset MPTP model of Parkinson's disease were investigated.
MPTP-treated marmosets showed no reduction in total sleep time, time spent in REM sleep, light or deep sleep and wake time after sleep onset (Verhave et al., 2011). However, MPTP significantly increased endogenous muscle tone during REM sleep ($p < 0.05$) (Fig. 3). We also determined the distribution of muscle tone as a percentage of the total time in REM sleep (Fig. 4). REM epochs were categorized according to muscle tone as either being absent or present in one of three predefined levels. Epochs with muscle tone more than 50% of the time were found to be rare in the control monkeys. However, they were significantly more frequently scored in animals treated with MPTP: MPTP, but not saline, increased the occurrence of epochs with muscle tone more than 10% of the time (Fig. 4: 32.8 ± 4.5 vs. 22.4 ± 2.9 % of REM epochs; $p < 0.05$). There were also significantly less epochs without atonia during the nights after MPTP treatment compared to the baseline values (Fig. 4: 38.3 ± 4.1 vs 66.3 ± 9.1 % of REM epochs; $p < 0.05$). Furthermore, discriminant analysis showed that after treatment, the number of epochs with 10% muscle tone during REM sleep classified 80% of the animals correctly and the epochs with 3 or more twitches added the remaining 20% of

this classification (Verhave et al., 2011). These two variables together classified the MPTP-treated monkeys up to a maximum of 100% ($p < 0.05$).
As the motor behavior in these MPTP-treated monkeys was disturbed to a mild extent, the Parkinson's disease induction could be described as a model of mildly Parkinsonian signs.

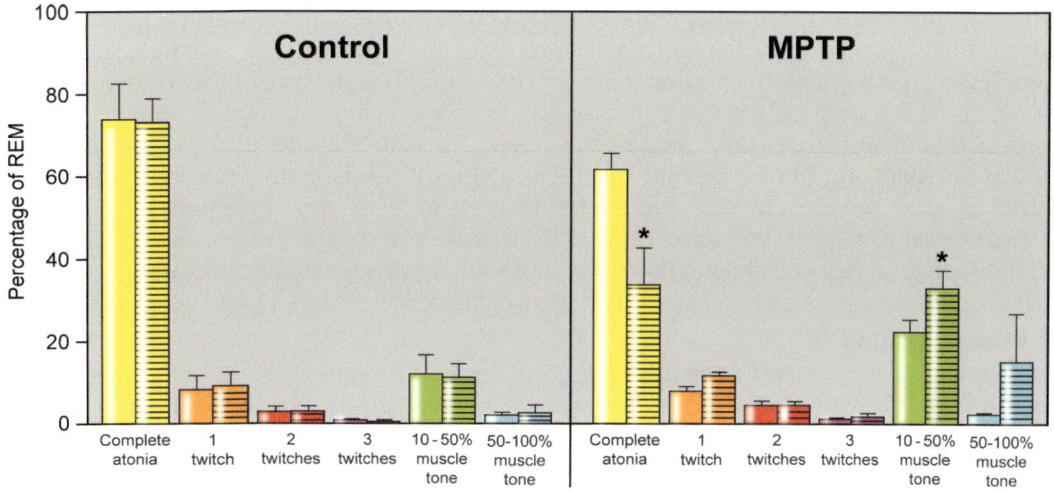

Fig. 4. Muscle tone during REM sleep in the marmoset monkey.
REM sleep epochs with tone as a percentage of REM sleep in the placebo control group (n=4) and the MPTP-treated group (n=5) before (baseline, solid bars) and after saline control or MPTP treatment (striped bars). Asterisks indicate significant differences between baseline value and after treatment ($p < 0.05$ Friedman) (Verhave et al., 2011).

In the paper of Verhave et al. (2011) it was explained that the MPTP induced changes in REM sleep muscle tone are presumably due to changes in dopamine neurotransmission. Reduction in dopamine in the *substantia nigra* caused by MPTP exposure results in a decrease dopamine signalling to its receptors localized within the *striatum* (Levey et al., 1993). Clinical conditions affecting dopamine, such as those seen in Parkinson's disease, also alter sleep architecture (Comella et al., 1993), which result in changes in REM sleep (Dahan et al., 2007) and muscle tone during REM sleep (Fantini et al., 2003; Garcia-Borreguero et al., 2002). Therefore, nigrostriatal neurons whose axons are located in the *striatum* are assumed to play a major role in the regulation of REM sleep. On the other hand, it has been suggested by Verhave et al. (2011) that the degenerative process in Parkinson's disease is initiated in the medulla, advances to the pons, and subsequently targets the midbrain (Braak et al., 2003). Thus, the presence of RBD might also reflect early involvement of non-dopamine medullary and/or pontine REM sleep-related structures (Iranzo et al., 2005). Therefore, it is suggested that these structures, which are closely connected to the *substantia nigra* pathways are affected by an imbalance of dopamine levels (Lai & Siegel, 1990) which would precede the actual neurodegenerative process. This is an important indication for the early onset of RBD during the neurodegenerative process leading to Parkinson's disease.
In conclusion, the MPTP-treated marmoset provides a new opportunity for quantitative studies on the mechanisms and intervention strategies of RBD and the premotor phase of Parkinson's disease.

5. Implications for the clinic

The current standard for diagnosing patients with Parkinson's disease remains the professional opinion of a neurologist based on a thorough neurological assessment. Earlier diagnosis of Parkinson's disease is becoming more and more important because of an ongoing shift in treatment, away from symptom control drugs and toward neuroprotective drugs that interfere with the cell death processes in order to stop or slow down the progressive pathophysiologic alterations in the brain. This is crucial because treatment should start at a very early phase of the disease to save as many neurons as possible. As the current treatment regimes don't stop or slow down the neurodegenerative process, research efforts are changing from symptom control strategies towards neuroprotection. From this point of view research models should be adapted to these new questions that ask for biomarkers for the early premotor stage of the disease and diagnostic tools to spot patients or individuals at risk and should, therefore, be based on early premotor indicators.

5.1 Neuroimaging

Neuroimaging can be used as an important tool for early diagnosis as well as for preclinical research into the early stages of the neurodegenerative diseases. However, it is not clear at what stage neuronal cell loss becomes evident in PET and SPECT imaging. At the onset of the disease manifestation, when more than 50% of the dopaminergic neurons in the *substantia nigra* are already lost, there is only a 30% reduction of putaminal F-DOPA measured by PET scan (Berg, 2006). As these techniques involve the exposure of subjects to radiation, they cannot be recommended for identifying individuals at risk for Parkinson's disease. An alternative could be MRI and MRS. In marmoset monkeys as well as in Parkinson's disease patients a reduction of the T2 relaxation time in the *substantia nigra* was found using MRI techniques (Kosta et al., 2006; van Vliet et al., 2008). The reduction of the T2 weighted signals, as was found in our MPTP-treated marmoset monkeys, is presumably caused by Parkinson's disease-related iron deposition. Iron creates magnetic field inhomogeneities that dephase nearby water protons resulting in a shortening of the T2 relaxation time (Kosta et al. 2006). Interestingly, iron deposition has been reported in the *substantia nigra* in MPTP models (Mochizuki et al., 1994; Temlett et al., 1994). Although the exact function of the increased iron levels is unknown, it is suggested that they contribute to oxidative stress in Parkinson's disease and MPTP models (Yantiri et al. 1999). Oxidative stress is known to be one of the features responsible for the initial triggering at the start of the neurodegenerative process (Philippens et al., 2010). In addition to the MRI measures, the NAA/tCR ratio, measured by MRS, is able to predict the disease state of the animal: a decrease in NAA/tCr ratio is associated with worsening of behavior after MPTP intoxication (van Vliet et al., 2008). This correlation suggests that NAA/tCr ratio measurement may be useful for studying the effects of neuroprotective drugs on the metabolic state of a neuron. A high correlation was found between NAA levels, measured with the MRS technique, and TH positive neurons, measured with the immunohistochemistry, in a mouse MPTP model (Boska et al., 2005) indicating that these parameters both predict neuronal damage.

5.2 Rapid eye movement behavior disorder

Another approach for detecting the early stage of Parkinson's disease is measuring premotor signs, such as the RBD, which is one of the most important indicators of developing

Parkinson's disease. The MPTP-treated marmoset model can be used for further studies into the mechanisms of RBD and sleep disturbances in the premotor symptom phase of Parkinson's disease, i.e., when patients can be diagnosed with RBD but not with Parkinson's disease (Gagnon et al., 2002; Iranzo et al., 2006; Schenck et al., 1996). However, the stringent criteria for RBD described in human studies (50-100% muscle tone per epoch) were not met by the parkinsonian marmosets in our study. The International Classification of Sleep Disorders (2005) describes RBD as the presence of REM sleep without atonia, and disruptive behavior during sleep. The atonia, normally observed during REM sleep, is interrupted by either short (phasic, 2-3 seconds) or long (tonic, 20-30 seconds) episodes of EMG activity (Gagnon et al., 2002; Iranzo et al., 2005; Lapierre & Montplaisir, 1992). Then again, a significant change in tonic activity is definitely apparent in our experimental animals, which suggests an RBD-like phenomenon. Indeed, an alternative and more suitable measure of RBD may be muscle activity as a percentage of REM sleep, given the variable outcome of polysomnogram measurements from 62 diagnosed patients (Mayer et al., 2008). This interpretation is supported by the parameters proposed by Mayer and colleagues (Mayer et al., 2008). For instance, the marmosets show a slight increase in phasic activity and a definite increase in tonic activity as a percentage of total REM sleep. The slight increase in phasic activity of EMG bursts or twitches (0.1-5 seconds) was seen in the epochs with one single twitch and the increase in tonic EMG was seen in the epochs with more than 10% tone of the time. This corresponds with EMG activity in at least one-third of the 30-second epochs.

5.3 Translational aspects

The translation of fundamental research into the clinic relies in the first place on appropriate animal models that show the pathological hallmarks and motor deficiencies of Parkinson's disease. It is of vital importance that these animal models actually mimic the clinical features of Parkinson's disease to the extent that the outcome is relevant. This can be determined by evaluating the marmoset MPTP model using scientifically-based criteria: face, predictive, construct and external validity as previously noted by Van der Staay and his colleagues (van der Staay et al., 2009).

Face validity: Based on the literature and our own findings, we can conclude that the marmoset model offers face validity in the sense that homologous neuro-anatomical structures are affected in this animal model and in Parkinson's disease as well (Jenner et al., 1984; Meredith et al., 2008). Changes induced in these structures result in neurodegeneration in the *substantia nigra* and reduced levels of dopamine in the *striatum*. The size of the lesion predicts the phenotype (van Vliet et al., 2008). Limited symptomatology in combination with the restricted damage of the dopamine neurons in the *substantia nigra* suggests that this model mimics an early Parkinson's disease patient (Tolosa et al., 2009).

Predictive validity: In the case of dopamine replacement therapy, predictive validity is certainly true for the marmoset model (Jenner, 2003b). However, for neuroprotection this model has not yet been very productive. Promising neuroprotective agents generated in the lab, have still not led to systematic treatment in patients (Olanow et al., 2008). This delay is mainly due to shortcomings of the models currently in use, the unknown cause of the disease and the difficulties for accurately estimating neuroprotection in the clinic.

Construct validity: Because the nature of the disorder is not well understood, construct validity is the most difficult scientific criterion to assess in modeling idiopathic Parkinson's disease. Animal models can only really mimic the pathology and the symptomatology of the disease but not its etiology. However, the use of MPTP with which neurodegeneration was first discovered in humans, represents the best toxin available for studying Parkinson's disease as its derived symptoms are indistinguishable from those of idiopathic Parkinson's disease (Ballard et al., 1985). The MPTP-treated marmoset is superior in behavioral assessment, as it shows a complete range of behavioral characteristics associated with Parkinson's disease (Eslamboli, 2005; Jenner, 2009; van Vliet et al., 2006). Additionally, the report of non-motor symptoms such as sleep impairments and neuroimaging markers brings this model even closer to human Parkinson's disease (van Vliet et al., 2008; Verhave et al., 2011). Therefore, the striking similarities between human Parkinson's disease and MPTP-induced Parkinsonism in non-human primates strongly supports to construct validity in the MPTP models.

External validity: The non-human primate model is very popular in scientific research resulting in substantial reports about the degeneration of dopamine neurons in combination with motor functional loss (Meredith et al., 2008; Philippens et al., 2010; Speciale, 2002). In the end, it is the scientific question that should be a predominant factor in deciding of which specific animal model to choose. In regard to the early onset of the disease, the marmoset monkey is in favor of other animal models. Parkinsonian behavior of MPTP non-human primates is comparable to human Parkinson's disease symptoms (Przedborski et al., 2001). Clinical assessment of Parkinson's disease symptoms is mostly done with the UPDRS (unified Parkinson's disease rating scale). Rating scales have been adapted for MPTP non-human primates, for instance the 'clinical score', a rating scale that includes cardinal clinical parkinsonian symptoms and some marmoset specific symptoms. Additionally, quantitative assessment of animal behavior is an often-used tool. In MPTP non-human primate models it has been shown that measurement of changes in general activity has direct application to the clinic as hypokinesia is a common feature of Parkinson's disease. Furthermore, the fine motor skills of patients are reduced owing to a combination of tremor, slowless of movement and disturbed motor planning. Assessment of these fine motor skills in MPTP non-human primates, e.g. hand-eye coordination, is also affected (reviewed by Emborg, 2004). Finally, sleep aspects can be measured in these monkeys for the identification of the early signs of Parkinson's disease (Verhave et al., 2011).

5.4 Further research

Today, patients, family members and physicians struggle with the fact that there is no cure or satisfactory treatment for Parkinson's disease. The nature of the disorder is suggested to be a combination of endogenous and exogenous factors starting years before the actual diagnosis. Therefore, it is our notion that research should be directed towards a combination of early diagnosis and development of neuroprotective treatments. As a first step, a shift should be made from diagnosis that is completely based on motor complications (Pahwa & Lyons, 2010) to early diagnosis that is supported by premotor symptoms. Relatively simple but informative diagnostic tools are the Parkinson's disease Sleep Scale (Dhawan et al., 2006) and the University of Pennsylvania Smell Identification Test (Deeb et al., 2010). Furthermore, these tests can be combined with neuroimaging techniques for subjects at risk. It is known that pathological changes in the brain, such as dopamine transporter density, are already present before motor signs appear. Furthermore, the NAA/tCr ratio correlates with the metabolic state of a neuron. These changes can be measured with neuroimaging techniques in human as well as in marmoset monkeys. However, insight into the dynamics of potential diagnostic tools for the early phase of the disease and the mechanisms for neuropathology and subsequently neuroprotection in early neurodegeneration will rely on disease models. We found that an RBD-like phenomenon also takes place in marmosets with moderate neurodegeneration. This underlines the fact that this mild MPTP model entails features of the premotor phase of Parkinson's disease. Therefore, the marmoset MPTP model for early Parkinson's disease offers a good opportunity to investigate neurodegeneration at different stages of pathology.

6. Conclusions

In order to halt or limit neurodegeneration, research should focus on a combination of early diagnosis supported by premotor symptoms and the further development of neuroprotective treatment. However, studying Parkinson's disease neuropathology related to disease manifestation in humans is limited to clinical trials and post-mortem material. In these circumstances, in the search for new targets for neuroprotective therapies, animal models represent a great asset in Parkinson's disease research. Insights into neuroprotection and the mechanisms of neuropathology in early neurodegeneration will rely on animal models to investigate the early stages of Parkinson's disease. Animal models should ideally mimic the main features of the disease pathology and additionally show the typical parkinsonian syndrome. The multi-factorial aspects of the disease dictate the need for Parkinson's disease-like animal models that couple disease manifestation to the underlying pathology.

The ultimate animal model for Parkinson's disease has not yet been developed; however, there are several experimental models used worldwide that reproduce Parkinson's disease-like neurodegeneration in combination with motor symptoms. One of these induction models is based on the neurotoxin MPTP that causes selective cell death in the dopamine neurons localised within the *substantia nigra* in humans, monkeys and mice, which indicate the high external validity. The marmoset MPTP model is congruent with the scientific criteria of face, predictive, construct and external validity. Besides motor deterioration and clinical parkinsonian signs, sleep and neuroimaging aspects can be relevant markers for moderate neurodegeneration in the marmoset MPTP model analogous to the clinical sleep problems and pathological changes in the brain, such as the REM sleep behavior disorder and affected NAA/tCr ratio, in the premotor phase of Parkinson's disease patients. Neuroimaging will give insight in the dynamic changes in the brain due to neurodegeneration and presents the opportunity to monitor the effect of a neuroprotective treatment over time. On the other hand, improvement in muscle tone during REM sleep can be seen as a novel diagnostic marker of early stages of Parkinson's disease and a useful marker for measuring neuroprotective effects in the marmoset disease model.

For the translation in the clinic, a combination of markers, such as genetic vulnerability, olfactory dysfunction, depression, RBD, neuroimaging abnormalities and slight motor signs, may be a helpful indicator for individuals at risk when developing Parkinson's disease. If treatment could be started at a stage when there are still neurons to protect, the quality of life of these patients could be improved.

7. Acknowledgment

The authors would like to thank Mr. Henk van Westbroek for the art work of the figures in this chapter. The studies described in this chapter were funded by TNO Defence, Security and Safety, The Netherlands (neuroimaging study) and by the U.S. Army Medical Research and Materiel Command, Award No. W81XH-05-1-0517 (sleep study).

8. References

Albanese, A.; Jenner, P.; Marsden, C.D. & Stephenson, J.D. (1988). Bladder hyperreflexia induced in marmosets by 1-methyl-4-phenyl-1,2,3,6-tetrahydropyridine. *Neurosci Lett*, 87, 46-50

Alexander, G.E. & Crutcher, M.D. (1990). Functional architecture of basal ganglia circuits: neural substrates of parallel processing. *Trends Neurosci*, 13, 266-271

Alexi, T.; Borlongan, C.V.; Faull, R.L.; Williams, C.E.; Clark, R.G.; Gluckman, P.D. & Hughes, P.E. (2000). Neuroprotective strategies for basal ganglia degeneration: Parkinson's and Huntington's diseases. *Prog Neurobiol*, 60, 409-470

Almirall, H.; Pigarev, I.; de la Calzada, M.D.; Pigareva, M.; Herrero, M.T. & Sagales, T. (1999). Nocturnal sleep structure and temperature slope in MPTP treated monkeys. *J Neural Transm*, 106, 1125-1134

Anderson, G.; Noorian, A.R.; Taylor, G.; Anitha, M.; Bernhard, D.; Srinivasan, S. & Greene, J.G. (2007). Loss of enteric dopaminergic neurons and associated changes in colon motility in an MPTP mouse model of Parkinson's disease. *Exp Neurol*, 207, 4-12

Annett, L.E.; Martel, F.L.; Rogers, D.C.; Ridley, R.M.; Baker, H.F. & Dunnett, S.B. (1994). Behavioral assessment of the effects of embryonic nigral grafts in marmosets with unilateral 6-OHDA lesions of the nigrostriatal pathway. *Exp Neurol*, 125, 228-246

Ballard, P.A.; Tetrud, J.W. & Langston, J.W. (1985). Permanent human parkinsonism due to 1-methyl-4-phenyl-1,2,3,6-tetrahydropyridine (MPTP): seven cases. *Neurology*, 35, 949-956

Barraud, Q.; Lambrecq, V.; Forni, C.; McGuire, S.; Hill, M.; Bioulac, B.; Balzamo, E.; Bezard, E.; Tison, F. & Ghorayeb, I. (2009). Sleep disorders in Parkinson's disease: the contribution of the MPTP non-human primate model. *Exp Neurol*, 219, 574-582

Bensimon, G.; Ludolph, A.; Agid, Y.; Vidailhet, M.; Payan, C. & Leigh, P.N. (2009). Riluzole treatment, survival and diagnostic criteria in Parkinson plus disorders: the NNIPPS study. *Brain*, 132, 156-171

Berg, D. (2006). Marker for a preclinical diagnosis of Parkinson's disease as a basis for neuroprotection, In: Oxidative stress and neuroprotection, ISBN 0303-6995, *J. Neural Transm.*, 71, 123-132

Berg, D. (2008). Biomarkers for the early detection of Parkinson's and Alzheimer's disease. *Neurodegener Dis*, 5, 133-136

Betarbet, R.; Sherer, T.B.; MacKenzie, G.; Garcia-Osuna, M.; Panov, A.V. & Greenamyre, J.T. (2000). Chronic systemic pesticide exposure reproduces features of Parkinson's disease. *Nat Neurosci*, 3, 1301-1306

Birkmayer, W. & Hornykiewicz, O. (1961). Der L-3, 4-Dioxyphenylalanin (= DOPA)-Effekt bel der Parkinson-Akinese. *Wien Klin Wochenschr*, 73, 787-788

Blanchet, P.J.; Calon, F.; Morissette, M.; Hadj Tahar, A.; Belanger, N.; Samadi, P.; Grondin, R.; Gregoire, L.; Meltzer, L.; Di Paolo, T. & Bedard, P.J. (2004). Relevance of the MPTP primate model in the study of dyskinesia priming mechanisms. *Parkinsonism Relat Disord*, 10, 297-304

Blandini, F.; Levandis, G.; Bazzini, E.; Nappi, G. & Armentero, M.T. (2007). Time-course of nigrostriatal damage, basal ganglia metabolic changes and behavioural alterations following intrastriatal injection of 6-hydroxydopamine in the rat: new clues from an old model. *Eur J Neurosci*, 25, 397-405

Boska, M.D.; Lewis, T.B.; Destache, C.J.; Benner, E.J.; Nelson, J.A. et al. (2005). Quantitative 1H magnetic resonance spectroscopic imaging determines therapeutic immunization efficacy in an animals of Parkinson's disease. *J Neurosci*, 25, 1691-700

Botella, J.A.; Bayersdorfer, F.; Gmeiner, F. & Schneuwly, S. (2009). Modelling Parkinson's disease in Drosophila. *Neuromolecular Med*, 11, 268-280

Bove, J.; Prou, D.; Perier, C. & Przedborski, S. (2005). Toxin-induced models of Parkinson's disease. *NeuroRx*, Jul, 2(3), 484-494

Braak, H.; Rub, U.; Gai, W.P. & Del Tredici, K. (2003). Idiopathic Parkinson's disease: possible routes by which vulnerable neuronal types may be subject to neuroinvasion by an unknown pathogen. *J Neural Transm*, 110, 517-536

Brownell, A.L.; Jenkins, B.G.; Elmaleh, D.R.; Deacon, T.W.; Spaelman, R.D. et al. (1998). Combined PET/MRS brain studies show dynamic and long-term physiological changes in a primate model of Parkinson disease. *Nat Med*, 4, 1308-12

Burns, R.S.; Chiueh, C.C.; Markey, S.P.; Ebert, M.H.; Jacobowitz, D.M. & Kopin, I.J. (1983). A primate model of parkinsonism: selective destruction of dopaminergic neurons in the pars compacta of the substantia nigra by N-methyl-4-phenyl-1,2,3,6-tetrahydropyridine. *Proc Natl Acad Sci U S A*, 80, 4546-4550

Castillo, M.; Kwock, L. & Mukherji, S.K. (1996). Clinical applications of proton MR spectroscopy. *AJNR Am J Neuroradiol*, Jan, 17(1), 1-15

Chan, D.K.; Woo, J.; Ho, S.C.; Pang, C.P.; Law, L.K.; Ng, P.W.; Hung, W.T.; Kwok, T.; Hui, E.; Orr, K.; Leung, M.F. & Kay, R. (1998). Genetic and environmental risk factors for Parkinson's disease in a Chinese population. *J Neurol Neurosurg Psychiatry*, 65, 781-784

Chen, C.C.; Chen, T.F.; Hwang, Y.C.; Wen, Y.R.; Chiu, Y.H.; Wu, C.Y.; Chen, R.C.; Tai, J.J.; Chen, T.H. & Liou, H.H. (2009). Different prevalence rates of Parkinson's disease in urban and rural areas: a population-based study in Taiwan. *Neuroepidemiology*, 33, 350-357

Comella, C.L.; Tanner, C.M. & Ristanovic, R.K. (1993). Polysomnographic sleep measures in Parkinson's disease patients with treatment-induced hallucinations. *Ann Neurol*, 34, 710-714

Dahan, L.; Astier, B.; Vautrelle, N.; Urbain, N.; Kocsis, B. & Chouvet, G. (2007). Prominent burst firing of dopaminergic neurons in the ventral tegmental area during paradoxical sleep. *Neuropsychopharmacology*, 32, 1232-1241

Dauer, W. & Przedborski, S. (2003). Parkinson's disease: mechanisms and models. *Neuron*, 39, 889-909

Deeb, J.; Shah, M.; Muhammed, N.; Gunasekera, R.; Gannon, K.; Findley, L.J. & Hawkes, C.H. (2010). A basic smell test is as sensitive as a dopamine transporter scan: comparison of olfaction, taste and DaTSCAN in the diagnosis of Parkinson's disease. *QJM*, Dec, 103(12), 941-52

Del Zompo, M.; Piccardi, M.P.; Ruiu, S.; Quartu, M.; Gessa, G.L. & Vaccari, A. (1993). Selective MPP+ uptake into synaptic dopamine vesicles: possible involvement in MPTP neurotoxicity. *Br J Pharmacol*, 109, 411-414

Dhawan, V.; Dhoat, S.; Williams, A.J.; Dimarco, A.; Pal, S.; Forbes, A.; Tobias, A.; Martinez-Martin, P. & Chaudhuri, K.R. (2006). The range and nature of sleep dysfunction in untreated Parkinson's disease (PD). A comparative controlled clinical study using the Parkinson's disease sleep scale and selective polysomnography. *J Neurol Sci,* 248, 158-162

Di Monte, D.A.; McCormack, A.; Petzinger, G.; Janson, A.M.; Quik, M. & Langston, W.J. (2000). Relationship among nigrostriatal denervation, parkinsonism, and dyskinesias in the MPTP primate model. *Mov Disord,* 15, 459-466

Dijkhuizen, R.M. & Nicolay, K. (2003). Magnetic resonance imaging in experimental models of brain disorders. *J Cereb Blood Flow Metab,* 23, 1383-402

Ehringer, H. & Hornykiewicz, O. (1960). Distribution of noradrenaline and dopamine (3-hydroxytyramine) in the human brain and their behavior in diseases of the extrapyramidal system. *J. Klin Wochenschr,* 38, 1236-1239

Emborg, M.E. (2004). Evaluation of animal models of Parkinson's disease for neuroprotective strategies. *J Neurosci Methods,* 139, 121-143

Eslamboli, A. (2005). Marmoset monkey models of Parkinson's disease: which model, when and why? *Brain Res Bull,* 68, 140-149

Fahn, S. (2005). Does levodopa slow or hasten the rate of progression of Parkinson's disease? *J Neurol,* 252, Suppl 4, IV37-IV42

Fahn, S. (2008). The history of dopamine and levodopa in the treatment of Parkinson's disease. *Mov Disord,* 23, Suppl 3, S497-508

Fantini, M.L.; Gagnon, J.F.; Filipini, D. & Montplaisir, J. (2003). The effects of pramipexole in REM sleep behavior disorder. *Neurology,* 61, 1418-1420

Ferini-Strambi, L. & Zucconi, M. (2000). REM sleep behavior disorder. *Clin Neurophysiol,* 111, S136-140

Fox, S.H.; Visanji, N.P.; Johnston, T.H.; Gomez-Ramirez, J.; Voon, V. & Brotchie, J.M. (2006). Dopamine receptor agonists and levodopa and inducing psychosis-like behavior in the MPTP primate model of Parkinson disease. *Arch Neurol,* 63, 1343-1344

Gagnon, J.F.; Bedard, M.A.; Fantini, M.L.; Petit, D.; Panisset, M.; Rompre, S.; Carrier, J. & Montplaisir, J. (2002). REM sleep behavior disorder and REM sleep without atonia in Parkinson's disease. *Neurology,* 59, 585-589

Garcia-Borreguero, D.; Caminero, A.B.; De La Llave, Y.; Larrosa, O.; Barrio, S.; Granizo, J.J. & Pareja, J.A. (2002). Decreased phasic EMG activity during rapid eye movement sleep in treatment-naive Parkinson's disease: effects of treatment with levodopa and progression of illness. *Mov Disord,* 17, 934-941

Garcia-Borreguero, D.; Larrosa, O. & Bravo, M. (2003). Parkinson's disease and sleep. *Sleep Med Rev,* 7, 115-129

Gatto, N.M.; Cockburn, M.; Bronstein, J.; Manthripragada, A.D. & Ritz, B. (2009). Well-water consumption and Parkinson's disease in rural California. *Environ Health Perspect,* 117, 1912-1918

Gerlach, M.; Riederer, P.; Przuntek, H. & Youdim, M.B.H. (1991). MPTP mechanisms of neurotoxicity and their implications for Parkinson's disease. *Eur J Pharmacol,* 208, 273-86

Gold, B.G. & Nutt, J.G. (2002). Neuroimmunophilin ligands in the treatment of Parkinson's disease. *Curr Opin Pharmacol,* 2, 82-86

Goldman, S.M.; Tanner, C.M.; Olanow, C.W.; Watts, R.L.; Field, R.D. & Langston, J.W. (2005). Occupation and parkinsonism in three movement disorders clinics. *Neurology,* 65, 1430-1435

Gujar, S.K.; Maheshwari, S.; Bjorkman-Burtscher, I. & Sundgren, P.C. (2005). Magnetic resonance spectroscopy. *J Neuroophthalmol*, Sep, 25(3), 217-26

Hantraye, P.; Varastet, M.; Peschanski, M.; Riche, D.; Cesaro, P.; Willer, J.C. & Maziere, M. (1993). Stable parkinsonian syndrome and uneven loss of striatal dopamine fibres following chronic MPTP administration in baboons. *Neuroscience*, 53, 169-178

Hardman, C.D.; Henderson, J.M.; Finkelstein, D.I.; Horne, M.K.; Paxinos, G. & Halliday, G.M. (2002). Comparison of the basal ganglia in rats, marmosets, macaques, baboons, and humans: volume and neuronal number for the output, internal relay, and striatal modulating nuclei. *J Comp Neurol*, 445, 238-255

Hilker, R.; Voges, J.; Weber, T.; Kracht, L.W.; Roggendorf, J.; Baudrexel, S.; Hoevels, M.; Sturm, V. & Heiss, W.D. (2008). STN-DBS activates the target area in Parkinson disease: an FDG-PET study. *Neurology*, 71, 708-713

Iranzo, A.; Santamaria, J.; Rye, D.B.; Valldeoriola, F.; Marti, M.J.; Munoz, E.; Vilaseca, I. & Tolosa, E. (2005). Characteristics of idiopathic REM sleep behavior disorder and that associated with MSA and PD. *Neurology*, 65, 247-252

Iranzo, A.; Molinuevo, J.L.; Santamaria, J.; Serradell, M.; Marti, M.J.; Valldeoriola, F. & Tolosa, E. (2006). Rapid-eye-movement sleep behaviour disorder as an early marker for a neurodegenerative disorder: a descriptive study. *Lancet Neurol*, 5, 572-577

Iravani, M.M.; Jackson, M.J.; Kuoppamaki, M.; Smith, L.A. & Jenner, P. (2003). 3,4-methylenedioxymethamphetamine (ecstasy) inhibits dyskinesia expression and normalizes motor activity in 1-methyl-4-phenyl-1,2,3,6-tetrahydropyridine-treated primates. *J Neurosci*, 23, 9107-9115

Jackson-Lewis, V.; Jakowec, M.; Burke, RE. & Przedborski, S. (1995). Time course and morphology of dopaminergic neuronal death caused by the neurotoxin 1-methyl-4-phenyl-1,2,3,6-tetrahydropyridine. *Neurodegeneration*, 4, 257-269

Jankovic, J. (2005). Motor fluctuations and dyskinesias in Parkinson's disease: clinical manifestations. *Mov Disord*, 20, Suppl 11, S11-16

Javitch, J.A.; D'Amato, R.J.; Strittmatter, S.M. & Snyder, S.H. (1985). Parkinsonism-inducing neurotoxin, N-methyl-4-phenyl-1,2,3,6 -tetrahydropyridine: uptake of the metabolite N-methyl-4-phenylpyridine by dopamine neurons explains selective toxicity. *Proc Natl Acad Sci U S A*, 82, 2173-2177

Jellinger, K.A. (2008). Neuropathological aspects of Alzheimer disease, Parkinson disease and frontotemporal dementia. *Neurodegener Dis*, 5, 118-121

Jenner, P.; Rupniak, N.M.; Rose, S.; Kelly, E.; Kilpatrick, G.; Lees, A. & Marsden, C.D. (1984). 1-Methyl-4-phenyl-1,2,3,6-tetrahydropyridine-induced parkinsonism in the common marmoset. *Neurosci Lett*, 50, 85-90

Jenner, P.; Zeng, B.Y.; Smith, L.A.; Pearce, R.K.; Tel, B.; Chancharme, L. & Moachon, G. (2000). Antiparkinsonian and neuroprotective effects of modafinil in the mptp-treated common marmoset. *Exp Brain Res*, 133, 178-88

Jenner, P. (2003a). The contribution of the MPTP-treated primate model to the development of new treatment strategies for Parkinson's disease. *Parkinsonism Relat Disord*, 9, 131-137

Jenner, P. (2003b). The MPTP-treated primate as a model of motor complications in PD: primate model of motor complications. *Neurology*, 61, S4-11

Jenner, P. (2009). From the MPTP-treated primate to the treatment of motor complications in Parkinson's disease. *Parkinsonism Relat Disord*, 15, Suppl 4, S18-23

Joshua, M.; Adler, A. & Bergman, H. (2009). The dynamics of dopamine in control of motor behavior. *Curr Opin Neurobiol,* 19, 615-620

Kauppinen, R.A. & Williams, S.R. (1994). Nuclear magnetic resonance spectroscopy studies of the brain. *Prog Neurobiol,* 44, 87-118

Kosta, P.; Agyropoulou, M.I.; Markoula, S. & Konitsiotis, S. (2006). MRI evaluation of the basal ganglia size and the iron content in patients with Parkinson's disease. *J Neurol,* Jan, 253(1), 26-32

Lai, Y.Y. & Siegel, J.M. (1990). Muscle tone suppression and stepping produced by stimulation of midbrain and rostral pontine reticular formation. *J Neurosci,* 10, 2727-2734

Langston, J.W.; Ballard, P.; Tetrud, J.W. & Irwin, I. (1983). Chronic Parkinsonism in humans due to a product of meperidine-analog synthesis. *Science,* 219, 979-980

Lapierre, O. & Montplaisir, J. (1992). Polysomnographic features of REM sleep behavior disorder: development of a scoring method. *Neurology,* 42, 1371-1374

Le Couteur, D.G.; Muller, M.; Yang, M.C.; Mellick, G.D. & McLean, A.J. (2002). Age-environment and gene-environment interactions in the pathogenesis of Parkinson's disease. *Rev Environ Health,* 17, 51-64

Levey, A.I.; Hersch, S.M.; Rye, D.B.; Sunahara, R.K.; Niznik, H.B.; Kitt, C.A.; Price, D.L.; Maggio, R.; Brann, M.R. & Ciliax, B.J. (1993). Localization of D1 and D2 dopamine receptors in brain with subtype-specific antibodies. *Proc Natl Acad Sci U S A,* 90, 8861-8865

Lima, M.M.; Andersen, M.L.; Reksidler, A.B.; Vital, M.A. & Tufik, S. (2007). The role of the substantia nigra pars compacta in regulating sleep patterns in rats. *PLoS ONE,* Jun 6, 2(6), e513

Luchtman, D.W.; Shao, D. & Song, C. (2009). Behavior, neurotransmitters and inflammation in three regimens of the MPTP mouse model of Parkinson's disease. *Physiol Behav,* 98, 130-138

Mandel, S.; Grünblatt, E.; Riederer, P.; Gerlach, M.; Levites, Y. & Youdim, M.B.H. (2003). Neuroprotective strategies in Parkinson's disease: An update on progress. *CNS Drugs,* 17 (10), pp. 729-762

Marek, K. & Jennings, D. (2009). Can we image premotor Parkinson disease? *Neurology,* 72, S21-26

Mayer, G.; Kesper, K.; Ploch, T.; Canisius, S.; Penzel, T.; Oertel, W. & Stiasny-Kolster, K. (2008). Quantification of tonic and phasic muscle activity in REM sleep behavior disorder. *J Clin Neurophysiol,* 25, 48-55

Meredith, G.E.; Totterdell, S.; Potashkin, J.A. & Surmeier, D.J. (2008). Modeling PD pathogenesis in mice: Advantages of a chronic MPTP protocol. *Parkinsonism Relat Disord,* 14, suppl 2, S112-117

Migliore, L. & Coppede, F. (2009). Genetics, environmental factors and the emerging role of epigenetics in neurodegenerative diseases. *Mutat Res,* 667, 82-97

Miletich, R.S.; BAnkiewicz, K.S.; Quareantelli, M.; Plunkett, R.J.; Frank, J.; Kopin, I.J. & Di Chiro, G. (1994). MRI detects acute degeneration of the nigrostriatal dopamine system after MPTP exposure in hemiparkinsonian monkeys. *Ann Neurol.,* 35, 689-97.

Miwa, T.; Watanabe, A.; Mitsumoto, Y.; Furukawa, M.; Fukushima, N. & Moriizumi, T. (2004). Olfactory impairment and Parkinson's disease-like symptoms observed in

the common marmoset following administration of 1-methyl-4-phenyl-1,2,3,6-tetrahydropyridine. *Acta Otolaryngol Suppl*, Aug, 553, 80-84
Mochizuki, H.; Imai, H.; Endo, K.; TYokomizo, K. ; Murata, Y.; Hattori, N. & Mizuno, Y. (1994). Iron accumulation in the substantia nigra of 1-methyl-4-phenyl-1,2,3,6-tetrahydropyridine (MPTP)-induced hemiparkinsonian monkeys. *Neurosci Lett.* 168, 251-3
Monaca, C.; Laloux, C.; Jacquesson, J.M.; Gele, P.; Marechal, X.; Bordet, R.; Destee, A. & Derambure, P. (2004). Vigilance states in a parkinsonian model, the MPTP mouse. *Eur J Neurosci*, 20, 2474-2478
Nicklas, W.J.; Vyas, I. & Heikkila, R.E. (1985). Inhibition of NADH-linked oxidation in brain mitochondria by 1-methyl-4-phenyl-pyridine, a metabolite of the neurotoxin, 1-methyl-4-phenyl-1,2,5,6-tetrahydropyridine. *Life Sci*, 36, 2503-2508
Nutt, J.G.; Burchiel, K.J.; Comella, C.L.; Jankovic, J.; Lang, A.E.; Laws, E.R. Jr.; Lozano, A.M.; Penn, R.D.; Simpson, R.K. Jr.; Stacy, M. & Wooten, G.F. (2003). Randomized, double-blind trial of glial cell line-derived neurotrophic factor (GDNF) in PD. *Neurology*, 60, 69-73
Nuytemans, K.; Theuns, J.; Cruts, M. & Van Broeckhoven, C. (2010). Genetic etiology of Parkinson disease associated with mutations in the SNCA, PARK2, PINK1, PARK7, and LRRK2 genes: a mutation update. *Hum Mutat*, Jul, 31(7), 763-80
Obinu, M.C.; Reibaud, M.; Blanchard, V.; Moussaoui, S. & Imperato, A. (2002). Neuroprotective effect of riluzole in a primate model of Parkinson's disease: behavioral and histological evidence. *Mov Disord*, 17, 13-19
Oerlemans, W.G. & de Weerd, A.W. (2002). The prevalence of sleep disorders in patients with Parkinson's disease. A self-reported, community-based survey. *Sleep Med*, 3, 47-149
Olanow, C.W.; Kieburtz, K. & Schapira, A.H. (2008). Why have we failed to achieve neuroprotection in Parkinson's disease? *Ann Neurol*, 64, Suppl 2, S101-110
Ondo, W.G.; Dat Vuong, K.; Khan, H.; Atassi, F.; Kwak, C. & Jankovic, J. (2001). Daytime sleepiness and other sleep disorders in Parkinson's disease. *Neurology*, 57, 1392-1396
Pahwa, R. & Lyons, K.E. (2010). Early diagnosis of Parkinson's disease: recommendations from diagnostic clinical guidelines. *Am J Manag Care*, 16 Suppl Implications, S94-99
Park, A. & Stacy, M. (2009). Non-motor symptoms in Parkinson's disease. *J Neurol*, 256, Suppl 3, 293-298
Parkinson, J. (1817). An essay on the shaking palsy. *Journal of clinical neuroscience*, 14, 223-230
ParkinsonStudyGroup (1993). Effects of tocopherol and deprenyl on the progression of disability in early Parkinson's disease. *N Engl J Med*, 328, 176-183
ParkinsonStudyGroup (2002). Dopamine transporter brain imaging to assess the effects of pramipexole vs levodopa on Parkinson disease progression. *Jama*, 287, 1653-1661
Pearce, R.K.; Collins, P.; Jenner, P.; Emmett, C. & Marsden, C.D. (1996). Intraventricular infusion of basic fibroblast growth factor (bFGF) in the MPTP-treated common marmoset. *Synapse*, 23, 192-200
Pearson, J.; Goldstein, M.; Markey, K. & Brandeis (1983). Human brainstem catecholamine neuronal anatomy as indicated by immunocytochemistry with antibodies to tyrosine hydroxylase. *Neuroscience*, 8, 3-32
Philippens, I.H.C.H.M.; Kersten, C.J.M.; Vanwersch, R.A.P. & Strijkstra, A.M. (2004). Sleep and sleep EEG spectra in marmoset monkeys. In: *Sleep-wake Research in the*

Netherland, Vol.15, Ruigt, G.S.F., et al. (Eds.), 49-51, ISBN 90-73675-13-8, Leiden, The Netherlands

Philippens, I.H.C.H.M. (2009). Non-human primate models for Parkinson's disease. *Drug Discovery Today: Disease Models,* Vol. 5, Issue 2, 105-111

Philippens, I.H.C.H.M.; 't Hart, B.A. & Torres, G. (2010). The MPTP marmoset model of Parkinsonism: a multi-purpose non-human primate model for neurodegenerative diseases. *Drug Discov Today,* 15(23-24), 985-990

Podell, M.; Hadjiconstantinou, M.; Smith, M.A. & Neff, N.H. (2003). Proton magnetic resonance imaging and spectroscopy identify metabolic changes in the straiatum in the MPTP feline model of parkinsonism. *Exp Neurol,* 179, 159-66

Postuma, R.B.; Lang, A.E.; Massicotte-Marquez, J. & Montplaisir, J. (2006). Potential early markers of Parkinson disease in idiopathic REM sleep behavior disorder. *Neurology,* 66, 845-851

Przedborski, S.; Jackson-Lewis, V.; Naini, A.B.; Jakowec, M.; Petzinger, G.; Miller, R, & Akram, M. (2001). The parkinsonian toxin 1-methyl-4-phenyl-1,2,3,6-tetrahydropyridine (MPTP): a technical review of its utility and safety. *J Neurochem,* 76, 1265-1274

Ravina, B.M.; Fagan, S.C.; Hart, R.G.; Hovinga, C.A.; Murphy, D.D.; Dawson, T.M. & Marler, J.R. (2003). Neuroprotective agents for clinical trials in Parkinson's disease: a systematic assessment. *Neurology,* 60, 1234-1240

Rechtschaffen, A. & Kales, A. (1968). *A manual of standardized terminology, techniques and scoring system for sleep stages of human subjects.* In. Los Angeles, Brain Information Service/Brain Research Institute, University of California.

Schapira, A.H. (2009). Etiology and pathogenesis of Parkinson disease. *Neurol Clin,* 27, 583-603

Schenck, C.H.; Bundlie, S.R. & Mahowald, M.W. (1996). Delayed emergence of a parkinsonian disorder in 38% of 29 older men initially diagnosed with idiopathic rapid eye movement sleep behaviour disorder. *Neurology,* 46, 388-393

Schmidt, N. & Ferger, B. (2001). Neurochemical findings in the MPTP model of Parkinson's disease. *J Neural Transm,* 108, 1263-1282

Schmidt, W.J. & Alam, M. (2006). Controversies on new animal models of Parkinson's disease pro and con: the rotenone model of Parkinson's disease (PD). *J Neural Transm,* Suppl, 273-276

Schule, B.; Pera, R.A. & Langston, J.W. (2009). Can cellular models revolutionize drug discovery in Parkinson's disease? *Biochim Biophys Acta,* 1792, 1043-1051

Sethi, K.D.; O'Brien, C.F.; Hammerstad, J.P.; Adler, C.H.; Davis, T.L.; Taylor, R.L.; Sanchez-Ramos, J.; Bertoni, J.M. & Hauser, R.A. (1998). Ropinirole for the treatment of early Parkinson disease: a 12-month experience. Ropinirole Study Group. *Arch Neurol,* 55, 1211-1216

Sherer, T.B.; Kim, J.H.; Betarbet, R. & Greenamyre, J.T. (2003). Subcutaneous rotenone exposure causes highly selective dopaminergic degeneration and alpha-synuclein aggregation. *Exp Neurol,* 179, 9-16

Shults, C.W.; Oakes, D.; Kieburtz, K.; Beal, M.F.; Haas, R.; Plumb, S.; Juncos, J.L.; Nutt, J.; Shoulson, I.; Carter, J.; Kompoliti, K.; Perlmutter, J.S.; Reich, S.; Stern, M.; Watts, R.L.; Kurlan, R.; Molho, E.; Harrison, M. & Lew, M. (2002.) Effects of coenzyme Q10 in early Parkinson disease: evidence of slowing of the functional decline. *Arch Neurol*, 59, 1541-1550

Smith, D.; Trennery, P.; Farningham, D. & Klapwijk, J. (2001). The selection of marmoset monkeys (Callithrix jacchus) in pharmaceutical toxicology. *Lab Anim*, 35, 117-130

Speciale, S.G. (2002). MPTP: insights into parkinsonian neurodegeneration. *Neurotoxicol Teratol*, 24, 607-620

Stephenson, R.; Siderowf, A. & Stern, M.B. (2009). Premotor Parkinson's disease: clinical features and detection strategies. *Mov Disord*, 24 Suppl 2, S665-670

Stiasny-Kolster, K.; Doerr, Y.; Moller, J.C.; Hoffken, H.; Behr, T.M.; Oertel, W.H. & Mayer, G. (2005). Combination of 'idiopathic' REM sleep behaviour disorder and olfactory dysfunction as possible indicator for alpha-synucleinopathy demonstrated by dopamine transporter FP-CIT-SPECT. *Brain*, 128, 126-137

Sydow, O. (2008). Parkinson's disease: recent development in therapies for advanced disease with a focus on deep brain stimulation (DBS) and duodenal levodopa infusion. *Febs J*, 275, 1370-1376

Tatton, W.G.; Kwan, M.M.; Verrier, M.C.; Seniuk, N.A. & Theriault, E. (1990). MPTP produces reversible disappearance of tyrosine hydroxylase-containing retinal amacrine cells, *Brain Res.*, 527, 21-31

Tandberg, E.; Larsen, J.P. & Karlsen, K. (1998). A community-based study of sleep disorders in patients with Parkinson's disease. *Mov Disord*, 13, 895-899

Temlett, J.A.; Landsberg, J.P.; Watt, F. & Grime, G.W. (1994). Increased iron in the substantia nigra compacta of the MPTP-lesioned hemiparkinsonian African green monkey: evidence from proton microprobe elemental microanalysis. *J Neurochem.*, 62, 134-46

Tolosa, E. & Poewe, W. (2009). Premotor Parkinson disease. *Neurology*, 72:S1

Tolosa, E.; Gaig, C.; Santamaria, J. & Compta, Y. (2009). Diagnosis and the premotor phase of Parkinson disease. *Neurology*, 72, S12-20

van der Staay, F.J.; Arndt, S.S. & Nordquist, R.E. (2009). Evaluation of animal models of neurobehavioral disorders. *Behav Brain Funct*, 5, 11

van Hilten, B.; Hoff, J.I.; Middelkoop, H.A.; van der Velde, E.A.; Kerkhof, G.A.; Wauquier, A.; Kamphuisen, H.A. & Roos, R.A. (1994). Sleep disruption in Parkinson's disease. Assessment by continuous activity monitoring. *Arch Neurol*, 51, 922-928

van Vliet, S.A.M.; Vanwersch, R.A.P.; Jongsma, M.J.; van der Gugten, J.; Olivier, B. & Philippens, I.H.C.H.M. (2006). Neuroprotective effects of modafinil in a marmoset Parkinson model: behavioral and neurochemical aspects. *Behav Pharmacol*, 17, 453-462

van Vliet, S.A.M.; Blezer, E.L.; Jongsma, M.J.; Vanwersch, R.A.P.; Olivier, B. & Philippens, I.H.C.H.M. (2008). Exploring the neuroprotective effects of modafinil in a marmoset Parkinson model with immunohistochemistry, magnetic resonance imaging and spectroscopy. *Brain Res*, 1189, 219-228

Verhave, P.S.; Vanwersch, R.A.P.; van Helden, H.P.; Smit, A.B. & Philippens, I.H.C.H.M. (2009). Two new test methods to quantify motor deficits in a marmoset model for Parkinson's disease. *Behav Brain Res*, 200, 214-219

Verhave, P.S.; Jongsma, M.J.; Van den Berg, R.M.; Vis, J.C.; Vanwersch, R.A.P.; Smit, A.B.; Someren, E.J.W. & Philippens, I.H.C.H.M. (2011). REM Sleep Behavior Disorder in the Marmoset MPTP Model of Early Parkinson's Disease. *Sleep*, in press

Visanji, N.P.; Gomez-Ramirez, J.; Johnston, T.H.; Pires, D.; Voon, V.; Brotchie, J.M. & Fox, S.H. (2006). Pharmacological characterization of psychosis-like behavior in the MPTP-lesioned nonhuman primate model of Parkinson's disease. *Mov Disord,* 21, 1879-1891

Waters, C.M.; Hunt, S.P.; Jenner, P. & Marsden, C.D. (1987). An immunohostochemical study of the acute nd long-term effects of 1-methyl-phenyl-1,2,3,6-tetrahydropyridine in the marmoset. *Neuroscience,* 23, 1025-39

Wichmann, T. & DeLong, M.R. (2003). Pathophysiology of Parkinson's disease: the MPTP primate model of the human disorder. *Ann N Y Acad Sci*, 991, 199-213

Willner, P. (1986). Validation criteria for animal models of human mental disorders: learned helplessness as a paradigm case. *Prog Neuropsychopharmacol Biol Psychiatry,* 10, 677-690

Xi, J. & Zhang, S.C. (2008). Stem cells in development of therapeutics for Parkinson's disease: a perspective. *J Cell Biochem*, 105, 1153-1160

Yantiri, F. & Anderson, J.K. (1999). The role of iron in Parkinson disease and 1-methyl-4-phenyl-1,2,3,6-tetrahydropyridine toxicity. *IUBMB Life*, 48,139-41

Yi, P.L.; Tsai, C.H.; Lu, M.K.; Liu, H.J.; Chen, Y.C. & Chang, F.C. (2007). Interleukin-1beta mediates sleep alteration in rats with rotenone-induced parkinsonism. *Sleep*, 30, 413-425

Zhang, Z.; Zhang, M.; Ai, Y.; Avison, C. & Gash, D.M. (1999). MPTP-Induced pallidal lesions in rhesus monkeys. *Exp Neurol.*, 155, 140-9

7

Cognitive and Psychiatric Aspects of Parkinson's Disease

Caspar Stephani
Department of Clinical Neurophysiology, University MedicalCenter Göttingen, Göttingen Germany

1. Introduction

Parkinson's disease (PD) is a neurodegenerative disorder affecting a variety of brain structures. Its prevalence in the general population is around 0.3% and increases considerably with age (de Lau & Breteler, 2006). The median age of onset is 60 years and the incidence is equal in both sexes (Katzenschlager et al., 2008). While initially symptoms are subtle severe disability often requiring permanent care is present in many patients within a time-frame of about ten years. On the other hand, there are patients who do not show relevant progression of PD over up to ten years (Hoehn & Yahr, 1967). Indeed, the most severe state of PD with regard to the Hoehn and Yahr (H&Y) scale may be reached after 6 to 40 years according to a variety of epidemiological studies (Poewe, 2006). Yet, overall the mortality rate of patients with PD is increased by a factor of 1.5-2.5 compared to the general population (Poewe, 2006).
The existence of at least two of the criteria resting tremor, bradykinesia and rigidity in an asymmetrical distribution leads the way to the diagnosis of this movement disorder. Accordingly, the pentamerous unified Parkinson's disease rating scale (UPDRS) mainly reflects the state of the motor symptoms of PD. Only the first item of the UPDRS takes into account psychiatric symptoms of the disease. However, cognitive decline as well as psychiatric disturbances are common in patients with PD and pose major problems. While the non-motor aspects of PD have been less well studied for a long time, they have received more attention in recent years. Nevertheless, therapy of these symptoms is less advanced compared to the numerous therapeutic options for the motor symptoms of PD. And not infrequently, treatment of motor symptoms and treatment of psychiatric and cognitive aspects of PD interfere with each other. For this chapter the literature on some factors of non-motor aspects of PD has been reviewed and is summarized here.

2. Cognitive and psychiatric comorbidities of Parkinson's disease

2.1 Dementia in PD

Epidemiology: Parkinson's disease is the second most common neurodegenerative disease and dementia is one of the main manifestations of PD. A large epidemiological study of 1449 patients with PD conducted in Germany found a point prevalence of dementia of 28.6% in this population (Von Reichmann et al., 2010). Accordingly, meta-analyses of prevalence studies on Parkinson's disease dementia (PDD) report point prevalence rates of 24.5% (Aarsland et al., 2005) or 30% (Marder, 2010). Hence, 30% may be an accurate estimate of the point prevalence of PDD. Additionally, it affects probably more than 50% of patients with PD in the course of the disease and cumulative prevalence rates reach 80% in some studies (Aarsland & Kurz, 2010). Indeed, compared to a control population the risk of developing dementia in PD is increased 6-fold (Buter et al., 2008). On the other hand, 3-4% of dementias in general are attributed to PD (Marder, 2010).

The most significant risk factors for developing PDD are a higher age of onset of PD as well as a higher degree of severity of parkinsonism. Also, the development of PDD often is preceded by the diagnosis of mild cognitive impairment (MCI). It has been suggested that deficits in semantic fluency and visuoconstruction indicate a higher risk for developing PDD compared to frontal executive dysfunctions (Aarsland & Kurz, 2010). An association between dementia and visual hallucinations in PD is established as well.

Pathophysiology: The pathophysiological mechanisms of PDD are not fully understood. As opposed to the motor symptoms cognitive deficits in PD normally do not improve with dopaminergic therapy. Therefore other pathology than the cerebral dopamine deficit is relevant in the pathophysiology of PDD. Postmortal analysis of brain of patients who had clinical symptoms of PDD shows a heterogeneous histological and immunochemical profile. Abundant cortical and nuclear Lewy bodies resembling the histopathological profile of Lewy body dementia (LBD) may be present. On the other hand, the pattern of post-mortem analysis may resemble that of Alzheimer's disease (AD). Lack of cortical amyloid, tau, or synuclein pathology in the presence of Lewy bodies in the substantia nigra was associated with less significant dementia underlining the importance of cortical pathology regarding PDD (Galvin et al., 2006). More knowledge on biomarkers of dementia has evolved in the last years with several studies that demonstrated specific findings in the cerebrospinal fluid of patients with PDD (CSF). Amyloid-beta (Aβ) peptides are the main components of amyloid-plaques which are found abundantly in patients with AD but also form part of the pathological changes in the brains of patients with PDD. Presence of the most prominent form of amyloid-beta - the Aβ-42 - in the CSF has been shown to be a reliable marker for dementias and particularly for AD. But discrimination between AD and PDD or LBD is not possible with this marker. However, the ratio between the subforms 42 and 37 of the Aβ protein have been proposed as biomarker for a differentiation between AD from PDD and LBD whereas the latter two forms of dementia may be differentiable by new subforms of the Aβ-protein that have been found in the CSF of patients with dementia (Bibl et al., 2006). Other proteins that can be detected in the CSF and whose concentration may indicate dementia are phospho-tau and alpha-synuclein. Regarding neurophysiological techniques a study analyzing the EEG of 50 patients with AD, 50 patients with LBD and 40 patients with PDD showed that patients with PDD or LBD had significantly slower posterior rhythms (5.6-7.9 Hertz) than patients with AD even in early stages of the disease (Bonanni et al., 2008). Neuroimaging studies demonstrate whole brain atrophy in PDD lacking confirmed specific changes that would differentiate between patients with PD and those with PDD. The co-occurrence of visual hallucinations and PDD has prompted pathoanatomical explanations relating both symptoms to Lewy body pathology in the temporal lobes (Harding et al., 2002). Another common mechanism of these manifestations of PD may be a cholinergic deficit supported by the therapeutic success that can be achieved by application of inhibitors of the acetylcholinesterase (Emre et al., 2004). A relation to the known protective effect of cigarette smoking on the incidence of PD may exist (Alves et al., 2004). Association of PDD with particular familial forms of PD have been demonstrated. But genetic risk factors for PDD exceeding these relatively rare forms of PD have not yet been found.

Phenomenology: Typically, patients with PDD exhibit deficits in different aspects of memory. A recent study showed that impaired attentional filtering as well as a reduced storage capacity is present in patients with PD even in the absence of dementia (Lee et al., 2010). However, no specific pattern of cognitive decline is characteristic for PDD and all major cognitive domains including memory, attention, constructional function, visuospatial function and execution are affected. Differentiation from AD and especially LBD is not reliably available based on the neuropsychological testing. Still, many studies suggest executive dysfunction as the predominating cognitive pattern in patients with PDD (Emre et al., 2007). Importantly, patients with dementia and PD show similar clinical signs compared to LBD even though postural instability is more common in PDD. Nevertheless, the frequency of falls does not differ between patients with PDD, LBD and AD. Visual and auditory hallucinations, as well as depression, sleep disturbances and cognitive fluctuation characterize PDD as well as LBD. Importantly, aside from the presence of extrapyramidal motor symptoms these criteria common in PDD and LBD are very useful in distinguishing PDD from AD (Galvin et al., 2006). The most significant predictor of developing PDD compared to patients with PD without dementia are visual hallucinations the occurrence of which at any point in the progress of PD increases the risk for developing dementia by a factor of twenty (Galvin et al., 2006). Typical clinical features that establish the diagnosis of PDD are found in table 1.

Diagnosis: Recently, a task force of 23 experts in the field of PD developed clinical diagnostic criteria for PDD. Features of this disorder were defined as well as the likelihood of its diagnosis based on the combination of symptoms (Emre et al., 2007; Goetz et al., 2008). According to the criteria in table 1 and 2 diagnosis of PDD is probable if 1) both core features are present, 2) at least two cognitive features and at least one behavioral feature are present, 3) none of the group III or group IV features are found. Diagnosis of PDD is possible if 1) both core features are present, 2) there is an atypical profile of cognitive impairment in one or more of the cognitive features like prominent or receptive-type aphasia, pure storage-failure type amnesia with preserved attention while behavioral symptoms may or may not be present. Possible PDD can be diagnosed also with one or more features of category II present in the absence of category IV features (Emre et al., 2007; Goetz et al., 2008).

Therapy: Currently, there are four relevant drugs with approval for the treatment of the symptoms of dementias. Donepezil, rivastigmine and galantamine are inhibitors of the acetylcholinesterase whereas memantine is an antagonist of the glutamatergic N-methyl-d-aspartate (NMDA)-receptor. These drugs are approved for the treatment of AD in the United States and/or within the European Union. Their indication for treatment of PDD has been established or is currently under approval. 20 studies regarding the treatment of PDD with inhibitors of the acetylcholinesterase were identified by a review published in 2010. The effects of donepezil were investigated in 12 studies, those of rivastigmine in 6 and galantamine was tested in 2 studies. 11 of these studies were open-label studies and 2 reported case series and all of these smaller studies with less than 40 patients showed

I. Core features	1. Diagnosis of Parkinson's disease according to Queen Square Brain Bank criteria	2. A dementia syndrome with insidious onset and slow progression, developing within the context of established Parkinson's disease and diagnosed by history, clinical, and mental examination, defined as: 1. Impairment in more than one cognitive domain 2. Representing a decline from premorbid level 3. Deficits severe enough to impair daily life (social, occupational, or personal care), independent of the impairment ascribable to motor or autonomic symptoms
II. Associated clinical features	**1. Cognitive features** **Attention:** Impairment in spontaneous and focused attention, poor performance in attentional tasks; performance may fluctuate during the day and from day to day Executive functions: Impairment in tasks requiring initiation, planning, concept formation, rule finding, set shifting or set maintenance; impaired mental speed (bradyphrenia) Visuo-spatial functions: Impairment in tasks requiring visual-spatial orientation, perception, or construction **Memory:** Impairment in free recall of recent events or in tasks requiring learning new material, memory usually improves with cueing, recognition is usually better than free recall **Language:** Core functions largely preserved. Word finding difficulties and impaired comprehension of complex sentences may be present	**2. Behavioral features** **Apathy:** Decreased spontaneity; loss of motivation, interest, and effortful behavior **Personality:** Changes in personality and mood including depressive features and anxiety **Hallucinations:** Mostly visual, usually complex, formed visions of people, animals or objects **Delusions:** Usually paranoid, such as infidelity, or phantom boarder (unwelcome guests living in the home) delusions **Excessive daytime sleepiness**

Table 1. Features favoring the diagnosis of dementia associated with Parkinson's disease (according to Emre et al., 2007 and Goetz et al., 2008)

III. Features which do not exclude PD-D, but make the diagnosis uncertain	• Co-existence of any other abnormality which may by itself cause cognitive impairment, but judged not to be the cause of dementia, e.g. presence of relevant vascular disease in imaging	• Time interval between the development of motor and cognitive symptoms not known
IV. Features suggesting other conditions or diseases as cause of mental impairment, which, when present make it impossible to reliably diagnose PD-D	• Cognitive and behavioral symptoms appearing solely in the context of other conditions such as: **Acute confusion due to** - Systemic diseases or abnormalities - Drug intoxication **Major Depression according to DSM IV**	• Features compatible with "Probable Vascular dementia" criteria according to NINDS-AIREN = dementia in the context of cerebrovascular disease as indicated by 1. focal signs in neurological exam such as hemiparesis, sensory deficits, and 2. evidence of relevant cerebrovascular disease by brain imaging AND a relationship between the two as indicated by the presence of one or more of the following: 1. onset of dementia within 3 months after a recognized stroke 2. abrupt deterioration in cognitive functions 3. fluctuating, stepwise progression of cognitive deficits

Table 2. Features not favoring the diagnosis of dementia associated with Parkinson's disease (according to Emre et al., 2007 and Goetz et al., 2008)

improvement in selected clinical outcome measures to some degree. Nevertheless, by nature the limitations of these studies' designs affect their representative value. Still, it may be an important clinical observation that improvement of hallucinations was observed among patients treated with rivastigmine, donepezil or galantamine in several of these studies while their were generally no changes in motor symptoms. 5 of the studies as of 2010 were randomized controlled trials of which only two had included more than 40 patients (van Laar et al., 2010). One of these studies investigated the effects of rivastigmine while the other investigated the effects of donepezil in patients with PDD. The latter study has not been published in a peer-reviewed journal as of April 2011 and results of the review are based on a poster presentation at an international conference in 2007 (van Laar et al., 2010). According to this preliminary review, this study included 550 patient with PDD who were randomized to one of three treatment arms receiving either 5 mg donepezil, 10 mg donepezil or placebo. A trend towards improvement but no significant effect on the primary cognitive outcome scales was the main result of this report. Nonetheless, significant improvement was present in several secondary outcome measures like the mini-mental state examination (MMSE), the brief test of attention (BTA) or the verbal fluency test from the Delis-Kaplan executive function system test battery (D-KEFS). Nausea and parkinsonian side effects were reported as most common adverse events. In the other placebo-controlled, randomized trial with 541 patients a moderate effect of 3-12 mg rivastigmine per day on cognitive outcome measures in patients with PD and mild to moderate dementia has been demonstrated. Primary efficacy variables were the scores for the cognitive part of the Alzheimer's disease assessment scale (ADAS-cog) and the scores for the Alzheimer's disease cooperative study-clinician's global impression of change (ADCS-CGIC) which both showed improvement in the group of patients treated with rivastigmine compared to the placebo-group. Importantly, both scales which originally are derived from use in patients with AD are regarded as valid and reliable for use in patients with PDD as well (Harvey et al., 2010). A decrease of 2.1 points in the ADAS-cog was found in the verum group while the score of this scale increased by 0.7 after 24 weeks of application of the placebo. This decline in cognitive performance has been attributed to the natural course of PDD. Significant but only weak improvement was found in several other scales of cognitive performance and activity level. The rate of side-effects like nausea (29%), vomiting (16.6%), tremor (10.2%) and dizziness (5.8%) was significantly increased in patients who had received rivastigmine compared to those who had received placebo leading to a drop out rate due to adverse effects of 17% in the treated group compared to 8% in the placebo group (Emre et al., 2004). In line with the cited observations of previous reports and open studies the rate of hallucinations in the group receiving rivastigmine was significantly lower than in the placebo group. In fact, presence of hallucinations tended to be a predictor of favorable cognitive outcome. An open-label extension study with a daily dose of 3-12 mg rivastigmine for another 24 weeks in 334 patients with PDD who previously had received rivastigmine or placebo largely confirmed the results of the original study. Hence, the efficacy as well as the profile of side effects of rivastigmine were reproduced in the group that had received placebo during the first part of the study (Poewe et al., 2005). Additionally, in a large meta-analysis on therapy of dementia in patients with PD it was concluded that rivastigmine could improve cognition and activities of daily living (Maidment et al., 2006). Memantine has been tested in several clinical trials in patients with PDD. In a first pilot study of this drug in PDD there was no beneficial effect on cognitive outcome measures while a good tolerability compared to application of inhibitors of the acetylcholinesterase was shown (Leroi et al., 2009). An early double-blind placebo controlled trial showed a positive effect in the clinical global impression of change scale as well as an improved speed on attentional tasks under treatment with memantine (Aarsland et al., 2009). But more recent evidence from a randomized, double-blind, placebo-controlled trial with 199 participants with PDD or LBD showed no clinical benefit in patients with PDD in any of the cognitive tests applied after 24 weeks of therapy whereas those with LBD improved moderately (Emre et al., 2010). Therefore, memantine may not be regarded as choice for the pharmacotherapy of PDD. Use of galantamine has been tested in one clinical trial which reported overall beneficial effects on several scales of cognitive performance as well as improvement of hallucinations, anxiety, apathy and sleep disturbances (Litvinenko et al., 2008). However, this was an open controlled trial. Still, not unlike in other forms of dementia the current therapeutic options to treat PD dementia are purely symptomatic. And unfortunately, the effect size of antidementive drugs tends to be small in the therapy of dementias may they be related to

PD or not. Finally it can be concluded that rivastigmine is currently the only FDA-approved drug to treat dementia associated with PD while donepezil can be considered as a treatment choice. When applying rivastigmine in patients with PDD slow titration should be adhered to in order to reduce the incidence of side effects like tremor or nausea. A transdermal patch of rivastigmine now available for treatment has been shown to be more tolerable compared to the capsule applied normally (Winbald et al., 2007). This may enable more frequent use and use of higher doses of rivastigmine in patients sensitive to side-effects of this drug. Whether rivastigmine or other inhibitors of the acetylcholinesterase is applicable for the primary treatment of hallucinations may be subject of future studies.

2.2 Depression in PD

Epidemiology: Depression is one of the most common diseases of humans and up to 21 million people in Europe are affected by uni- or bipolar depression (Olesen et al., 2006). In the western world it is among the most common causes of incapacity to work among employees under the age of 50 years. Depression may also be the most common psychiatric comorbidity in patients with PD. Reported prevalence rates of depression in PD vary between 3 and 90% depending on the population studied. Whereas earlier reports suggested prevalence rates of 40-50% (Zesiewicz & Hauser, 2002) more recent studies tend to report a lower prevalence of moderate to severe depression of 5-20% (Tandberg et al., 1996; Schrag et al., 2001). In fact, these figures are in line with a recent meta-analysis which calculated an average prevalence of depression in PD of 17%. Regarding prevalence rates the population under investigation needs to be exactly defined. In exemplum prevalence rates tend to be smaller in population studies as compared to inpatient or outpatient cohorts (Reijnders et al., 2008). Minor depression was found in 22% of the patients within this meta-analysis. Finally, a recent large nationwide study in Germany with 315 participating neurological settings recruited a random sample of 1,449 outpatients with PD who performed a standardized clinical assessment in order to evaluate the frequency of dementia, depression, and other neuropsychiatric symptoms in PD on a selected study day. Depression as defined by a score of ≥14 in the Montgomery Asberg depression rating scale (MADRS) was diagnosed in 23.8% of all patients. Though not directly related to age prevalence of depression increased from 14.7% in patients with PD in HY stage I-II to 44.9% in patients with HY status IV-V (Riedel et al., 2010). Given that there are about 1.2 million patients suffering from PD in Europe 250.000 to 600.000 of these patients may be affected by any type of depression.

Pathophysiology: The major mechanism that underlies the antidepressant effect of most antidepressant drugs is an increase of the concentration of neurotransmitters in the synaptic cleft by inhibition of axonal reuptake mechanisms or inhibition of intrasynaptic fermentation. The most relevant neurotransmitters targeted by antidepressants are the monoamines dopamine, noradrenaline and serotonine. The discovery of the mechanisms of action of these antidepressants has considerably influenced the pathophysiologic theory of transmitter deficiency in depression still valid today (Kalia, 2005; Schildkraut, 1965). However, as opposed to the pathophysiologic models of PD there is no specific neuropathoanatomical correlate for depression. Several systems of transmitters and cortical areas are thought to be altered in patients with depression. Hypometabolism in a FDG-PET has been demonstrated in the dorsal and ventral prefrontal cortex, as well as in the anterior cingulate cortex and the inferior parietal region in patients with depression (Mayberg, 2002). Increased cerebral blood-flow was found in the orbital cortex, the medial thalamus and the amygdala (Drevets, 2000). Studies with post-mortal cerebral tissue of patients who had suffered from depression indeed have shown cell atrophy in the dorsolateral prefrontal cortex and the orbitofrontal cortex as well as cell loss in the subgenual prefrontal cortex (Rajkowska, 2000). Other studies report on hippocampal volume loss in patients with major depression being related to the duration of the disease suggesting a possible link between the pathophysiology of neurodegenerative disorders and depression (Bremner et al., 2000). Cell loss or cell atrophy in depressed patients have been partially attributed to elevated cellular "stress" particularly mediated by corticosteroids. Reduced neuronal plasticity substantiated by decreased levels of the brain derived neurotrophic factor (BDNF) which plays an important for neuronal plasticity has been suggested to be causative for neuronal cell atrophy or cell loss. Interestingly, antidepressant treatment was found to upregulate the neuronal expression of the BDNF among others. Therefore, a neuroprotective effect of antidepressants on neuroanatomical structures which are affected by depression has been proposed (Duman et al., 2000). Regarding another neurotransmitter system, loss in cortical cholinergic function has been shown in a PET-study in patients with PD dementia and depression (Bohnen et al., 2007). Also there is a degeneration of several subcortical nuclei in PD a finding that resembles results from patients with depression only (Lisanby et al., 1993). Twin studies indicate hereditarity of major depression of 30-40 %. Still, there is no single genetic locus with a high association to depression whereas several polymorphisms of serotonine-transport genes or genes of the mono-amino-oxidase (MAO) have been linked to depression. Generally, depression is regarded as a polygenetic disease (Ebmaier et al., 2006; Hamet & Tremblay, 2005). These mechanisms have been recognized in the pathogenesis of major depression in the absence of PD but probably represent the most relevant mechanisms that lead to depression in patients with PD as well (Lemke et al., 2004).

Phenomenology: Not unlike other patients with depression patients with PD and depression present loss of interests, depressed mood, anhedonia, hopelessness, pessimism, feeling of worthlessness, loss of weight, insomnia, less often hypersomnia, suicidal ideas. Symptoms like hypomimia, bradyphrenia, disturbance of libido or sleep which are common in depression are common symptoms of PD without coexisting depression as well and may pose problems regarding their differentiation. Importantly, depression is thought to precede the occurrence of motor symptoms in PD not infrequently.

Apathy has been proposed as a symptom or syndrome distinct from depression in PD. Apathy is a condition which is characterized by a primary lack of motivation and involves behavioral, cognitive and affective deficits while there is no relevant affective component i.e. no feelings of sadness, depressed mood or feelings of worthlessness. Problems with the initiation and sustaining of activities have been described as being characteristic for apathy (Pluck & Brown, 2002). Even though symptoms of apathy and depression overlap apathy can occur in the absence of depression as has been demonstrated particularly in patients with progressive supranuclear palsy (PSP) (Litvan et al., 1996).

Diagnosis: The most common diagnostic manuals which define criteria for diagnosing a major depressive episode are the diagnostic and statistical manual of mental disorders (DSM-IV) as well as the tenth edition of the classification of diseases and related health problems (ICD-10). In the DSM-IV five or more of nine defined depressive symptoms of which one has to be either depressed mood or loss of interest/pleasure have to be present for at least 2 weeks and must represent a change from previous states. Besides 1) depressed mood most of the day (indicated by feeling or expression of sadness) and 2) reduced interest or pleasure in activities the other predefined symptoms which should each be present nearly every day are 3) significant weight loss or weight gain (change >5% of the body weight within one month), 4) insomnia or hypersomnia most of the day, 5) psychomotoric retardation or agitation, 6) fatigue/loss of energy, 7) the feeling of worthlessness or inappropriate guilt, 8) reduced concentration or ability to think, 9) recurrent thoughts of death/suicidal ideation/a plan for committing suicide or a suicide attempt. Significant clinical distress and impairment in the absence of a recognized medical condition accounting for the depressive symptoms are further criteria that need to be checked in order to diagnose a major depressive episode (American Psychiatric Association, 2010a). In the ICD-10 the depressive episodes can be categorized into mild, moderate or severe forms. While using a catalogue of criteria comparable with that of the DSM-IV diagnosis of a mild depressive episode requires 2 to 3 of the criteria, while a moderate depressive episode is diagnosed when 4 or more criteria are fulfilled. In contrast to a moderate depressive episode, presence of suicidal thoughts or plans as well as presence of several somatic symptoms indicate a severe depressive episode (World Health Organization, 2007a). Depressions often are classified based on depression scales like the Hamilton depression scale (HAM-DS) or Beck's depression inventory or the Montgomery Asberg depression rating scale (Gotham et al., 1986). These scales differ regarding the significance of somatic and psychic symptoms and the HAM-DS is probably the most frequently used inventory in patients with PD and depression (Dissanayaka et al., 2007; Schrag et al., 2007).

Therapy: Despite the existence of a broad spectrum of antidepressants there is scarce evidence for the efficacy of antidepressants in patients with PD. Studies utilizing selective serotonin reuptake inhibitors (SSRIs) like citalopram, sertraline and paroxetine or tricyclic antidepressants imipramine, desipramine, amitriptyline and nortriptyline or bupropion have been conducted. In a large literature review effect sizes between antidepressant and placebo treatment did not differ in patients with PD and depression being in line with previous meta-analyses (Weintraub et al., 2005). Within this review only 11 studies performed between 1965 and 2003 with a treatment duration of about 12 weeks on average utilizing SSRIs in the majority were found suitable for meta-analysis. Only two of these studies were placebo-controlled trials. Sample size was 30 patients on average. Generally, the effect size of antidepressant as well as placebo treatment was regarded as considerable. Therefore, nonspecific treatment effects were suggested as likely reason for the positive effects reported in several open-label studies. In accordance, the effect size found was similar to that of placebo arms of randomized, placebo-controlled trials in elderly patients with depression and without PD. Finally, the completion rates of open-label studies with antidepressants were about 87% in general and 86% in patients receiving SSRIs thus deeming poor tolerance of antidepressants in patients with PD an unlikely cause of the ineffective antidepressive action (Weintraub et al., 2005). In the meantime two rather small placebo controlled trials with each about 50 participants have demonstrated superiority of selected antidepressants. In one study citalopram as well as desipramine proofed to be more affective than placebo 30 days after initializing treatment as demonstrated by significant improvement in the Montgomery Asberg depression rating scale (MADRS). Additionally, treatment with desipramine resulted in a significant antidepressant effect after 14 days as well. On the other hand, side-effects were reported twice as often in patients with desipramine compared to patients who received citalopram being often in accordance with the anticholinergic profile of tricyclic drugs. Still, with 15 or less patients in each group sample sizes were low (Devos et al., 2008). In another recent placebo controlled trial application of 48.5 mg of nortriptyline on average and 28.4 mg of paroxetine on average each was compared to placebo in 52 patients with PD and depression. The primary outcome variable in this study was change in the Hamilton depression rating scale (HAM-D). While nortriptyline was superior to placebo 2 and 8 weeks after initializing treatment paroxetine was not. Also the responder rate defined as a change of ≥50% in the HAM-D was significantly higher in the group treated with nortriptyline (Menza et al., 2009). Other studies have evaluated the antidepressant effect of antiparkinsonian medication. Most recently it has been shown that depressive symptoms in PD can be treated with the dopamine agonist pramipexole (Barone et al., 2010). Of 287 patients with mild to moderate PD on stable antiparkinsonian therapy 139 received 0.125 - 1.0 mg pramipexole three times a day and 148 received placebo each over 12 weeks. Significant therapeutic effects of pramipexole on Beck's depression inventory as well as in the UPDRS motor scores were found. Therefore, pramipexole may be a favorable primary choice for patients with PD and depression.

2.3 Psychoses in PD

Epidemiology: Hallucinations, illusions and delusions are the main psychotic symptoms in PD. Among these hallucinations are the most common with visual hallucinations being much more frequent than acoustic hallucinations. Tactile hallucinations are less frequent and prevalence rates are not well-established. Olfactory hallucinations should be regarded as unusual in PD and there are occasional reports on this type of phenomenon. Hallucinations occur in up to 40% of patients with PD if minor visual hallucinations like sensation of the presence of another person are included (Fénelon et al., 2000). Within the parkinsonian disorders visual hallucinations occur predominantly in PD and dementia with Lewy bodies. They are much less likely to occur in patients with progressive supranuclear palsy (PSP), multiple system atrophy (MSA) or vascular Parkinsonism and in fact this symptom has been proposed as a useful predictor for the differential diagnosis of these groups of parkinsonian syndromes (Williams et al., 2008).

Pathophysiology: In a post-mortem study of 788 brains of patients with history of parkinsonism a history of visual hallucinations predicted the existence of Lewy body pathology with 93%. On the other hand visual hallucinations were present in 50% of patients with PD and 73% of patients with LBD (Williams et al., 2008). Visual hallucinations were identified as a symptom of advanced stages of Lewy body parkinsonism and occurred in the second half of the duration of PD from onset to death in almost every patient in this study. In a longitudinal study with 5-year clinical follow up patients were divided into two groups: those who experienced hallucinations within 3 months after initiating levodopa therapy and those who experienced such hallucinations after 1 year or later. In everyone of the 12 patients who had experienced hallucinations during the first 3 months of levodopa treatment the primarily made diagnosis of PD had to be revised either due to a newly diagnosed underlying psychiatric illness or due to existence of LBD or AD with extrapyramidal signs (Goetz et al., 1998a). Therefore, very early occurrence of hallucinations should prompt a control of a diagnosis of PD. With regard to the dopamine hypothesis of schizophrenia and the fact that antipsychotic drugs all include an antidopaminergic effect it may be reasoned that the occurrence of psychosis in PD is due to the dopaminergic treatment. Indeed, it has been suggested that treatment with levodopa may "kindle" psychotic symptoms in PD (Moskovitz et al., 1978). Still, other diseases which are treated with dopaminergic agents like hyperprolactinemia do not carry an increased risk for hallucinations (Williams & Lees, 2005). Additionally, intravenous infusion of levodopa was not able to induce hallucinations in patients who experienced spontaneous hallucinations on a daily basis rendering a simple association of hallucinations to levodopa serum-levels unlikely (Goetz et al., 1998b). And importantly, hallucinations have been described in patients with PD before introduction of levodopa into therapy of PD (Diederich et al., 2009). Probably, the pathophysiology of PD itself is mainly responsible for the increased risk of hallucinations in patients with PD. Similarly, other neurodegenerative disorders like AD or LBD harbor a higher risk for the occurrence of hallucinations in the absence of dopaminergic treatments. Additionally, there appears to be a difference between the levodopa-equivalent dose between patients with hallucinations and those without hallucinations (Diederich et al., 2009). Pathophysiologically, the existence of Lewy bodies in the basolateral nucleus of the amygdala as well as in the parahippocampus and other inferior temporal regions has been identified as possible correlate of visual hallucinations (Harding et al., 2002). A correlation between cholinergic dysfunction and visual hallucinations has been recently established when the short-latency afferent inhibition - a neurophysiologic measure of inhibitory intracortical mechanisms depending on cholinergic function - was shown to be significantly reduced compared to patients with PD and compared to healthy controls without visual hallucinations (Manganelli et al., 2009).

Phenomenology: In accordance with previous statements early presence of visual hallucinations is a predictor for early mortality (Williams & Lees, 2005). Additionally, there is a correlation between visual hallucinations and cognitive dysfunction which may reflect its association with advanced disease state. Nevertheless, cognitive function of patients without visual hallucinations appears not to differ from those with minor hallucinations whereas patients with major visual hallucinations show deficits in verbal fluency tasks which are not found in patients without visual hallucinations (Llebaria et al., 2010).

In one study with 216 patients hallucinations were divided into three groups. First, minor forms of hallucinations including the feeling of the presence of somebody or something, which was also the most frequent hallucination, were grouped together. With regard to this type of hallucination, patients perceived the presence of a living or deceased relative, another person, an animal or an unidentified sensation. Within the group of the minor symptoms hallucinations of passage were identified as distinctive phenomena and were described as a brief impression of a person or animal (frequently a cat or a dog) passing by. Illusions were a second group of symptoms and were described as impression of a transformation of an object e.g. into an animal (Fénelon et al., 2000). Formed visual hallucinations and auditory hallucinations formed the other major groups of hallucinations in PD in this study. With a prevalence of approximately 10% auditory hallucinations in PD are less common than visual hallucinations and frequently do not occur alone but in association with visual hallucinations (Inzelberg et al., 1998; Fénelon et al., 2000). Auditory hallucinations are perceived as externally generated human voices. They may be incomprehensible or may be commenting familiar voices. In contrast to auditory hallucinations in schizophrenia they predominantly do not have an affective component, are not imperative and are not paranoid in character in PD (Inzelberg et al., 1998). Tactile hallucinations have been rarely reported. One study described eight patients with PD and tactile hallucinations which were always associated with simultaneously or non-simultaneously occurring visual or auditory hallucinations. Those tactile hallucinations predominantly included the sensation of contact with animals like spiders, cockroaches, grubs, mites, ants or rats. Often sensation of contact with these small animals were also subject of simultaneous visual hallucinations. They occurred predominantly in the evening or at night and were perceived as unpleasant. Interestingly and in accordance with the descriptions of visual hallucinations insight into the non-realistic nature of the phenomena was maintained or recovered within a few seconds (Fénelon et al., 2002).

Diagnosis: Only 20% percent of patients with PD spontaneously report the occurrence of hallucinations or other psychotic symptoms (Fénelon & Alves, 2010). Therefore, these symptoms should be actively asked for when examining patients and/or persons associated with the patient's care. There is no generally accepted scale for evaluation of psychotic symptoms in PD. An expert group recently suggested criteria for the diagnosis of PD associated with psychosis. First, at least one of the symptoms of hallucinations, illusions, delusions or false sense of presence has to be present. Second, the primary diagnosis of PD has to be established according to the UK Brain Bank criteria for PD. Third, the onset of PD has to precede the onset of the psychotic symptoms mentioned first. Fourth, the symptoms occur recurrently or continuously for at least one month. Fifth, other possible causes of parkinsonism and psychiatric disorders have to be excluded. Sixth, it should be specified if symptoms occurred a)with or without insight, b)with or without preexisting dementia and c) if they were associated with a specific treatment for PD (Ravina et al., 2007).

Therapy: Upon occurrence of psychotic symptoms in PD possible reversible causes have to be excluded. First, any association to changes of the patients antiparkinsonian treatment has to be reviewed. If there is no recent change in medication which could explain the onset of psychotic symptoms modification of the patients' medication should follow a distinct sequence which ranks the psychotic potential of different classes of drugs used in the treatment of patients with PD. According to the guidelines of the German Neurological Association 1) anticholinergic substances and tricyclic antidepressants which carry anticholinergic side-effects should be discontinued. 2) budipine, amantadine and inhibitors of the mono-amino-oxidase-B (MAO-B) should be reduced or discontinued, 3) dopamine-agonists should be reduced or discontinued, 4) inhibitors of the catechyl-O-methyl-transferase (COMT) should be reduced or discontinued, 5) therapy with levodopa may be reduced to its lowest effective dose if reduction/discontinuation of one or more of the previously listed substances did not to lead to relief from psychotic symptoms (Eggert et al., 2008). Secondary, a relation to the treatment with other drugs e.g. antibiotics that can increase the likelihood of psychotic symptoms should be assessed. Third, acute infection or imbalance of serum electrolytes should be excluded. Restitution of the dopaminergic deficit caused by cell loss of the neurons of the pars compacta of the substantia nigra is the leading mechanisms of most antiparkinsonian drugs. On the other hand antipsychotic drugs all act antidopaminergic based on the dopamine-hypothesis of psychosis. Most of the classic antipsychotic drugs especially of the butyrophenon group exhibit a high affinity to several D (=dopamine)-receptors especially the D2-receptors. Therefore most antipsychotic drugs can not be used in PD. However, for therapy of psychosis or hallucinations in PD the group of atypical antipsychotics is much better tolerated from patients with PD due to a more favorable mechanism of action. A fast dissociation of atypical neuroleptics from the D2-receptor has been proposed as possible explanation for the comparatively good tolerability in patients with PD therefore being first-line therapeutics in Parkinson patients with psychotic symptoms (Kapur & Seeman, 2001). Notably, quetiapine or clozapine are the preferred antipsychotic drugs in patients with PD. Clozapine is the drug of choice for the treatment of psychosis in patients with PD and is used in a low-dose range of 25-100 mg/d.

It acts predominantly on the D4-dopaminergic receptor and therefore has less impact on the striatonigral dopaminergic system which exhibits predominantly D1- and D2-receptors. Several studies have proven the effectiveness of clozapine in treating psychotic symptoms in PD. One rater-blinded study compared quetiapine and clozapine use in 27 patients with PD and psychosis. Both drugs were effective in treating psychosis based on the clinical global impression of change scale (CGIC). Whereas clozapine was more efficient in treating delusions it induced leucopenia in one case (Merims et al., 2006). Clozapine has proven its efficacy in a randomized, double-blind, placebo-controlled trial with 60 patients who received either placebo or clozapine in a dose of 50 mg or less for 4 weeks while the antiparkinsonian medication was left stable. A significant improvement in all clinical rating scales was demonstrated and importantly there was no deterioration of motor symptoms. But one case of leucopenia occurred (The Parkinson Study Group, 1999). Side-effects of clozapine are sleepiness, dysarthria, weight gain which are dose-dependent and less common in patients with PD psychosis as compared to patients with schizophrenia where much higher doses of up to 1000 mg per day are used. However, the risk of agranulocytosis of clozapine requires regular blood counts and depending on individual legislations the patient needs to be carefully instructed regarding benefits and risks and informed consent may be obtained before starting a treatment with clozapine. Quetiapine is the second atypical antipsychotic used in patients with PD. Its effect is probably mainly mediated by antagonistic effects on 5HT2-, D1- and D2-receptors with a higher selectivity for 5HT2-receptors. Common side effects of quetiapine include sedation, hypotension, increase in weight and change of blood sugar and lipids. Moreover, there have been case reports of agranulocytosis, prolactin elevation and rhabdomyolysis under therapy with quetiapine (Stephani & Trenkwalder, 2010). Whereas the efficacy of clozapine has been proven by blinded studies a double-blind study which compared quetiapine use to placebo in patients with PD and psychosis over a three-month interval found no significant effect in any clinical scale evaluated (Rabey et al., 2006). The number of patients in this study was rather small due to a significant drop-out rate which may have influenced the results. Indeed, the result of this trial contrasts with the clinical experience which favors a beneficial role of quetiapine for treatment of psychosis in PD. And currently the use of quetiapine for the treatment of psychotic symptoms in patients with PD is widely accepted despite the inconclusive evidence on the topic. It has been proposed that this discrepancy of negative studies and positive clinical evaluation may be due to the sedative (side-)effect of quetiapine rather than a direct anti-hallucinatory effect (Diederich et al., 2009). Doses of up to 300 mg quetiapine a day are currently applied in patients with PD. Aside from pharmacotherapy, patients experiencing visual hallucinations naturally often use coping strategies. These have been categorized into visual techniques, cognitive techniques and interactive techniques (Diederich et al., 2003). Visual techniques include focusing on the hallucination or defocusing. With cognitive techniques the patient should try to actively remain conscious about the hallucinatory or illusionary nature of the psychotic symptom. Interactive techniques would describe any technique that requires participation of others. Patients may be asked for application of such techniques and may be instructed on if required. However, there are no controlled studies on the effectiveness of this kind of therapeutic approach.

2.4 Impulse control disorders

The chapter on mental and behavioral disorders of the 10th revision of the international statistical classification of diseases and related health problems (ICD-10) lists 4 specific habit and impulse control disorders which are pathological gambling (F63.0), pyromania (F63.1), kleptomania (F63.2) and trichotillomania (F63.3). Whereas pathological gambling is a well-known impulse control disorder in patients with PD there is no report of pyromania in patients with PD available. Anecdotal reports of kleptomania and trichotillomania in PD exist but there is no study on their frequency in patients with PD compared to controls. In addition to pathologic gambling there are other specific psychiatric disorders that have been found to exist in patients with PD and that are not listed in the group of impulse control disorders in the ICD-10 but share characteristics with disorders of the impulse control. Hypersexuality is currently neither directly classified in the DSM-IV of the American psychiatric association nor in the ICD-10. Excessive sexual drive (F52.7) is classified in the latter within the subsection of sexual dysfunctions and comprises those deviations classically named satyriasis and nymphomania. Similarly, binge-eating can be a impulse control disorder-like psychiatric comorbidity in patients with PD. Binge-eating most closely corresponds to the symptom of overeating (F50.4) among the non-organic eating disorders classified in the ICD-10. Oniomania which is compulsive shopping again is not a specified symptom in the current psychiatric classifications and therefore may be ranked within the category of "other impulse control disorders" (F63.8) of the ICD-10. These disorders have been also described as repetitive and reward-seeking behaviors or behavioral addictions concepts that considerably overlap with that of compulsive or impulsive control disorders. These disorders are regarded as dopamine replacement related-disorders therefore being extrinsically generated and not directly depending on PD itself (Wolters et al., 2008).

2.4.1 Pathological gambling

According to the ICD-10 of the World Health Organization (WHO) pathological gambling consists of "frequent, repeated episodes of gambling that dominate the patient's life to the detriment of social, occupational, material, and family values and commitments" (World Health Organization, 2007b). Pathological gambling was found to have a lifetime prevalence of 0.42% in a large US cohort (Petry et al., 2005). In patients with PD this trait was reported in more than 7% of those who were on a dopamine agonist (Voon et al., 2006a). The overall lifetime prevalence of pathologic gambling in PD has been reported to be 3.4% and the point prevalence was reported with 1.7% (Voon et al., 2006b). Similarly, in a prospective study of 388 consecutive PD clinic patients a prevalence of pathological gambling of 4.4% in general. and of 8% in patients treated with dopamine agonists was demonstrated (Grosset et al., 2006). Pathological gambling as a psychiatric comorbidity of PD can be largely attributed to therapy with dopamine agonists or levodopa and has been recognized in patients with restless legs syndrome treated with dopamine agonists as well (Pourcher et al., 2010). Confirmatory, there is no evidence for an increased prevalence of this trait in untreated patients with PD (O'Sullivan & Lees, 2007). A younger age of onset of PD, a higher novelty seeking personality profile and an impaired planning capacity each compared to patients with PD but without impulse control or compulsive behaviors have been recognized as factors associated with the occurrence of pathological gambling in PD. A positive personal or immediate family history of alcohol use disorders is a risk factor for developing pathological gambling indicating a genetic predisposition (Voon et al., 2007). Pathophysiologically, a functional magnetic resonance imaging (fMRI) study with 12 female patients with restless legs syndrome without pathological gambling who were under chronic therapy with dopamine agonists showed that the ventral striatal activation upon receipt or omission of rewards in a gambling task during dopaminergic treatment differed significantly from that while off treatment with dopamine agonists (Abler et al., 2009). The diagnosis of pathological gambling currently is often based on the criteria of the DSM-IV. These indicate persistent and recurrent maladaptive gambling behavior as indicated by five (or more) of the following: the patient 1) "is preoccupied with gambling", 2) "needs to gamble with increasing amounts of money in order to achieve the desired excitement", 3) "has repeated unsuccessful efforts to control, cut back, or stop gambling", 4) "is restless or irritable when attempting to cut down or stop gambling", 5) "gambles as a way of escaping from problems or of relieving a dysphoric mood", 6) "after losing money gambling, often returns another day to get even", 7) "lies to family members, therapist, or others to conceal the extent of involvement with gambling", 8) "has jeopardized or lost a significant relationship, job, or educational or career opportunity because of gambling", 9) "relies in other to provide money to relieve a desperate financial situation caused by gambling". Additionally, a manic episode as possible underlying cause needs to be excluded (American Psychiatric Association, 2010b). A history of illegal acts like forgery, fraud theft, embezzlement to finance gambling is currently a 10th possible criterion for the diagnosis of pathological gambling but is not included in the proposed revision for the DSM-5 which is scheduled to be released 2013. Importantly, the work group for this revision also proposes to reclassify the diagnosis from an impulse-control disorder into a substance-related disorder (American Psychiatric Association, 2010b). The therapy of choice of pathological gambling in PD is the discontinuation of the dopamine agonist and replacement by an adequate dose of levodopa. In fact, 15 patients with PD and pathological gambling were followed up for 21 months on average. In all of them the treatment with dopamine agonists had been discontinued and was replaced by levodopa. All of them reported cessation of the pathological gambling even though one patient reported to have a continuing urge to gamble (Macphee et al., 2009). If levodopa itself is the suspected cause of pathological gambling dose reduction will be necessary.

2.4.2 Hypersexuality

In a large multicentre study the prevalence of compulsive sexual behavior in patients with PD was 3.5% (Weintraub et al., 2010). Others found lifetime prevalence rates of 2.4% in patients with PD with a point prevalence of 2.0%. The lifetime prevalence increased to 7.2% in patients on therapy with dopamine agonist (Voon et al., 2006b). Importantly, hypersexuality occurs nearly exclusively in male patients according to most reports. However, this symptom has been also recognized in women with PD (Cooper et al., 2009). There is a proposal for operational diagnostic criteria of symptoms defining hypersexuality. 1) maladaptive preoccupation with sexual thoughts, 2) inappropriately or excessively requesting sex from spouse or partner, 3) habitual promiscuity, 4) compulsive masturbation, 5) use of telephone sex lines or pornography, 6) paraphilias are symptoms that can define hypersexuality if one or more of them persist for at least one month and if symptoms are not exclusively due to a period of hypomania or mania. Additionally, this must cause at least one of the following 1) marked distress, 2) unsuccessful attempts to control thoughts or behavior or marked anxiety or distress due to such attempts, 3) significant time consuming 4) interference with social or occupational functioning (Voon et al., 2006b). If none of the last 4 symptoms are found while the other symptoms of hypersexuality are present subsyndromal hypersexuality may be diagnosed. Dopaminergic drugs are a significant risk factor for the occurrence of hypersexuality in

PD. They are present in 90% of those patients with PD developing the disorder. Additionally, symptoms may resolve as soon as dopamine agonists are discontinued while continuing treatment with levodopa. Also association with other obsessive or addictive symptoms is frequent (Klos et al., 2005). An association to depression has been described and it is not clear whether there is any functional dependency between both symptoms. Therapeutically, the medical history of the patients needs to be controlled for any temporal relation of the occurrence of pathological gambling to installation of a dopamine agonist therapy. If applicable a treatment with such a dopamine agonist should be reduced or replaced by an equivalent dose of levodopa. Persisting symptoms may then even warrant other therapeutic options like general reduction of the dopaminergic treatment. There is no evidence for specific pharmacologic treatments of hypersexuality in PD.

2.4.3 Obsessive eating

The prevalence of obsessive eating or binge-eating among patients with PD was 1% in a recent analysis while subthreshold binge eating was diagnosed in about 8% (Zahodne et al., 2011). However, in a cross-sectional study with 3000 patients with PD binge eating was diagnosed in 5.6% (Antonini & Cilia, 2009). The weight gain often is significant and an average gain of 13 ± 7 kg has been found in 7 patients with this disorder (Nirenberg & Waters, 2005). As in other impulse control disorders in PD the major risk factor is the use of a dopamine agonist of which pramipexole based on the existing literature has been most often associated with obsessive eating. Other risk factors include a young age of onset of PD, a personal or direct family history of addictive behavior as well as a novelty seeking and impulsive personality profile. A mechanism based on stimulation of the mesolimbic dopaminergic reward system which is probably common to the impulse control disorders recognized in PD has been proposed as being causative for obsessive eating. Again, discontinuation of dopamine agonists is effective based on evidence from case reports (Nirenberg & Waters, 2005; Khan & Rana, 2010).

2.4.4 Oniomania

This symptom also known as compulsive shopping is characteristic of manic episodes of psychiatric patients. In the absence of uni- or bipolar disorders it is currently not further specified in the classification systems of mental diseases. Still, its prevalence in a large study of patients with PD was described with 7.2% (Antonini & Cilia, 2009). A current prevalence of oniomania of 0.7% was reported in another study demonstrating the tentativeness of the current data (Voon et al., 2006b). Still, in general the prevalence of oniomania appears to be lower than that of pathologic gambling or hypersexuality (Ceravolo et al., 2010). Due to a scarcity of data specific risk factors for oniomania are not established. Most studies report general risk factors for developing impulse control disorders in PD with oniomania among them. Most significant risks for developing an oniomania are the younger age of onset of PD and a personal or family history of addictive behavior (Ceravolo et al., 2010; Voon et al., 2006b). Diagnosis of oniomania in PD requires exclusion of a general hypomanic or manic episode. Oniomania is time-consuming and distressing and results in financial, family-related or social problems (McElroy et al., 1994). The therapy again relies on the adjustment of the patients antiparkinsonian medication especially in the withdrawal from dopamine agonists. Additionally, the patients access to money or shopping opportunities may be regulated if possible.

3. Conclusion

Cognitive and psychiatric consequences of Parkinson's disease have a major impact on patients as well as caregivers. They affect the majority of patients with Parkinson's disease to some extent. Dementia, depression and psychotic symptoms are very common traits of advanced parkinsonism and especially affect elderly patients. Still they remain untreated not infrequently. Impulse control disorders are less common in Parkinson's disease and are related to the medical treatment and early onset parkinsonism. Their possibly devastating implications require awareness of the treating physician. Therapeutic options for the cognitive and psychiatric aspects of Parkinson's disease will benefit from future research efforts.

4. Acknowledgment

This work has been supported by the grant ZN 2187 of the Niedersachsen-Israel Research Cooperation Program, and by the DFG, grant NI 683/6-1.

5. References

Aarsland, D., Ballard, C., Walker, Z., et al. (2009). Memantine in patients with Parkinson's disease dementia or dementia with Lewy bodies: a double-blind, placebo-controlled, multicentre trial. *Lancet Neurology*, Vol. 8, pp. 613-618.

Aarsland, D. & Kurz, M.W. (2010). The epidemiology of dementia associated with Parkinson's disease. *Brain pathology*, Vol. 20, pp. 633-639.

Aarsland, D., Zaccai, J. & Brayne, C. (2005). A systematic review of prevalence studies of dementia in Parkinson's disease. *Movement Disorders*, Vol. 20, pp. 1255–1263.

Abler, B., Hahlbrock, R., Unrath, A., et al. (2009). At-risk for pathological gambling: imaging neural reward processing under chronic dopamine agonists. *Brain*, Vol. 132, pp. 2396-2402.

Alves, G., Kurz, M., Lie, S.A., et al. (2004). Cigarette smoking in Parkinson's disease: influence on disease progression. *Movement Disorders*, Vol. 19, pp. 1087-1092.

American Psychiatric Association (2010a). DSM-5 Development. *Available from* http://www.dsm5.org/ProposedRevisions/Pages/proposedrevision.aspx?rid=427#

American Psychiatric Association (2010b). DSM-5 Development. *Available from* http://www.dsm5.org/ProposedRevisions/Pages/proposedrevision.aspx?rid=210#

Antonini, A. & Cilia, R. (2009). Behavioural adverse effects of dopaminergic treatments in Parkinson's disease: incidence, neurobiological basis, management and prevention. *Drug safety*, Vol. 32, pp. 475-488.

Barone, P., Poewe, W., Albrecht, S., et al. (2010). Pramipexole for the treatment of depressive symptoms in patients with Parkinson's disease: a randomized, double.-blind, placebo-controlled trial. *The Lancet Neurology*, Vol. 9, pp. 573-580.

Bibl, M., Mollenhauer, B., Esselmann, H., et al. (2006). CSF amyloid-β-peptides in Alzheimer's disease, dementia with Lewy bodies and Parkinson's disease dementia. *Brain*, Vol. 129, pp. 1177-1187.

Bohnen, N.I., Kaufer, D.I., Hendrickson, R., et al. (2007). Cortical cholinergic denervation is associated with depressive symptoms in Parkinson's disease and parkinsonian dementia. *Journal of Neurology Neurosurgery and Psychiatry*, Vol. 78, pp. 641-643.

Bonanni, L., Thomas, A., Tiraboschi, P., et al. (2008). EEG comparisons in early Alzheimer's disease, dementia with Lewy bodies and Parkinson's disease with dementia patients with a 2-year follow-up. *Brain*, Vol. 131, pp. 690-705.

Bremner, J.D., Narayan, M., Anderson, E.R., et al. (2000). Hippocampal volume reduction in major depression. *American Journal of Psychiatry*, Vol. 157, pp. 115-117.

Buter, T.C., van der Hout, A., Matthews, F.E., et al. (2008). Dementia and survival in Parkinson disease. *Neurology*, Vol. 70, pp. 1017-1022.

Ceravolo, R., Frosini, D., Rossi, C., et al. (2010). Spectrum of addictions in Parkinson's disease: from dopamine dysregulation syndrome to impulse control disorders. *Journal of Neurology*, Vol. 257, Supplement 2, pp. S276-S283.

Cooper, C.A., Jadidian, A., Paggi, M., et al. (2009). Prevalence of hypersexual behavior in Parkinson's disease patients: not restricted to males and dopamine agonist use. *International Journal of General Medicine*, Vol. 30, pp. 57-61.

De Lau, L.M.L. & Breteler, M.M.B. (2006). Epidemiology of Parkinson's disease. *The Lancet Neurology*, Vol. 5, pp. 525-535.

Devos, D., Dujardin, K., Poirot, I., et al. (2008). Comparison of desipramine and citalopram treatments for depression in Parkinson's disease: a double-blind, randomized, placebo-controlled study. *Movement Disorders*, Vol. 23, pp. 850-857.

Diederich, N.J., Pieri, V. & Goetz, C.G. (2003). Coping strategies for visual hallucinations in Parkinson's disease. *Movement Disorders*, Vol. 18, pp. 831–832.

Diederich, N.J., Fénelon, G., Stebbins, G., et al. (2009). Hallucinations in Parkinson's disease. *Nature Reviews Neurology*, Vol. 5, pp. 331-342.

Dissanayaka, N.N.W., Sellbach, A., Matheson, S., et al. (2007). Validity of Hamilton depression inventory in Parkinson's disease. *Movement Disorders*, Vol. 22, pp. 399-403.

Drevets, W.C. (2000). Neuroimaging studies of mood disorders. *Biological Psychiatry*, Vol. 48, pp. 813-829.

Duman, R.S., Malberg, J., Nakagawa, S., et al. (2000). Neuronal plasticity and survival in mood disorders. *Biological Psychiatry*, Vol. 48, pp. 732-739.

Ebmaier, K.P., Donaghey, C. & Steele, D. (2006). Recent developments and current controversies in depression. *The Lancet*, Vol. 367, pp. 153-167.

Eggert, K.M., Oertel W.H., Reichmann H., et al. (2008). Parkinson-Syndrome: Diagnostik und Therapie. In: *Leitlinien für Diagnostik und Therapie in der Neurologie*, Diener H.C. & Putzki N., pp. 82-112, Georg Thieme Verlag, Stuttgart.

Emre, M., Aarsland, D., Albanese, A., et al. (2004). Rivastigmine for dementia associated with Parkinson's disease. *The New England Journal of Medicine*, Vol. 351, pp. 2509-2518.

Emre, M., Aarsland, D., Brown, R., et al. (2007). Clinical diagnostic criteria for dementia associated with Parkinson's disease. *Movement Disorders*, Vol. 22, pp. 1689-1707.

Emre, M., Tsolaki, M., Bonucelli, U., et al. (2010). Memantine for patients with Parkinson's disease dementia or dementia with Lewy bodies: a randomised, double-blind, placebo-controlled trial. *Lancet Neurology*, Vol. 9, pp. 969-977.

Fénelon, G., Mahieux, F., Huon, R., et al. (2000). Hallucinations in Parkinson's disease-Prevalence, phenomenology and risk factors. *Brain*, Vol. 123, pp. 733-745.

Fénelon, G., Thobois, S., Bonnet, A.M., et al. (2002). Tactile hallucinations in Parkinson's disease. *Journal of Neurology*, Vol. 249, pp. 1699-1703.

Fénelon, G. & Alves, G. (2010). Epidemiology of psychosis in Parkinson's disease. *Journal of the Neurological Sciences*, Vol. 289, pp. 12-17.

Galvin J.E., Pollack, J. & Morris J.C. (2006). Clinical phenotype of Parkinson disease dementia. *Neurology*, Vol. 67, pp. 1605-1611.

Goetz, C.G., Vogel, C., Tanner, C.M. et al. (1998a). Early dopaminergic drug-induced hallucinations in parkinsonian patients. *Neurology*, Vol. 51, pp. 811-814.

Goetz, C.G., Pappert, E.J., Blasucci, L.M., et al. (1998b). Intravenous levodopa in hallucinating Parkinson's disease patients: high-dose challenge does not precipitate hallucinations. *Neurology*, Vol. 50, pp. 515-517.

Goetz, C.G., Emre, M. & Dubois, B. (2008). Parkinson's disease dementia: definitions , guidelines, and research perspective in diagnosis. *Annals of Neurology*, Vol. 64, Supplement, S81-S92.

Gotham, A.M., Brown, R.G. & Marsden, C.D. (1986). Depression in Parkinson's disease: a quantitative and qualitative analysis. *Journal of Neurology Neurosurgery and Psychiatry*, Vol. 49, pp. 416-421.

Grosset, K.A., Macphee, G., Pal, G., et al. (2006). Problematic gambling in dopamine agonists: not such a rarity. *Movement Disorders*, Vol. 21, pp. 2206-2208.

Hamet, P. & Tremblay, J. (2005). Genetics and genomics of depression. *Metabolism Clinical and Experimental*, Vol. 54, pp. 10-15.

Harding, A.J., Broe, G.A. & Halliday, G.M. (2002). Visual hallucinations in Lewy body disease relate to Lewy bodies in the temporal lobe. *Brain*, Vol. 125, pp. 391–403.

Harvey, P.D., Ferris, S.H., Cummings, J.L., et al. (2010). Evaluation of dementia rating scales in Parkinson's disease dementia. *American Journal of Alzheimer's Disease & other dementias*, Vol. 25, pp. 142-148.

Hoehn, M.M. & Yahr, M.D. (1967). Parkinsonism: onset, progression and mortality. *Neurology*, Vol. 17, pp. 427–442.

Inzelberg, R., Kipervasser, S. & Korczyn, A.D. (1998). Auditory hallucinations in Parkinson's disease. *Journal of Neurology, Neurosurgery and Psychiatry*, Vol. 64, pp. 533-535.

Kalia, M. (2005). Neurobiological basis of depression: an update. *Metabolism Clinical and Experimental*, Vol. 54, pp. 24-27.

Kapur, S. & Seeman, P. (2001). Does fast dissociation from the dopamine D2 receptor explain the action of atypical antipsychotics? A new hypothesis. *American Journal of Psychiatry*, Vol. 158, pp. 360-369.

Katzenschlager, R., Head, J., Schrag, A., et al. (2008). Fourteen-year final report of the randomized PDRG-UK trial comparing three initial treatments in PD. *Neurology*, Vol. 71, pp. 474–80.

Khan, W. & Rana, A.Q. (2010). Dopamine agonist induced compulsive eating behaviour in a Parkinson's disease patient. *Pharmacy World & Science*, Vol. 32, pp. 114-116.

Klos, K.J., Bower, J.H., Josephs, K.A., et al. (2005). Pathological hypersexuality predominantly linked to adjuvant dopamine agonist therapy in Parkinson's disease and multiple system atrophy. *Parkinsonism and Related Disorders*, Vol. 11, pp. 381-386.

Lee, E.Y., Cowan, N., Vogel, E.K., et al. (2010). Visual working memory deficits in patients with Parkinson's disease are due to both reduced storage capacity and impaired ability to filter out irrelevant information. *Brain*, Vol. 133, pp. 2677-2689.

Lemke, M.R., Fuchs, G., Gemende, I., et al. (2004). Depression and Parkinson's disease. *Journal of Neurology*, Vol.251, Supplement 6, pp. 24-27.

Leroi, I., Overshott, R., Byrne, E.J., et al. (2009). Randomized controlled trial of memantine in dementia associated with Parkinson's disease. *Movement Disorders*, Vol. 24, pp. 1217-1221.

Lisanby, S.H., McDonald, W.M., Massey, E.W., et al. (1993). Diminished subcortical nuclei in Parkinson's disease by MR imaging. *Journal of Neural Transmitters Supplement*, Vol. 40, pp. 13-21.

Litvan, I., Mega, M.S., Cummings, J.L., et al (1996). Neuropsychiatric aspects of progressive supranuclear palsy. *Neurology*, Vol. 47, pp. 1184–1189.

Litvinenko, I.V., Odinak, M.M., Mogil'naya, V.I., et al. (2008). Efficacy and safety of galantamine (reminyl) for dementia in patients with Parkinson's disease (an open controlled trial). Neuroscience and Behavioral Physiology, Vol. 38, pp. 937-945.

Llebaria, G., Pagonabarraga, J., Martínez-Corral, et al. (2010). Neuropsychological correlates of mild to severe hallucinations in Parkinson's disease. *Movement Disorders*, Vol. 25, pp. 2785-2791.

Macphee, G.J.A., Copeland, C., Stewart, D., et al. (2009). Clinical follow up of pathological gambling in Parkinson's disease in the West Scotland study. *Movement Disorders*, Vol. 24, pp. 2430-2431.

Maidment, I., Fox, C. & Boustani, M. (2006). Cholinesterase inhibitors for Parkinson's disease dementia. *Cochrane Database Systematic Reviews*, Vol. 25, CD004747.

Manganelli, F., Vitale, C., Santangelo, G., et al. (2009). Functional involvement of central cholinergic circuits and visual hallucinations in Parkinson's disease. *Brain*, Vol. 132, pp. 2350-2355.

Marder, K. (2010). Cognitive impairments and dementia in Parkinson's disease. *Movement Disorders*, Vol. 25, pp. S110-S116,

Mayberg, H. (2002). Depression II. *American Journal of Psychiatry*, Vol. 159, p. 1979.

McElroy, S.L., Keck, P.E., Pope, H.G., et al. (1994). Compulsive buying: a report of 20 cases. *Journal of Clinical Psychiatry*, Vol. 55, pp. 242-248.

Menza, M., Dobkin, R.D., Marin, H., et al. (2009). A controlled trial of antidepressants in patients with Parkinson disease and depression. *Neurology*, Vol. 72, pp. 886-892.

Merims, D., Meirav, B., Chava, P., et al. (2006). Rater-blinded, prospective comparison: quetiapine versus clozapine for Parkinson's disease psychosis. *Clinical Neuropharmacology*, Vol. 29, pp. 331-337.

Moskovitz, C., Moses, H. & Klawans, H.L. (1978). Levodopa-induced psychosis: a kindling phenomenon. *American Journal of Psychiatry*, Vol. 135, pp. 669-675.

Nirenberg, M.J. & Waters, C. (2005). Compulsive eating and weight gain related to dopamine agonist use. *Movement Disorders*, Vol. 21, pp. 524-529.

Olesen, J., Baker, M., Freund, T., et al. (2006). Consensus document on European brain research. *Journal of Neurology Neurosurgery and Psychiatry*, Vol. 77, Supplement 1, pp. i1-49.

O'Sullivan, S.S. & Lees, A.J. (2007). Pathological gambling in Parkinson's disease. *The Lancet Neurology*, Vol. 6, pp. 384-386.

Petry, N.M., Stinson, F.S. & Grant, B.F. (2005). Comorbidity of DSM-IV pathological gambling and other psychiatric disorders: results from the National Epidemiologic Survey on Alcohol and Related Conditions. *Journal of Clinical Psychiatry,* Vol. 66, pp. 564–74.

Pluck, G.C. & Brown, R.G. (2002). Apathy in Parkinson's disease. *Journal of Neurology, Neurosurgery and Psychiatry,* Vol. 73, pp. 636-642.

Poewe, W. (2006). The natural history of Parkinson's disease. *Journal of Neurology,* Vol. 253, Supplement 7, pp. 2-6.

Poewe, W., Wolters, E., Emre, M., et al. (2005). Long-term benefits of rivastigmine in dementia associated with Parkinson's disease: an active treatment extension study. *Movement Disorders,* Vol.21, pp. 456-461.

Pourcher, E., Rémillard, S. & Cohen, H. (2010). Compulsive habits in restless legs syndrome patients under dopaminergic treatment. *Journal of the Neurological Sciences,* Vol. 290, pp. 52-56.

Rabey, J.M., Prokhorov, T., Miniovitz, A., et al. (2006). Effect of quetiapine in psychotic Parkinson's disease patients: a double-blind labeled study of 3 months' duration. *Movement Disorders,* Vol. 22, pp. 313-318.

Rajkowska, G. (2000). Postmortem studies in mood disorders indicate altered numbers of neurons and glial cells. *Biological Psychiatry,* Vol. 48, pp. 766-777.

Ravina, B., Marder, K., Fernandez, H.H., et al. (2007). Diagnostic criteria for psychosis in Parkinson's disease: report of an NINDS, NIMH work group. *Movement Disorders,* Vol. 22, pp. 1061-1068.

Reijnders, J.S.A.M., Ehrt, U., Weber, W.E.J., et al. (2008). A systematic review of prevalence studies of depression in Parkinson's disease. *Movement Disorders,* Vol. 23, pp.183-189.

Riedel, O., Klotsche, J., Spottke, A., et al. (2010). Frequency of dementia, depression, and other neuropsychiatric symptoms in 1,449 outpatients with Parkinson's disease. *Journal of Neurology,* Vol. 257, pp. 1073-1082.

Schildkraut, J.J. (1965). The catecholamine hypothesis of affective disorders: a review of supporting evidence. *American Journal of Psychiatry,* Vol. 122, pp. 509-522.

Schrag, A., Barone, P., Brown, R.G., et al. (2007). Depression rating scales in Parkinson's disease: Critique and recommendations. *Movement disorders,* Vol. 22, pp. 1077-1092.

Schrag, A., Jahanshahi, M. & Quinn, N.P. (2001). What contributes to depression in Parkinson's disease? *Psychological Medicine,* Vol. 31, pp. 65-73.

Stephani, C. & Trenkwalder, C. (2010). Rhabdomyolysis after low-dose quetiapine in a patient with Parkinson's disease with drug-induced psychosis: a case report. *Movement Disorders,* Vol. 25, pp. 782-783.

Tandberg, E., Larsen, J.P., Aarsland, D., et al. (1996). The occurrence of depression in Parkinson's disease: a community-based study. *Archives of Neurology,* Vol. 53, pp. 175-179.

The Parkinson Study Group (1999). Low-dose clozapine for the treatment of drug-induced psychosis in Parkinson's disease. *The New England Journal of Medicine,* Vol. 340, pp. 757-763.

Van Laar, T., De Deyn, P.P., Aarsland, D., et al. (2010). Effects of cholinesterase inhibitors in Parkinson's disease dementia: a review of clinical data. *CNS Neuroscience & Therapeutics,* (Epub ahead of print).

Von Reichmann, H., Deuschl, G., Riedel, O., et al. (2010). The German Study on the epidemiology of Parkinson's disease with dementia (GEPAD): more than Parkinson. *MMW Fortschritte der Medizin*, Vol. 152, Supplement 1, pp. 1-6.

Voon, V., Hassan, K., Zurowski, M., et al. (2006a) Prospective prevalence of pathologic gambling and medication association in Parkinson disease. *Neurology*, Vol. 66, pp. 1750–52.

Voon, V., Hassan, K., Zurowski, M., et al. (2006b). Prevalence of repetitive and reward-seeking behaviors in Parkinson disease. *Neurology*, Vol. 67, pp. 1254–57.

Voon, V., Thomsen, T., Miyasaki, J.M., et al. (2007). Factors associated with dopaminergic drug-related pathological gambling in Parkinson disease. *Archives of Neurology*, Vol. 64, pp. 212-216.

Weintraub, D., Loester, J., Potenza, M.N., et al. (2010). Impulsive control disorders in Parkinson's disease: a cross-sectional study of 3090 patients. *Archives of Neurology*, Vol. 67, pp. 589-5995.

Weintraub, D., Morales, K.H., Moberg, P.J., et al. (2005). Antidepressant studies in Parkinson's disease: A review and meta-analysis. *Movement Disorders*, Vol. 20, pp. 1161-1169.

Williams, D.R. & Lees, A.J. (2005). Visual hallucinations in the diagnosis of idiopathic Parkinson's disease: a retrospective autopsy study. *The Lancet Neurology*, Vol. 4, pp. 605-610.

Williams, D.R., Warren, J.D. & Lees, A.J. (2008). Using the presence of visual hallucinations to differentiate Parkinson's disease from atypical parkinsonism. *Journal of Neurology, Neurosurgery and Psychiatry*, Vol. 79, pp. 652-655.

Winbald, B., Cummings, J., Andreasen, N., et al. (2007). A six-month double-blind, randomized, placebo-controlled study of a transdermal patch in Alzheimer's disease: Rivastigmine patch versus capsule. *International Journal of Geriatric Psychiatry*, Vol. 22, pp. 456-467.

Wolters, E.C., van der Werf, Y.D. & van den Heuvel, O.A. (2008). Parkinson's disease-related disorders in the impulsive-compulsive spectrum. *Journal of Neurology*, Vol. 255, Supplement 5, pp. 48-56.

World Health Organization (2007a). ICD-Version 2007. *Available from* http://apps.who.int/classifications/apps/icd/icd10online/?gf30.htm+f322

World Health Organization (2007b). ICD-Version 2007. *Available from* http://apps.who.int/classifications/apps/icd/icd10online/?gf60.htm+f630

Zahodne, L.B., Susatia, F., Bowers, D., et al. (2011). Binge eating in Parkinson's disease: prevalence, correlates and the contribution of deep brain stimulation. *Journal of Neuropsychiatry and Clinical Neuroscience*, Vol. 23, pp. 56-62.

Zesiewicz, T.A. & Hauser, R.A. (2002). Depression in Parkinson's disease. *Current Psychiatry Reports*, Vol. 4, pp. 69-73.

8

The Psychosocial Impact of Parkinson's Disease on the Wider Family Unit: A Focus on the Offspring of Affected Individuals

David Morley
University of Oxford
United Kingdom

1. Introduction

The psychosocial effects of Parkinson's disease (PD) on those affected by the condition are well documented (e.g. Calne et al., 2008; Frisina et al., 2008; Morley et al., 2007a; Ravina et al., 2007; Schrag et al., 2003; Slawek et al., 2005). A significant body of literature has also emerged investigating the impact of PD on affected individual's spouses and carers (e.g. Carter et al., 1998; Dyck, 2009; Lökk, 2008; Morley et al., 2007b; O'Connor & McCabe, 2010; Schrag et al., 2006). Perhaps surprisingly however, the impact of parental PD on the psychosocial adjustment and quality of life of both young and grown up children has, until recently, received little attention. Although Parkinson's disease is commonly regarded as a disease of the elderly a significant number are diagnosed before the age of fifty, and in approximately 5-10% the condition is apparent prior to age forty (Clarke & Moore, 2007). There is, therefore, the potential for children of a range of ages, young to adult, to be affected in a variety of ways by their parent's condition.

Previous studies focusing on children's response to a range of parental conditions and disabilities identify a number of recurrent themes. For example, children report elevated levels of depression and anxiety (Black et al., 2003; Forehand et al., 1988; Somers, 2007; Visser-Meily, et al., 2005; Yahav et al., 2007). Additionally, many experience changing roles and heightened responsibility (Caton et al., 1998; Strunin & Boden, 2004; Yahav et al., 2007). The provision of information for children regarding their parent's condition is also frequently raised (Caton et al., 1998; Cross & Rintell, 1999; Mukherjee et al, 2002). Previous studies also indicate that not all parental conditions affect children similarly. For example, some have suggested that children of parents with spinal cord injury appear well-adjusted to their parent's condition (Alexander et al., 2002; Buck & Hohmann, 1981). Additionally, children of parents with inflammatory bowel disease report some positive as well as negative responses to their parent's condition (Mukherjee et al, 2002).

The aims of this chapter are to present the emerging body of literature that focuses specifically on the impact of parental Parkinson's. The development of a questionnaire, the Parental Illness Impact Scale, (Schrag et al., 2004a; Morley et al., 2010a) to measure this impact has significantly aided research and allowed the field to move forward from earlier qualitative work. The development of this questionnaire is briefly outlined in the coming chapter. Research that has followed indicates that the children of people with Parkinson's

(PWP) can be affected in a number of ways. Evidence highlights potential difficulties in areas such as emotional well-being, changing roles, concerns for the future and relationships with friends. A number of these factors appear associated with key demographic variables such as a child's age or the duration of their parent's Parkinson's (Schrag et al., 2004b; Morley, 2008). There is also evidence that certain family structure variables may be implicated in children's response to their parent's condition. For example, research indicates that children without the support of siblings show inferior adjustment to parental illness when compared to those with brothers and sisters (Morley et al., 2010b). Issues surrounding sources of support and the provision of information for children regarding their parent's condition are also frequently raised (Schrag et al., 2004b; Morley et al., 2005; Morley, 2008; Morley et al., 2011). Emotional well-being has also been assessed and children of PWP appear at heightened risk of depression when compared to the normal population (Schrag et al., 2004b; Morley et al., 2005; Morley, 2008). Over the coming pages these research findings will be discussed in greater detail, and the chapter will conclude by discussing limitations in current research and making recommendations for future investigations.

2. Early research investigating the impact of parental Parkinson's

The report compiled for the United Kingdom Parkinson's Disease Society by Roger Grimshaw (1991) was, to the best of the author's knowledge, the first to focus specifically on the offspring of parents with Parkinson's disease. As the first of its kind the importance of this work should not be underestimated, particularly in light of it being a catalyst for later research. In his research Grimshaw took a qualitative approach and focused on the perspectives of pre-adolescent children aged 5-12, and young people aged 16-24.

The work of Grimshaw (1991) built on a number of factors identified in previous research with families of those affected by chronic illness and disability such as that by Thurman (1985) and Rolland (1988). Such factors included, for example, the examination of styles of communication and those resources upon which families are able to draw when dealing with change. The research of Thurman and Rolland placed emphasis on the differing stages that individuals and families pass through, and also on the importance of gaining insight into how changes have specific impact at particular points in the lives of both parents and their children. Grimshaw, however, extended this and identified the need to view childhood as an 'active and responsive phase' in an individual's social development. Furthermore, he suggested the family is set in a far wider social context, as a 'social institution concerned with dependence', be that in relation to the elderly, the sick or more junior members. That a sense of obligation on the part of children to parents arises as a consequence of this 'social arrangement' is regarded as a foreseeable outcome. The equivalent concern of parents in not becoming a burden to their offspring is similarly viewed. In viewing the family unit in such a manner, Grimshaw postulated that it is important not to disregard aspects such as the gender of individual members and the affect this might have on how each might respond. Similarly issues of ethnic variations between families, the role of material circumstances, and accessibility of appropriate services are all areas that need to be taken into consideration. The final report of Grimshaw highlighted a number of pertinent factors when children are confronted with parental Parkinson's. These included children's changing roles, both domestic and emotional, within the family of a parent with PD, as well as relationships with both the well and unwell parent. Clear issues regarding children's social and emotional development and well-being, their level of independence, perceptions of disease, and fears for the future were documented.

The data collected by Grimshaw was qualitative in nature and achieved via family case studies through semi-structured interviews. This approach aimed to gain a greater understanding of the processes through which parents and children react to change and then develop new ways of living. Importance was attached to concentrating not solely on the negative experiences of children, but also on displaying how their experiences and perceptions uncover a variety of issues that have been confronted, some successfully, others less so. However, as Grimshaw himself acknowledged, a qualitative approach does not allow generalisations to be made regarding outcomes for a broader population. The qualitative nature of this research is therefore a major limitation, as is the selective nature and small size of the sample, which consisted of just thirteen participants. A major challenge for investigating this area further therefore was the development of a tool that allowed for greater generalistaion and the work of Grimshaw proved to be a catalyst for further investigation into the impact of parental Parkinson's.

3. Development of the Parental Illness Impact Scale (PIIS)

The Parental Illness Impact Scale (PIIS) evolved as a direct result of the previously discussed findings of Grimshaw (1991), firstly in an attempt to expand on this work, and secondly to take a quantitative rather than qualitative approach in investigating the impact of parental Parkinson's. The PIIS has been central to recent research, the findings of which will be discussed in a later section. Here the aim is to briefly outline the development and validation of the scale which to date has been subject to two major phases.

3.1 Initial development and validation of the PIIS

The initial development of the PIIS (Schrag et al., 2004a) was based on the qualitative data generated by Grimshaw (1991). Through a basic content analysis of the findings of this study, the original PIIS was constructed around a quality of life (QoL) model. As a concept it is generally agreed that QoL is multidimensional in nature, and is composed of differing domains. For example, one model of QoL put forward by Felce and Perry (1995) proposes the five principle dimensions of physical well-being, material well-being, social well-being, development and activity, and emotional well-being. Such dimensions are generally reflected in most models and regarded as significant in how an individual perceives their own QoL. It is worth noting however that despite the many advances in QoL research, there is still a degree of disagreement and no overriding consensus on a universally agreed definition (Dijkers, 2007; Moons et al., 2006). Recently there has been a move towards the inclusion of spirituality, religion, and personal beliefs as an additional dimension (O'Connell & Skevington, 2005; WHOQOL SRPB Group, 2006), although it has been suggested that this requires further investigation due to difficulties in its measurement (Molzhan, 2007; Moreira-Almeida & Koenig, 2006).

The preliminary version of the PIIS was comprised of 75 questions, 53 answerable on a 5-point Likert scale, and a further set of 22 dichotomous questions focusing on the provision of information and support. The questionnaire was administered to 89 children of parents with Parkinson's disease and subjected to psychometric analysis resulting in a questionnaire of 60 items, 38 answerable on a 5-point Likert scale, and 22 dichotomous questions. The authors concluded that the instrument demonstrated adequate psychometric properties. A number of limitations were identified, in particular weaknesses in the method of item generation, the self-selecting sample and the relatively small size of this sample. It was also recommended that the instrument be further validated with children of alternative parental conditions.

3.2 Further development and validation of the PIIS

The second phase of development of the PIIS aimed to address a number of the limitations of the original instrument as well as incorporate the recommendations of Schrag et al (2004a). The revised PIIS (PIIS-R; Morley et al., 2010a) was subject to a number of recognised procedures in the development of scientifically sound questionnaires. Key informant interviews and a literature review were conducted to ensure all relevant themes were incorporated in the revised instrument. Pre-testing was conducted through a 17 member expert panel and cognitive interviews with eight adolescent and adult children. The revised instrument was administered to 169 children of people with Parkinson's disease, multiple sclerosis and stroke, and subsequently subjected to a psychometric analysis. An outline of the structure of the PIIS-R along with reliability coefficients is given in Table 1.

Subscale	Number of Questions	Reliability (Cronbach's α)
Burden of Daily Help	8	.84
Emotional Impact	4	.83
Social Impact	6	.83
Communication & Understanding	7	.75
Impact on Personal Future	3	.84
Friends Reactions	3	.79
Parent / Child Relationship	3	.56
Global Well-Being	3	.73
PIIS-R Total	37	.92

Table 1. The Revised Parental Impact Scale: Outline Structure

The item reduction technique of principal components analysis was performed and resulted in 8 subscales, comprised of 37 items. The revised instrument showed good concurrent and discriminant validity through correlations with established measures of quality of life and psychosocial well-being. Internal consistency (Cronbach's α .92) was high, and test-retest reliability values for subscales (r = .58 - .78) and total score (r = .78) were moderate to high. Whilst these results suggest the PIIS-R is a robust tool with which to measure the impact of parental illness, the authors acknowledged that a number of limitations still remain. The sample was again self-selected due to the mode of recruitment, and therefore responses on which the development of the PIIS-R was based may not have been representative of the target population. The sample was also largely of White-British origin, and therefore the reliability of the scale needs to be further assessed in alternative community samples. The authors also recommended that analysis of the psychometric properties of the PIIS-R continue with further administration, preferably in even larger samples. Longitudinal data would also provide the opportunity for further properties, such as predictive validity and sensitivity to change, to be assessed.

4. Current research findings

The administration of the PIIS and PIIS-R in conjunction with other validated questionnaires has generated the first quantitative data assessing the potential impact on children on having a parent with Parkinson's. This section summarises key findings in relation to QoL and emotional well-being that should be of relevance to both clinicians and service providers, as well as provide some direction for future research.

4.1 Quality of life

As previously stated, the PIIS and subsequent revised version were constructed broadly around a QoL model. Studies to date indicate that the QoL of the offspring of parents with Parkinson's can be affected in a number of ways and dependent on a number of key factors, and particularly a number of demographic variables which are outlined below.

4.1.1 Age of child

In the first quantitative assessment of offspring of PWP, Schrag et al. (2004b) reported significant associations between childrens' age and a number of factors relating to QoL as measured by the PIIS. Results suggested that the younger the child the greater their perceived burden of daily help, and the greater the degree of difficulty in relationships with friends. Conversely, and as might be expected, the older the child the greater the recognition of the effects of PD on both their well and unwell parent. The authors of this study also make comparisons between a group aged 12-24 and those aged 25 and above, the results largely supporting the associations reported above. The younger sample reported a significantly heightened sense of burden in relation to their contribution to daily help in the parental home. As might be expected they also reported far greater difficulty in dealings with friends. The older sample reported a significantly heightened impact on family functioning.
Morley (2008) further assessed associations between age and QoL incorporating the PIIS-R. Results confirmed those of Schrag et al. (2004b) in relation to perceived burden of daily help and relationships with friends. Findings also suggested that the perceived impact on children's personal future increases as they get older. This is perhaps unsurprising since, with increasing age, children may become progressively more aware and realistic about their parent's condition. They are also better equipped educationally and emotionally to deal with the realistic prospects of their parent's condition (Lewandowski, 1992). What this data highlights is that children may require different types of support at different ages, and this needs to be considered in the management of their adjustment to parental Parkinson's.

4.1.2 Parental disease duration

Schrag et al. (2004b) reported a reduction in overall QoL as parental disease duration increases. Such a pattern was also evident in three particular subscales of the PIIS. Longer disease duration was associated with worsening communication and understanding, reduced development and independence, and increased impact on family functioning. Morley (2008) reported similar findings with longer disease duration again associated with inferior communication and understanding and deteriorating parent / child relationships. Such results reflect the progressive nature of PD and its impact on the child and highlight the need for ongoing support as the parental condition advances.

4.1.3 Sibling support

To the best of the author's knowledge just one study to date has focused on the availability of siblings as a factor in adjustment to parental neurological illness. Morley et al. (2010b) assessed the importance of sibling support within the family unit on adolescent and adult children's response to parental Parkinson's, multiple sclerosis (MS), and stroke. Participants without siblings reported significantly greater emotional impact, elevated social impact, inferior communication and understanding with their affected parent, and heightened concerns for their personal future, as measured by the PIIS-R (Morley et al., 2010a). Total QoL scores were also significantly lower for children without the support of siblings. It is reasonable to speculate that these results reflect an inability to access support from siblings. This fits well with the Compensatory Siblings Hypothesis (Boer et al., 1992) where siblings use each other as a resource to make up for deficiencies in the parent-child relationship. This theory, however, is controversial and is contradicted by the Congruence Hypothesis (Sanders, 2004). Consistent with social learning theory the Congruence Hypothesis' contends that it is positive interactions between children and their parents that fosters positive interactions between the siblings themselves.

Results from this study should be met with a degree of caution. Although a sample of 168 adolescent and adult children participated, only 16 were 'only children'. Additionally, participants came from a range of parental neurological conditions and there are, therefore, limitations as to what can be concluded specifically in relation to parental PD. The results, however, stress the importance of recognising that children without the support of brothers or sisters may be at greater risk of responding negatively to their parent's condition, and this should be considered in the management of family adjustment to the parental condition.

4.2 Availabilty of information and support

The PIIS and the revised instrument incorporate a number of dichotomous questions focusing on the availability of support and information. Schrag et al. (2004b) reported that more than half of their sample (53.9%) felt they did not have enough information about PD, with an even greater proportion (67.4%) feeling they did not know enough about what would happen to their parent as their Parkinson's progressed. Nearly half of all participants (49.4%) felt that more information would lessen feelings of uncertainty and insecurity, with the same percentage relying solely on their parents as a source of information about PD. Morley (2008) reported similar results with 37.5% feeling they did not have enough information about their parent's PD and over half (53.8%) not knowing enough about what will happen to their affected parent in the future. This study also found 61.1% relying solely on their parents as a source of information about PD. These results and those of previous studies with alternative parental conditions (i.e. Caton, et al., 1998; Cross & Rintell, 1999; Mukherjee, 2002) emphasise the need to have appropriate and accessible information available for children of all ages of parents with PD.

Regarding provision of help Schrag et al. (2004b) reported 69.7% of participants wanting greater levels of help from local services, and 48.3% feeling it would be helpful if they had some influence over help provided. Of those families who participated in the study 55.1% had outside help available to help care for their parent with PD. Only 40% of families had access to support from local services, whilst approximately 60% thought more support should be provided. Again, Morley (2008) largely mirrors these results with 61% feeling greater levels of help should be provided by services and 40.5% suggesting it would help to be able to talk to relevant services about the care provided for their affected parent. Just 40.8% of families were receiving external help. Such results highlight the need for services to firstly be available where required and secondly to engage with affected families regarding the level and nature of their provision.

4.3 Emotional well-being

Emotional well-being has been assessed in two studies to date, with both indicating elevated levels of depression in the offspring of PWP compared to levels in the general population. Incorporating the Beck Depression Inventory (Beck et al., 1961) for adults and Birleson Depression Self Rating Scale (Birleson, 1981) for adolescent participants, Schrag, et al. (2004b) reported 17.2% of 12-24 year olds and 21.7% of participants aged 25 and above as mildly to moderately depressed. Morley (2008) reported 12.5% of adolescent and 17.7% of adult children experiencing mild to moderate depression. Prevalence of depression in adults in the general population is estimated at 5%-10% (Singleton et al., 2003) and in adolescents at 4%-8% (Hazell, 2002; Son & Kirchner,2000). As has been reported in other studies, the key to the effective treatment of depression remains its recognition and treatment in both adolescents and adults (Rowe et al., 2004; Kessler et al, 1999). It is therefore important that children confronted with parental PD, be they young or adult, are recognised as being at increased risk of mental health problems, as is supported by the levels of self-reported depression reported in studies of alternative chronic progressive conditions such as multiple sclerosis (Pakenham & Bursnall, 2006; Steck, et al., 2006; Yahav, et al., 2005, 2007).

5. Future research

The following section attempts to identify current limitations and some key areas for future research that should facilitate further recognition of the impact of parental Parkinson's, help in developing practical strategies to assist in its management and inform the development of evidence based guidelines.

5.1 Longitudinal study

There is a limit to what can be concluded from cross-sectional studies such as those currently undertaken with children of parents with PD. Longitudinal study is required in order in order to assess families over time and follow the course of social, emotional, physical and practical adjustment. This is particularly important with chronic progressive conditions such as Parkinson's, as it is likely that the impact on the child and the pressures they face, such as the decision to leave home, will become more profound as their affected parent's condition advances. A longitudinal approach might also highlight differences not evident from current cross-sectional studies. For example, current data shows minimal differences between males and females in their response to parental PD. Research suggests, however, that females rely emotionally on their parents more than males (Moore, 1987), and it may be that the impact of parental PD has a greater impact on females over time. As their parent's condition deteriorates emotional support is likely to be less forthcoming and the parent themself may rely on the child for some of their emotional needs. Longitudinal study would also provide an avenue for the development of interventions, as well as the identification of those families and illness groups most 'at risk'. Despite significant advances in understanding a range of parental conditions, only in the assessment of parental affective disorder has longitudinal study made a significant contribution to the literature (i.e. Beardslee et al., 1993; Weisman et al., 1997), although important new longitudinal data is emerging regarding parental stroke (Sieh, et al., 2010; van de Port et al., 2007). Longitudinal research should therefore remain an important priority for those investigating parental PD and alternative conditions.

5.2 Comparative data

There is a limit to what can be concluded from current studies of parental PD in the absence of comparative data from adolescent and adult children with healthy parents. Few studies across a range of parental conditions have incorporated control groups to date, although some recent studies, such as those investigating adolescent children of parents with cancer (Harris & Zakowski, 2003), and adolescent children of parents with multiple sclersois (Yahav et al., 2005, 2007) have done so. This is another challenge for future research in this field. In the absence of control groups it is difficult to draw firm conclusions on a number of issues which are of importance when assessing the impact of parental illness.

5.3 Assessment of younger children

There is a further need to assess the impact of parental PD on younger children, and not solely adolescent and adult children. Although the numbers of these children are likely to be small, the implications for children below the age of 11 are likely to be just as profound, if not more so, than for older children. Support groups and workshops, such as that provided for younger children of parents with cancer (Greening, 2009) and multiple sclerosis (Mutch, 2005), may well be a valuable tool in helping younger children understand what is happening to their parent with Parkinson's. Such groups allow children to meet with other children confronted with parental illness and encourage them to discuss their fears and emotional concerns in a supportive environment. Additionally, they can be provided with information to help them better understand the nature of their parent's condition.

5.4 Assessment of alternative groups

There remain further important demographic factors and groups that need to be addressed in a comprehensive examination of factors influencing the QoL of children with Parkinson's. The need to examine different cultures is an important issue (Grimshaw, 1991). In doing so it is important to recognise that different cultures may require very different support. This is particularly so for those cultures where a far greater emphasis is placed on the social support network of the family. A comparison between ethnic minority groups and their support needs, and those of more individualised Western cultures would be an informative line of research. A further, and likely highly significant group currently not assessed are single-parent families where the parent is chronically ill, this being of particular relevance to the caring role played by children (Becker et al., 1998). The importance of investigating this group is further highlighted by research that has shown that child and adolescent rates of mental disorder are twice that in single parent families when compared with two parent families (Meltzer et al., 2000).

6. Conclusion

This chapter has presented the emerging body of research investigating adolescent and adult children's response to parental Parkinson's. It is hoped that it has highlighted the potential needs of these children and that these needs should not go unrecognised. There is, however, much further research to be done. The needs of younger chidren have yet to be assessed and longitudinal study will facilitate the development of effective interventions and information resources. Such research will help to inform evidence-based guidelines. The recognition of the needs of the offspring of PWP is lacking in current clinical guidelines for

PD due to lack of research evidence. This is in stark contrast to other chronic conditions such as MS, where a significant body research has allowed the needs of children to be included in relevant guidelines (Morley et al., 2011). It is therefore vital that further research should become a priority if we are to adequately meet the needs of children touched by the effects of parental Parkinson's.

7. References

Alexander, C. J., Hwang, K., Sipski, M.L. (2002). Mothers with spinal cord injury: impact on marital, family, and children's adjustment. *Archives of Physical Medicine & Rehabilitation,* Vol. 83, No. 1, (January 2002), pp. 24-30, ISSN 0003-9993

Beardslee, W.R., Keller, M.B., Lavori, P.W., Staley, J., Sacks, N. (1993). The impact of parental affective disorder on depression in offspring: a longitudinal follow-up in a non-referred sample. *Journal of the American Academy of Child & Adolescent Psychiatry,* Vol. 32, No. 4, (July 1993) pp. 723-730, ISSN 1527-5418

Beck, A.T., Ward, C.H., Mendelson, M., Mock, J.E., Erbaugh, J.K. (1961). An inventory for measuring depression. *Archives of General Psychiatry,* Vol. 4, No.6, (June 1961), pp. 561-571, ISSN 0003-990X

Becker, S., Aldridge, J., Dearden, C. (1998). *Young Carers and Their Families,* Oxford: Blackwell Science, ISBN 0632049669

Birleson, P. (1981). The validity of depressive disorder in childhood and the development of a self-rating scale: A Research Report. *Journal of Child Psychology & Psychiatry & Allied Disciplines,* Vol 22, No. 1, (January 1981), pp. 73-88, ISSN 0021-9630

Black, D.W., Gaffney, G.R., Schlosser, S., Gabel, J. (2003). Children of parents with obsessive-compulsive disorder -- a 2-year follow-up study. *Acta Psychiatrica Scandivanica,* Vol. 107, No. 4, (April 2003), pp. 305-313, ISSN 1600-0447

Boer, F., Goedhart, A.W., Treffers P.D.A. (1992). Siblings and their parents. In: *Children's Sibling Relationships: Developmental and Clinical Issues.* Boer, F., Dunn, J. & Dunn, J.F. (Eds.), pp. 41-54, Hillsdale, N.J: Lawrence Erlbaum Associates, ISBN 0805811079

Buck, F.M., Hohmann, G.W. (1981). Personality, behaviour, values, and family relations of children of fathers with spinal cord injury. *Archives of Physical Medicine & Rehabilitation,* Vol. 62, No. 9, (September 1981), pp. 432-438, ISSN 0003-9993

Calne, S.M., Lidstone, S.C., Kumar, A. (2008). Psychosocial issues in young-onset Parkinson's disease: Current research and challenges. *Parkinsonism & Related Disorders,* Vol. 14, No. 2, (March 2008), pp. 143-150, ISSN 1353-8020

Carter, J., Stewart, B.J., Archibold, P.G., Inoue, I., Jaglin, J., Lannon, M., Rost-Ruffner, E., Tennis, M., McDermott, M.P., Amyot, D., Barter, R., Cornelius, L., Demong, C., Dobson, J., Duff, J., Erickson, J., Gardiner, N., Gauger, L., Gray, P., Kanigan, B., Kiryluk, B., Lewis, P., Mistura, K., Malapira, T., Pay, M., Sheldon, C., Winfield, L., Wolfington-Shallow, K., Zoog, K. (1998). Living with a person who has Parkinson's disease: The spouse's perspective by stage of disease. *Movement Disorders,* Vol. 13, No. 1, (January 1998), pp. 20-28, ISSN 1531-8257

Caton, C.L.M., Cournos, F., Felix, A., Wyatt, R.J. (1998). Childhood experiences and current adjustment of offspring of indigent patients with Schizophrenia. *Psychiatric Services,* Vol. 49, No. 1, (January 1998), pp. 86-90, ISSN 1557-9700

Clarke, C.E., Moore, A.P. (2007). Parkinson's Disease. *Clinical Evidence (Online),* Accessed 07-04-11, Available from:
www.ncbi.nlm.nih.gov/pmc/articles/PMC2943804/

Cross, T., Rintell, D. (1999). Children's perceptions of parental MS. *Psychology Health & Medicine,* Vol. 4, No. 4, (November 1999), pp. 355-360, ISSN 1465-3966

Dijkers, M. (2007). "What's in a name?" The indiscriminate use of the "Quality of life" label, and the need to bring about clarity in conceptualizations. *International Journal of Nursing Studies,* Vol. 44, No. 1, (January 2007), pp. 153-155, ISSN 0020-7489

Dyck, C. (2009). Who cares for the caregiver? *Parkinsonism & Related Disorders,* Vol. 15, Suppl. 3, pp. S118-121, (December 2009), ISSN 1353-8020

Felce, D., Perry, J. (1995). Quality of Life: Its Definition and Measurement. *Research in Developmental Disabilities,* Vol. 16, No. 1, (January - February 1995), pp. 51-74, ISSN 0891-4222

Forehand, R., Steele, R., Armistead, L., Morse, E., Simon, P., Clark, L. (1988). The Family Health Project: psychosocial adjustment of children whose mothers are HIV infected. *Journal of Consulting and Clinical Psychology,* Vol. 66, No. 3, (June 1998), pp. 513-520, ISSN 0022-006X

Frisina, P.G., Borod, J.C., Foldi, N.S., Tenenbaum, H.R. (2008). Depression in Parkinson's disease: Health risks, etiology, and treatment options. *Neuropsychiatric Disease & Treatment,* Vol. 4, No. 1, (February 2008), pp. 81-91, ISSN 1178-2021

Grimshaw, R. (1991). *Children of parents with Parkinson's disease.* A research report for the Parkinson's Disease Society.

Greening, K. (1999). Support groups for children of patients with cancer. *Cancer Practice,* Vol. 7, No. 4, (July 1999), pp. 208-211, ISSN 1523-5394

Harris, C.A., Zakowski, S.G. (2003). Comparisons of distress in adolescents of cancer patients and controls. *Psycho-oncology,* Vol. 12, No. 2, (March 2003), pp. 173-182, ISSN 1009-1611

Hazell, P. (2002). Depression in children and adolescents. *Clinical Evidence,* Vol. 8, No. (December 2002), pp. 330-339, ISSN 1752-8526

Kessler, D., Lloyd, K., Lewis, G., Gray, D.P. (1999). Cross sectional study of symptom attribution and recognition of depression and anxiety in primary care. *British Medical Journal,* Vol. 318, No. 7181, (February 1999), pp. 436-440, ISSN 0959-8138

Lewandowski, L. (1992). Needs of children during the critical illness of a parent or sibling. *Critical Care Nursing Clinics of North America,* Vol. 4, No. 4, (December 1992), pp. 573-585, ISSN 0899-5885

Lökk, J. (2008). Caregiver strain in Parkinson's disease and the impact of disease duration. *European Journal of Physical & Rehabilitation Medicine,* Vol. 44, No. 1, (March 2008), pp. 39-45, ISSN 1827-1804

Meltzer, H., Gatward, R., Goodman, R., Ford, T. (2000). The mental health of children and adolescents in Great Britain. Office for National Statistics. London: The Stationary Office, ISBN 1 85774 384 9

Molzhan, A.E. (2007). Spirituality in later life: effect on quality of life. *Journal of Gerontological Nursing*, Vol. 33, No.1, (January 2007), pp. 32-39, ISSN 0098-9134

Moons, P., Budts, W., De Geest, S. (2006). Critique on the conceptualisation of quality of life: a review and evaluation of different conceptual approaches. *International Journal of Nursing Studies*, Vol. 43, No. 7, (September 2006), pp. 891-901, ISSN 0020-7489

Moore, D. (1987). Parent-adolescent separation: The construction of adulthood by late adolescents. *Developmental Psychology*, Vol. 23, No. 2, (March 1987), pp. 298-307, ISSN 0012-1649

Moreira-Almeida, A., Koenig, H.G. (2006). Retaining the meaning of the words religiousness and spirituality: a commentary on the WHOQOL SRPB group's "a cross-cultural study of spirituality, religion, and personal beliefs as components of quality of life" (62: 6, 2005, 1486-1497). *Social Science & Medicine*, Vol. 63, No. 4, (August 2006), pp. 843-845, ISSN 0277-9536

Morley, D., Selai, C. Jahanshahi, M., Thompson, A. (2005). Assessing the impact of parental illness on adolescent and adult children. *Abstracts of the 12th Annual Conference of the International Society for Quality of Life Research*, pp. 1987, San Francisco, California, USA, October 19-25, 2005

Morley, D., Selai, C., Thompson, A. (2007a). Quality of life and psychosocial well-being in people with multiple sclerosis and Parkinson's disease. *Abstracts of the 14th Annual Conference of the International Society for Quality of Life Research*, pp. 114, Toronto, Ontario, Canada, October 10-13, 2007

Morley, D., Selai, C., Thompson, A. (2007b). Comparing caregiver anxiety across chronic and acute neurological conditions. *Proceedings of the 27th Conference of the Stress & Anxiety Research Society*, pp. 189-195, Rethymnon, Crete, Greece, July 13-15, 2007

Morley, D. (2008). The Impact of Parental Neurological Illness on Adolescent & Adult Children: Quality of Life, Psychosocial Factors, & Relationship with Parent Well-Being. PhD Thesis, University of London

Morley, D., Selai, C., Schrag, A., Thompson, A. Jahanshahi, M. (2010a). Refinement and validation of the Parental Illness Impact Scale. *Parkinsonism & Related Disorders*, Vol. 16, No. 3, (March 2010), pp. 181-185, ISSN 1353-8020

Morley, D., Selai, C., Thompson, A. (2010b). Sibling support and adjustment to parental neurological illness. *Abstracts of the 17th Annual Conference of the International Society for Quality of Life Research*, pp. 143-144, London, United Kingdom, October 27-30, 2010

Morley, D., Selai, C., Schrag, A., Jahanshahi, M., Thompson, A. (2011). Adolescent and adult children of parents with Parkinson's disease: incorporating their needs in clinical guidelines. *Parkinson's Disease*, 2011:951874, (April 2011), pp.1-6, ISSN 2042-0080.

Mukherjee, S., Sloper, P., Lewin, R. (2002). The meaning of parental illness to children: the case of inflammatory bowel disease. *Child: Care, Health & Development,* Vol. 28, No. 6, (November 2002), pp. 479-485, ISSN 1365-2214

Mutch, K., (2005). Information for young people when multiple sclerosis enters the family. *British Journal of Nursing,* Vol. 14, No. 14, (July-August 2005), pp. 758-767, ISSN 0966-0461

O'Connell, K.A., Skevington, S.M. (2005). The relevance of spirituality, religion and personal beliefs to health-related quality of life: themes from focus groups in Britain. *British Journal of Health Psychology,* Vol. 10, No. 3, (September 2005), pp. 379-398, ISSN 2044-8287

O'Connor, E,J., McCabe, M.P. (2010). Predictors of quality of life in carers for people with a progressive neurological illness: a longitudinal study. *Quality of Life Research,* DOI: 10.1007/s11136-010-9804-4. ISSN 1573-2649

Pakenham, K.I., Bursnall, S. (2006). Relations between social support, appraisal and coping and both positive and negative outcomes for children of a parent with multiple sclerosis and comparisons with children of healthy parents. *Clinical Rehabilitation,* Vol. 20, No. 8, (August 2006), pp. 709-723, ISSN 1477-0873

Ravina, B., Camicioli, R., Como, P.G., Marsh, L., Jankovic, J., Weintraub, D., Elm, J. (2007). The impact of depressive symptoms in early Parkinson's disease. *Neurology,* Vol. 69, No. 4, (July 2007), pp. 342-347, ISSN 0028-3878

Rolland, J.S. (1988). A Conceptual Model of Chronic and Life Threatening Illness and its Impact on Families. In: *Chronic Illness and Disability – Families in Trouble Series, Volume 2,* Chilman, C.S., Cox, F.M., Nunnally, E.W. (Eds.), pp.17-68, Sage, London, ISBN 0803927045,

Rowe, L., Tonge, B., Melvin, G. (2004). When should GPs prescribe SSRIs for adolescent depression? *Australian Family Physician,* Vol. 33, No. 12, (December 2004), ISSN 1005-1008

Sanders, R. (2004). The quality of sibling relationships. In: *Sibling Relationships: Theory and Issues for Practice,* Sanders, R. (Ed.) New York: Palgrave, pp. 82-108, ISBN 0-333-96411-X

Schrag, A., Hovris, A., Morley, D., Quinn, N., Jahanshahi, M. (2003). Young- versus older-onset Parkinson's disease: Impact of disease and psychosocial consequences. *Movement Disorders,* Vol. 18, No. 11, (November 2007), pp. 1250-1256, ISSN 1531-8257

Schrag, A., Morley, D., Quinn N, Jahanshahi, M. (2004a). Development of a measure of the impact of chronic parental illness on adolescent and adult children: The Parental Illness Impact Scale (Parkinson's disease). *Parkinsonism & Related Disorders,* Vol. 10, No. 7, (October 2004), pp. 399-405, ISSN 1353-8020

Schrag, A., Morley, D., Quinn N, Jahanshahi, M. (2004b). Impact of Parkinson's disease on patients' adolescent and adult children. *Parkinsonism & Related Disorders* 10, Vol. 10, No. 7, (October 2004), pp. 391-397, ISSN 1353-8020

Schrag, A., Hovris, A., Morley, D., Quinn, N., Jahanshahi, M. (2006). Caregiver burden in Parkinson's disease is closely linked to psychiatric symptoms, falls, and disability.

Parkinsonism & Related Disorders, Vol. 12, No. 1, (January 2006), pp. 35-41, ISSN 1353-8020

Sieh, D. S., Meijer, A.M., Visser-Meily, J.M. (2010). Risk factors for stress in children after parental stroke. *Rehabilitation Psychology,* Vol. 55, No. 4, (November 2010), pp. 391-397, ISSN 0090-5550

Singleton, N., Bumpstead, R., O'Brien, M., Lee, A., Meltzer, H. (2003). Psychiatric Morbidity among adults living in private households, 2000. *International Review of Psychiatry,* Vol. 15, No. 1-2, (February-May 2003) pp. 65-73, ISSN 1369-1627

Slawek, J., Derejko, M., Lass P. (2005). Factors affecting the quality of life of patients with idiopathic Parkinson's disease: a cross-sectional study in an outpatient clinic attendees. *Parkinsonism & Related Disorders,* Vol. 11, No. 7, (November 2005), pp. 465-468, ISSN 1353-8020

Somers, V. (2007). Schizophrenia: the impact of parental illness. *British Journal of Social Work,* Vol. 37, No. 8, (December 2007), pp. 1319-1334, ISSN 1468-263X

Son, S.E,. Kirchner, J.T. (2000). Depression in children and adolescents. *American Family Physician,* Vol. 62, No. 10, (November 2000), pp. 2297-2308, ISSN 0002-838X

Steck, B., Amsler, F., Grether, A., Dillier, A.S., Baldus, C., Haagen, M., Diareme, L., Tsiantis, J., Kappos, L., Burgin, D., Romer, G. (2006). Mental health problems in children of somatically ill parents, e.g. multiple sclerosis. *European Child & Adolescent Psychiatry,* Vol. 16, No. 3, (April 2006), pp. 199-207, ISSN 1435-165X

Strunin, L., Boden, L.I. (2004). Family consequences of chronic back pain. *Social Science & Medicine,* Vol. 58, No. 7, (April 2004), pp. 1385-1393, ISSN 0277-9536

Thurman, S.K. (1985). *Children of Handicapped Parents: Research and Clinical Perspectives,* London, Academic Press, ISBN 0126907803

van de Port, I.G., Visser-Meily, A.M., Post. M.W., Lindeman, M.E. (2007). Long-term outcome in children of patients after stroke. *Journal of Rehabilitation Medicine,* Vol. 39, No. 9, (November 2007), pp. 703-707, ISSN 1650-1977

Visser-Meily, A., Post,M., Meijer, A.M., Maas, C., Ketelaar, M., Lindeman, E. (2005). Children's adjustment to a parent's stroke: determinants of health status and psychological problems, and the role of support from the rehabilitation team. *Journal of Rehabilitation Medicine,* Vol. 37, No. 4, (July 2005), pp. 236-241, ISSN 1650-1977

Weisman, M., Warner, V, Wickramaratne, P., Moreau, D., Olfson, M. (1997). Offspring of depressed parents: ten years later. *Archives of General Psychiatry,* Vol. 54, No. 10, (October 1997), pp. 932-940, ISSN 0003-990X

WHOQOL SRPB Group. (2006). A cross-cultural study of spirituality, religion, and personal beliefs as components of quality of life. *Social Science & Medicine,* Vol. 62, No. 6 (March 2006), pp. 1486-1497, ISSN 0277-9536

Yahav, R., Vosburgh, J., Miller, A. (2005). Emotional responses of children and adolescents to parents with multiple sclerosis. *Multiple Sclerosis,* Vol. 11, No. 4, (August 2011), pp. 464-468, ISSN 1477-0970

Yahav, R., Vosburgh, J., Miller, A. (2007). Separation-individuation processes of adolescent children of parents with multiple sclerosis. *Multiple Sclerosis,* Vol. 13, No. 1, (January 2007), pp. 87-94, ISSN 1477-0970

9

The Negative Impact of Apathy in Parkinson's Disease

Iracema Leroi
Lancashire Care Foundation NHS Trust/University of Manchester
United Kingdom

1. Introduction

Apathy is one of the most common neuropsychiatric complications of neurodegenerative disorders such as Alzheimer (AD) and Parkinson disease (PD). Apathy can be broadly defined as a clinical syndrome characterised by a change from baseline in three key domains: level of interest, level of initiative and emotional reactivity. It is one of the most under-diagnosed and poorly managed aspects of the neurodegenerative disorders. In PD particularly, the consequences of apathy may be significant and may impact negatively on long-term prognosis, exacerbate the motor and physical aspects of the disease, add to carer burden and stress, be associated with greater functional decline and disability, and impair quality of life (QOL). This chapter will outline these various outcomes and their relation to apathy in PD.

2. Background to apathy in PD

The prevalence of apathy in PD has been reported as ranging from about 17% to over 40% (Pluck and Brown, 2002). This wide range is likely a result of differences in populations studied (e.g. community versus clinic), types of apathy rating scales used, and discrepancies in, or lack of, the use of validated diagnostic criteria. In a cross-sectional validation study of newly proposed diagnostic criteria for apathy, the frequency of apathy in the PD subgroup was 27% (Mulin et al., 2011).

The definition of apathy has evolved over the past few years as the multi-dimensional nature of the syndrome is increasingly being recognised. A common conceptualisation of apathy, as proposed by Starkstein et al. (2001) among others, is that it constitutes a lack or reduction of goal-directed behaviour, as manifested in the dimensions of: (1) loss of or diminished initiative; (2) loss of or diminished interest; and (3) diminished or blunted emotions. The syndrome of apathy, while very common in neurodegenerative disorders, may also occur in other medical, neurologic or psychiatric conditions. The diagnostic criteria for apathy have followed the definition. Most recently, an international task force proposed a new set of criteria which have now been validated in several conditions, including AD and PD (Robert et al. 2009; Mulin et al., 2010). According to these criteria, a diagnosis of apathy can be made in the presence of four or more weeks of a loss of or reduction in motivation in at least two of three proposed apathy dimensions of emotional reactivity, interest and initiative. This change in behaviour should be sufficient to cause clinically significant impairment in functioning in various spheres.

Aside from diagnostic criteria, apathy can also be rated using a number of different validated apathy rating scales. These scales were reviewed by the Movement Disorder Society (MDS) and the recommendation for PD was that the Apathy Scale (AS) (Starkstein et al., 1992) or the Apathy Evaluation Scale (AES; clinician version, AES-C) (Marin, 1991) were the most robust scales for use in PD (Leentjens et al., 2008). PD-specific apathy rating scales which have recently been developed include the Apathy Inventory (AI) (Robert al., 2002), which can be either patient- or informant-rated, as well as the Lille Apathy Scale (LARS) (Sockeel et al., 2006). The LARS is a 33-item scale comprised of nine domains underscoring the apathy syndrome. Scores can range from an optimal score (no apathy) of +36 to the most severe score of -36, and the cut-off score for moderate apathy is -16. Principal component analysis of data derived from a study of 159 PD participants (51 with apathy as per the LARS cut-off) revealed a four-factor solution describing apathy dimensions. These were: intellectual curiosity, action initiation, emotion and self-awareness (Dujardin et al., 2007). Gallagher et al. (2008) used the LARS to determine how useful the Unified Parkinson's Disease Rating Scale, Part I (UPDRS) (Fahn & Elton, 1987) is as an apathy screening and diagnostic instrument by rating both scales in 74 PD sufferers. Using the LARS cut-off, 20% of the sample had apathy and they found that the UPDRS apathy item was sensitive (73%) in detecting apathy in PD but did not have sufficient diagnostic quality. Finally, the apathy domain of the informant-based Neuropsychiatric Inventory (NPI) (Cummings et al., 1994), has also been validated for identifying apathy, as either a "present/absent", or in terms of magnitude (frequency x severity). On this scale, a domain score for magnitude of symptoms of ≥ 4 indicates "clinically significant" pathology although no clear cut-off score for apathy per se has been established. A clinician-rated version of the NPI (NPI-C) is currently being developed and may be useful in the assessment and diagnosis of apathy (de Medeiros et al., 2010).

The underlying pathophysiology of apathy is related to specific disease-related degenerative brain changes that impact on motivation, and possibly, reward pathways. In particular, deficits in the frontal-subcortical circuit involving the anterior cingulated cortex (ACC) are likely to result in an apathy syndrome, or in specific dimensions of the syndrome (Robert et al., 2009; Devinsky et al., 1995). Neurotransmitter deficits which may play a role in apathy include: dopamine, which is important in reward and motivation; serotonin (5-HT), which may also have a role in PD-related depression in PD; and acetylcholine, a key neurotransmitter whose loss is related to dementia in PD (Czernecki et al., 2002; Leentjens et al., 2006).

The syndrome of apathy may occur as a sole behavioural complication of PD, or, as is frequently the case, may be co-morbid with other psychiatric complications such as depression or anxiety (Pluck and Brown, 2002; Aarsland et al, 1999). In our own cross-sectional study of a sample of 99 PD participants without dementia, the proportion of the 26 participants with apathy (on AES-C) who also experienced moderate to severe depression (Hospital Anxiety and Depression Rating Scale (HADS), depression sub-score ≥ 11) was 45%, which was significantly higher than in the PD participants with no apathy. Furthermore, HADS anxiety ratings were also significantly higher in those with apathy compared to those with no apathy (Leroi et al., 2009). The co-occurrence of apathy and depression in PD may be a diagnostic challenge, however, it is important to distinguish these syndromes in order to ensure that management strategies for depression, which are commonly prescribed, do not worsen or leave apathy symptoms untreated. If properly validated scales for apathy and depression are used in the diagnosis, it is possible to parse out the diagnostic entities with a degree of accuracy (Marin et al., 1993; Dujardin et al., 2007).

3. Impact of apathy on prognosis in PD

The question of whether the presence of apathy in PD impacts on prognosis is an important one since it has implications for early and robust detection and management of apathy. Unfortunately, very few long-term prospective studies have examined this question and the handful of cross-sectional studies linking apathy to disease severity are not entirely adequate to address the question of causation. Nonetheless, a few shorter-term follow-up studies have been done, in PD as well as AD, and suggest that the presence of apathy may have negative implications for the disease course, particularly once dementia is already established. Apathy in PD may also as a risk factor for the conversion into dementia from the non-demented state (Starkstein et al., 2006; Robert et al., 2006a; Dujardin et al. 2009). One of the only PD studies to address this question longitudinally is a study of apathy in a cohort of 40 non-demented PD patients who were followed up for a median of 18 months. Those with apathy (n=20) had a higher rate of conversion to dementia in PD over this period compared to those who had no apathy (n=20) at the start of the study (Dujardin et al., 2009). These findings are consistent with a longer study in AD patients for up to four years which revealed that apathy sufferers had a more severe overall prognosis and declined more rapidly compared to those without apathy (Starkstein et al., 2006). Another study, of shorter duration, found that in those with apathy and the amnestic form of mild cognitive impairment (MCI) converted to dementia in AD at a higher rate after one year compared to those without apathy (Robert al., 2006a).

4. Impact of apathy on the physical aspects of PD

PD is primarily a movement disorder affecting gait, speed and flexibility of movement. As the disease progresses, these symptoms become worse rendering the PD sufferer less active and increasingly prone to the complications of immobility. Furthermore, other, non-motor aspects of the disease such as postural instability, swallowing difficulties, bladder and bowel problems, cognitive impairment and depression may also contribute to a greater disease burden and increase the risk of developing medical complications. If apathy is present as well, effects of both the motor and the non-motor aspects of the disease may be exaggerated. In particular, the apathy dimensions of lack of initiative and interest may result in the PD sufferer withdrawing from their usual physical activities and hobbies, including activities of daily living and becoming increasingly sedentary. This may exacerbate existing problems such as constipation, and may also lead to secondary physical complications including urinary and respiratory infections, deep vein thrombosis and increased frailty. Loss of appetite, weight loss and poor nutritional status may also be associated with the presence of apathy and these conditions also add risk of developing medical complications and hastening decline (Benoit et al, 2008).

5. Impact of apathy on cognitive function in PD

Cognitive impairment in PD can broadly be categorised into dopaminergically-driven executive-type cognitive changes, which appear early on in the course of the disease, and more widespread, cholinergically-driven dementia-type cognitive changes, which occur as the disease advances (Williams-Gray et al., 2007). Executive dysfunction, including impairments in planning, verbal fluency, working memory, and attention, may progress to the point whereby functional abilities are affected. At this stage, it can be considered "mild cognitive impairment" (MCI) in PD. The more widespread cognitive impairments that lead to a full dementia syndrome typically appear after about 11 years of PD and may occur in over 80% of PD sufferers if they live with the disease for long enough (Hely et al., 2008).

A characteristic aspect of cognitive impairment in PD is "bradyphrenia", or slowness of thinking, which may be underscored by various aspects of the disease, including deficits in attention and interest, fatigue, slowness of thinking, poor persistence in tasks, mild memory problems, as well as apathy. Specifically, the lack of initiative and interest, which are key dimensions of PD-related apathy, may contribute to the development of bradyphrenia.

The cognitive changes that frequently accompany apathy syndromes are gradually being understood, however there have only been a few studies specifically examining this issue in PD. Whether these cognitive changes are the consequence or an impact of apathy, rather than apathy being a behavioural manifestation of the cognitive changes is not entirely clear (Duffy and Campbell, 1994). At best this relationship can be considered "bidirectional". Some of the studies examining cognitive changes in apathy in PD have used such tools as the Mini-mental State Exam (MMSE) (Folstein et al., 1975). The overall finding are that those with apathy are more cognitively impaired globally compared to those who do not have apathy (e.g. Landes et al., 2001; Starkstein et al., 2001, 2005; Aarsland et al., 2001; Senanarong et al., 2005). Studies using more specific neuropsychological test batteries reveal a strong association between apathy and frontal-type cognitive functions, even in the non-demented state. In our own cross-sectional study of a cohort of 99 non-demented PD sufferers, 46%of the variance predicting working memory impairment, an aspect of frontal-executive dysfunction, was accounted for by the presence of apathy, as well as older age and the presence of motor complications (Andrews et al., 2009). Working memory deficits in apathy in PD are of particular interest since both these functions may be underpinned by deficits in the ACC. In addition to working memory deficits, this same study also found significantly greater impairments in global cognitive impairment, as per the MMSE, as well as verbal fluency, even when accounting for differences in age, age on onset and duration of disease, and depression and anxiety. Interestingly, although attentional shift was initially worse in the apathy group, this difference was no longer evident once the co-variates were accounted for. These findings are supported by studies of cognitive impairment in AD and MCI, which have also found significantly worse word list learning, verbal fluency, set shifting and naming in those with apathy compared to those without apathy (Kuzis et al., 1999; Sperry et al., 2001; Robert et al., 2006b; McPherson et al., 2002; Pluck and Brown, 2002; Starkstein et al., 1992).

6. Impact of apathy on quality of life in PD

Measurements of the *subjective* experience of living with a chronic, neurodegenerative disease have increasingly become a focus of clinical and research interest in PD. The concept of "quality of life", or, more accurately, "health-related quality of life" (Hr-QOL) is a multidimensional construct embodying aspects of cognitive, emotional and physical functioning (Schrag, 2000). Several studies have used Hr-QOL scales to assess the impact of PD on individuals. These have shown that PD patients generally score lower than age-matched controls with other diseases and that key factors associated with poor Hr-QOL include depression, social isolation, physical functioning, sleep impairment, pain and discomfort, amongst other factors (Schrag, 2006). Depression in particular is an important factor determining Hr-QOL in PD, and this would suggest that a behavioural syndrome such as apathy, which is closely linked to depression, would also impact on this outcome.

6.1 PD study of apathy and quality of life

To date, one of the only studies directly examining the impact of apathy on Hr-QOL in PD is our own cross-sectional study of 97 non-demented community dwelling PD sufferers (Leroi et al., 2011a) who were assessed with the Parkinson's Disease Quality of Life Scale-8 item version (PDQ-8)(Jenkinson et al., 1997), which is a well-validated abbreviated version of the PDQ-39 (Peto et al., 1995). This study found that in those without frank dementia in PD, lower self-reported Hr-QOL was associated with *less* cognitive impairment and younger age, rather than the profile typical of those with apathy, namely, older age and more cognitive impairment (Leroi et al., 2011a*)*. These findings can be explained in that the younger and more active the PD sufferer is, the greater the impact of a diagnosis of a chronic degenerative disease may be. In contrast, those who are older, no longer working, and who may have lower expectations of life, may be less affected in terms of HRQoL. Interestingly, these findings are supported by a study of AD sufferers in care homes who had apathy. It found that in those with apathy, self-reported QOL was lower in those with less cognitive impairment, based on MMSE scores (Gerritson et al., 2005).

Data from the PD study mentioned above (Leroi et al., 2011a) were further analysed in order to compare "low" and "high" Hr-QOL in PD using the median split method. The median score on the PDQ-8 was 20.8. Those who scored above this median (n=48) were considered as to have poorer Hr-QOL (higher PDQ-8 score is worse Hr-QOL), and those who scored below this median (n=51) were considered as having better Hr-QOL. Table 1 shows a comparison of the mean scores across various demographic and clinical factors. From this analysis, it was clear that "level of motivation" or apathy as determined by the AES-C score differed between the two groups, with significantly higher apathy scores (AES-C) in the "high" PDQ-8 group. This comparison also revealed that those who were in the "high" PDQ-8 group (worse Hr-QOL) were no different in age to the low group, but differed significantly on several disease variables, including the "high" group having younger onset of disease, longer duration and more motor complications, in the form of dyskinesias, "on/off" phenomena and dystonias. Psychiatrically, the two groups differed, with higher anxiety, depression and overall psychiatric burden scores, the latter as reflected by the NPI "total" score, in the "high" scoring group. Cognitively, the two groups did not differ on global cognition (MMSE total), attention (serial 7's; Trail Making Test-B), short-term memory (5 minute recall from the MMSE) or verbal fluency (FAS test), however, as is consistent with Leroi et al. (2011a), the "high" group were significantly better than the "low" group on measures of working memory (n-back).

The above findings, however, contrast with other studies in PD, in which more severe levels of cognitive impairment or dementia, depression, and more advanced disease stage are associated with worse levels of self-reported Hr-QOL (Schrag 2006). The impact of disease variables may depend on stage of disease, with advanced disease and the presence of dementia having a greater impact compared to early disease (Schrag 2006). Indeed, these are the conditions that are associated with more severe and more prevalent apathy syndromes. It is possible that the presence of dementia may alter the impact of apathy on self-reported Hr-QOL due to apathy's effect on insight and the ability to reflect on experiences affecting the self. Our own data found that in comparing PDQ-8 in a cohort of PD-apathy sufferers (NPI ≥ 4) without cognitive impairment (n=24) to those with PDD and apathy (n=9), the PDD group had worse Hr-QOL (mean PDQ-8 in PD, 23.26 (SD 9.51); mean PDQ-8 in PDD, 34.02 (SD 12.67); $t=-2.64$, $p=.01$).

Patient measures (n=99)	**Low PDQ-8 (better Hr-QOL) (n=51)**	**High PDQ-8 (worse Hr-QOL) (n=48)**	**Statistic (t test or Mann-Whitney U)**	**Significance (*p*-value)**
	Mean (SD)			
Apathy Evaluation Scale -Clinicians' version (total score)	26.92 (12.38)	33.30 (15.68)	-2.24	.03
Demographic factors:				
Age at assessment (years)	64.51 (9.67)	62.39 (11.46)	0.99	.33
Clinical factors:				
Unified PD Rating Scale: motor subscale	27.00 (12.10)	30.79 (11.40)	-1.55	.12
Unified PD Rating Scale: complications of therapy subscale	2.37 (2.56)	5.15 (3.48)	U=589.50	<.001
Duration of PD (months)	82.47 (52.35)	110.35(75.09)	-2.14	.04
Age of onset of motor symptoms	57.71 (11.05)	52.78 (11.83)	2.12	.04
Psychiatric measures:				
Hospital Anxiety & Depression Rating Scale- depression subscore	5.02 (3.56)	7.67 (3.65)	U=609.50	<.001
Hospital Anxiety & Depression Rating Scale- anxiety subscore	4.59 (3.62)	8.15 (4.38)	U=704.50	<.001
Neuropsychiatric Inventory total	8.12 (11.09)	15.13 (13.99)	U=743.50	.002
Cognitive measures:				
MMSE Serial sevens	4.27 (1.00)	4.09 (1.33)	0.79	.43
MMSE 5-minute recall	2.49 (0.83)	2.48 (0.86)	0.07	.95
Trails B error score	5.53 (9.31)	7.66 (10.39)	-1.05	.30
n-back	16.83 (3.51)	15.02 (3.62)	2.43	.02
FAS	40.84 (14.06)	41.17 (12.44)	-0.12	.90

Table 1. Comparison of high- and low-PDQ-8 groups across various demographic and clinical variables in the PD participant groups.

7. Impact of apathy on disability in PD

The notion of "disability" in PD is increasingly recognised as being important however there is almost no literature on the specific association between apathy and disability in PD. Disability, like quality of life or carer burden, is a multidimensional construct, likely underpinned by a variety of different factors, both generic and PD-specific. The general definition of "disability" as defined by the "Americans with Disabilities Act of 1990 is "a physical or mental impairment that substantially limits one or more major life activities" (http://www.ada.gov/cguide). With regards to PD, "disability" loosely refers to "functional impairment" and is most commonly associated with the core aspects of the disease, namely, severity of motor impairments (tremor, instability, rigidity, bradykinesia). Non-motor aspects of PD have also been shown to be key contributors to overall functional impairment, or disability. In particular, some studies have shown that the presence of or severity of depression is associated with increased disability (Weintraub et al., 2004; Holroyd et al., 2005). One of the most comprehensive studies on this topic was by Weintraub et al. (2004). This study found that using a bivariate analysis, the key associated features with disability were the presence of psychosis, depression (presence and severity), age, duration of PD, cognitive impairment, apathy, sleepiness and aspects of motor impairment. Assessing these factors with a multivariate analysis, 37% of the variance in UPDRS ADL score was accounted for by severity of depression and worsening cognition, and 54% of the variance in Schwab-England score was accounted for by the same two factors plus increasing severity of PD. The limitation of this study was that it was undertaken in a mostly male, veteran population in the USA and did not have a control group of comparable motor severity in PD. Hence, the generalisability to the general PD population is limited. To date there have been relatively few studies investigating the specific impact of apathy on disability in PD, however, it is likely that apathy-induced disability has a further impact by increasing carer burden and levels of distress.

7.1 PD study of apathy and disability

In PD, the most robust way to measure disability is using a PD-specific activities of daily living (ADL) scale from the UPDRS, as well as a more general disability scale, the Schwab-England scale (Schwab & England, 1969). Disability captures the notion that the ability to undertake ADL is an important measure of disease severity and may not be dependent on duration of disease or stage according to the Hoehn-Yahr scale. The UPDRS ADL subscale is a 13-item scale that rates degree of ability to carry out daily tasks such as dressing and using a cutlery on a scale of 0-4 per item. It has a range of 0-52, with higher scores indicating greater impairment. It was designed specifically for assessing those with a diagnosis of PD and encompasses such items as the ability to eat and drink, move, toilet, dress, undertake hygiene routines, and communicate. The Schwab-England scale rates ADL ability on a scale of 0-100% with 100% being completely independent and with no disability. This scale is a useful *global* measure of independence and performance on ADL.

Using the UPDRS ADL scale, as well as the Schwab-England scale, we undertook a cross-sectional study of 99 non-demented PD sufferers with apathy, as determined by the AES-C

(Leroi et al., 2011a). These participants were consecutively recruited from neurology clinics in the UK and all met criteria for idiopathic PD. We found that disability on these measures was significantly higher in those with both apathy and PD (n=26) compared to those without apathy and PD (n=73). Mean disability ratings are shown Table 2. Furthermore, apathy was strongly and significantly associated with higher levels of disability rated on both these scales (UPDRS-ADL, rho=0.36; p<0.001; Schwab-England, rho=-0.55; p<0.001). In a subsequent multivariate regression analysis, apathy, together with later stage of disease and more cognitive impairment, accounted for 56% (p<.001) of the variance predicting disability.

	Mean (SD)		
	Apathy (n=26)	**Control (n=73)**	**Statistic**
Unified PD Rating Scale: ADL subscale	18.23 (4.10)	13.35 (4.97)	t=4.50; p<.001
Schwab-England scale	63.46 (12.39)	82.00 (9.26)	t=-8.93; p<.001

Table 2. Disability ratings compared between the two non-demented PD groups: with and without apathy

Further analysis of these data using the median split method was undertaken to explore the relationship of various demographic and clinical (motor, psychiatric and cognitive) factors between those with *high* levels of disability (mean UPDRS ADL score equal to or above the median cut-off of 15; n=53) and those with *low* levels of disability (mean UPDRS ADL score below the median cut-off of 15; n=46). Table 3 shows the comparison between the two groups of the mean scores across various factors. The mean apathy score (AES-C) was significantly higher in the "high" disability group (p=.004) in spite of there being *no* significant difference in age and several disease variables such as duration of disease, age of onset and dopaminergic load. However, the more disabled group did have worse motor scores (higher UPDRS motor score)(p<.001), worse motor complications (higher UPDRS complications of therapy score)(p=.03), and more severe stage of disease (Hoehn-Yahr score)(p=.001).

Interestingly, and in contrast to previous findings in the literature, there was no difference between groups on level of self-rated depression and anxiety, as assessed by the HADS. With regards to cognitive variables, there was no difference in complex attention (serial 7's), and short-term memory (5 minute recall from the MMSE). In contrast, there was greater impairment in verbal fluency (FAS test)(p=.04) and time for attentional shift/visual scanning (Trail-making Test-B time)(p=.006) in the high disability group. Finally, as expected, this group was also significantly more impaired on working memory (n-back; p=.001). These findings underscore the significant impact that apathy and cognitive impairment have on disability in PD.

Participant measures (n=99)	Low ADL Mean (SD) (n=53)	High ADL Mean (SD) (n=46)	Statistic (t test or Mann-Whitney U)	Significance (*p*-value)
	Mean (SD)			
	Measure of motivation:			
Apathy Evaluation Scale-Clinicians' version	26.17 (12.07)	33.78 (15.63)	U=817.00	.004
	Demographic factor:			
Age at assessment (years)	62.04 (10.50)	64.65 (10.78)	t=-1.22	.23
	Disease factors:			
Unified PD Rating Scale: motor	24.00 (10.10)	34.47 (11.27)	t=-4.72	<.001
Unified PD Rating Scale: complications of therapy	2.92 (2.74)	4.48 (3.71)	U=917.00	.03
Duration of PD (months)	84.87 (59.96)	105.83 (69.61)	t=-1.61	.11
Age of onset of motor symptoms (years)	54.92 (11.41)	55.54 (12.03)	t=-0.26	.79
Hoehn-Yahr scale	2.09 (0.67)	2.55 (0.65)	t=-3.44	.001
Levodopa equivalent daily dose (mg)	798.19 (641.38)	821.10 (507.66)	U=1132.00	.54
	Psychiatric measures:			
Hospital Anxiety & Depression Scale: depression subscore	5.81 (4.13)	6.78 (3.37)	U=979.00	.12
Hospital Anxiety & Depression Scale: anxiety	6.73 (4.73)	5.76 (3.84)	U=1089.50	.45
	Cognitive measures:			
Mini-mental State Exam 5-minute recall	2.55 (0.77)	2.41 (0.91)	U=1133.00	.47
Trail Making Test-B time to complete (sec)	134.41 (86.64)	175.46 (88.31)	U=793.56	.006
Trail Making Test- B error score	5.12 (9.02)	7.89 (10.49)	U=956.50	.13
n-back	17.06 (3.38)	14.55 (3.55)	t=3.48	.001
FAS	43.47 (14.71)	38.22 (10.58)	t=2.01	.04

Table 3. Comparison of high- and low-disability (ADL) groups across various demographic and clinical variables in the PD participant groups.

8. Impact of apathy on carer burden in PD

Caring for someone with a chronic, prolonged and degenerative disorder such as PD can be associated with significant stress, strain and perceived burden in the carer. This is similar to the well-established effects that such caring may have on informal carers of any chronic and serious disease, and it has been shown that mortality of these carers is actually increased if emotional or mental strain results (Schulz and Beach, 1999). In PD, the complexity of the disease, which involves not only physical, but also cognitive and behavioural impairment, means that the caring role is even more challenging. Carers in PD have to be responsible for managing the household, the family finances, and other activities of daily living, as well as the physical care needs of the patient. These responsibilities generally increase as the disease progresses, and one study showed that while in the earlier stages of PD the carer performed an average of 11 care-related activities per day, in the later stages of PD, this increased to up to 30 per day (Carter et al., 1998). The manifestations of such carer burden in PD carers include depression, limitations in social life and low quality of life (Schrag et al., 2006).

Patient factors that have been shown to be associated with carer burden and stress include: severity of motor functioning; presence of mental dysfunction, particularly depression and cognitive impairment (Aarsland et al., 1999); and functional status (Martinez-Martin et al., 2007; Aarsland et al., 1999). However, the specific impact on carer burden of apathy has not been as well studied other than in those with significant cognitive impairment and dementia (Aarsland, 2007).

8.1 PD study of apathy and carer burden

Over the past few years, the issue of assessing carer burden and distress has been recognized as being much more complicated than previously appreciated. Since PD is a long-term condition which impacts on multiple facets of functioning, it follows that the effect on carers cannot be easily modelled. However, a simplified and commonly used method for assessing subjective carer burden is using a well-validated scale, the 29-item Zarit Burden Interview (Zarit et al., 1980). In this questionnaire, responses range from 0 (never) to 4 (nearly always) and it rates the impact on the carer's physical, emotional and socioeconomic status. Higher scores reflect greater carer burden. Our own study used a modified version (22-item) of this measure to examine the impact of apathy on carer burden in a cohort of 71 non-demented PD patients and their carers (Leroi et al., 2011b). The carers in this group were mostly male (60.6%) and had a mean age of 62.7 (SD 10.9) years. They had known the PD sufferer for a mean length of time of 39.8 (SD 14.4) years. The mean ZBI score in the group overall was 23.8 (SD 14.0) years. Apathy was defined in the PD sufferer as being a score of ≥14 on the modified Apathy Scale (Starkstein et al., 1992). Findings from this study revealed that carer burden in those with apathy was significantly greater compared to those without apathy (p=.004). This was supported by the finding of a strong correlation between level of apathy and carer burden (rho=0.41; p=<.001).

9. Conclusion

The discussion above has highlighted the significant negative impact that the presence of apathy can have in PD, whether or not dementia is present. In particular, apathy can have an adverse effect on prognosis of the disease, cognitive and physical functioning, quality of life, disability and carer burden. However, this evidence has been gained mostly from cross-sectional studies which are limited in their ability to determine causality between apathy and these various outcomes. Longer, more detailed prospective studies are needed to examine these issues further in order to emphasize the need for more robust detection of and intervention into apathy in order to offset the negative outcomes.

10. References

Aarsland D, Larsen JP, Karlsen K, Lim NG, Tandberg E. (1999). Mental symptoms in Parkinson's disease are important contributors to caregiver distress. *International Journal of Geriatric Psychiatry,* Vol. 14, pp. 866 - 874

Aarsland D, Cummings JL, Larsen JP. (2001). Neuropsychiatric differences between Parkinson's disease with dementia and Alzheimer's disease. *International Journal of Geriatric Psychiatry,* Vol. 16, pp. 184-191

Aarsland, D, Bronnick, K, Ehrt, U, De Deyn, P P, Tekin, S, et al. (2007). Neuropsychiatric symptoms in patients with Parkinson's disease and dementia: frequency, profile and associated care giver stress. *Journal of Neurology, Neurosurgery and Psychiatry,* Vol. 78, pp. 36-42

Andrews MA, Leroi I, McDonald K, Elliott R, Byrne EJ, Burns A. (2010). Cognitive Dysfunction in Apathy and Impulsivity in Parkinson's Disease. *XVII World Congress of Parkinson's Disease and Related Disorders,* Miami, December 13-16, 2010

Benoit M, Andrieu S, Lechowski L et al. (2008). Apathy and depression in Alzheimer's disease are associated with functional defict and psychotropic prescription. *International Journal of Geriatric Psychiatry,* Vol. 23, pp. 409-414

Carter JH, Stewart BJ, Archbold PG, Inoue I, Jaglin J, Lannon M et al. (1998). Living with a person who has Parkinson's disease: the spouse's perspective by stage of disease. Parkinson's Study Group. *Movement Disorders.* Vol. 13(1), pp. 20-8

Cummings JL, Mega M, Gray K, Rosenberg-Thompson S, Carusi DA, Gornbein J. (1994). The Neuropsychiatric Inventory: comprehensive assessment of psychopathology in dementia. *Neurology,* Vol.44, pp. 2308–2314

Czernecki V, Pillon B, Houeto JL, Pochon JB, Levy RL, Dubois B.(2002). Motivation, reward, and Parkinson's disease: influence of dopatherapy. *Neuropsychologia,* Vol. 40, pp. 2257–2267

de Medeiros, Robert P, Gauthier S, Stella F, Politis A et al. (2010). The Neuropsychiatric Inventory-Clinician rating scale (NPI-C): reliability and validity of a revised assessment of neuropsychiatric symptoms in dementia. *International Psychogeriatrics.* Vol. 22(6), pp. 984-94

Devinsky O, Morrell MJ, Vogt BA.(1995). Contributions of anterior cingulate cortex to behaviour. *Brain,* Vol. 118(Pt 1), pp. 279-306

Duffy JD, Campbell JJ. (1994). The regional prefrontal syndromes: a theoretical and clinical overview. *Journal of Neuropsychiatry and Clinical Neuroscience,* Vol. 6, pp. 379-387

Dujardin K, Sockeel P, Devos D et al.(2007). Characteristics of apathy in Parkinson's disease. *Movement Disorders,* Vol 22, pp. 778-784

Dujardin K , Sockeel P, Delliaux M, Deste´e A, Defebvre L. (2009). Apathy may herald cognitive decline and dementia in Parkinson's disease. *Movement Disorders,* Vol. 24, pp. 2391-2397

Fahn S, Elton RL, UPDRS Development Committee. (1987) . Unified Parkinson's Disease Rating Scale. In: Fahn S, Marsden CD, Calne DB, Goldstein M, eds. *Recent Developments in Parkinson's Disease*. Florham Park, NJ: Macmillan; pp.153-163

Folstein MF, Folstein SE, McHugh PR. (1975). "Mini-Mental State": a practical method for grading

the cognitive state of patients for the clinician. *Journal of Psychiatric Research,* Vol. 12, pp. 189–198

Gallagher DA, Lees AJ, Schrag A. (2008). Unified Parkinson's Disease Rating Scale (UPDRS) part I as a screening and diagnostic instrument for apathy in patients with Parkinson's disease. *Parkinsonism and Related Disorders,* Vol.14, pp. 586-587

Gerritson DL, Jongenelis K, Steverink N et al. Down and drowsy? Do apathetic nursing home residents experience low quality of life? (2005). *Aging and Mental Health,* Vol. 9, pp. 135-141

Hely MA, Reid WGJ, Adena MA, Halliday GM Morris JGL. (2008).The Sydney multicenter study of Parkinson's disease: The inevitability of dementia at 20 years. *Movement Disorders,* Vol. 23, pp. 837-844.

Holroyd S, Currie LJ, Wooten GF.(2005). Depression is associated with impairment of ADL, non motor function in Parkinson disease. *Neurology,* Vol. 64, pp. 2134-2135

Jenkinson C, Fitzpatrick R, Peto V, Greenhall R, Hyman N. (1997). The PDQ-8: development and validation of a short-form Parkinson's disease questionnaire. *Psychology and Health,* Vol. 12, pp. 805–814

Kaufer DI, Cummings JL, Christine D, Bray T, Castellon S et al. (1998). Assessing the impact of neuropsychiatric symptoms in Alzheimer's disease: The Neuropsychiatric Inventory Caregiver Distress Scale. *Journal of the American Geriatrics Society,* Vol. 46, pp. 210-215

Kuzis G, Sabe L, Tiberti C, Dorrego F, Starkstein SE. (1999). Neuropsychological correlates of apathy and depression in patients with dementia. *Neurology,* Vol. 52, pp. 1403–1407

Landes AM, Sperry SD, Strauss ME, Geldmacher DS. (2001). Apathy in Alzheimer's disease. *Journal of the American Geriatrics Society,* Vol. 49, pp. 1700–1707

Leentjens AFG, Scholtissen B, Vreeling FW, Verhey FRJ. (2006). The serotonergic hypothesis for depression in Parkinson's disease: an experimental approach. *Neuropsychopharmacology,* Vol. 31, pp. 1009-1015

Leentjens AF, Dujardin K, Marsh L, Martinez-Martin P, Richard IH, Starkstein SE, et al. (2008). Apathy and anhedonia rating scales in Parkinson's disease: critique and recommendations. *Movement Disorders,* Vol. 23, pp. 2004-2014

Leroi I, Andrews MA, McDonald K, Byrne EJ, Burns A. (2009). Predictors of the impulsive and apathetic behavioural phenotypes in Parkinson's disease. *Movement Disorders Society Annual Meeting,* Paris, June 7-9, 2009.

Leroi I, Ahearn DJ, Andrews M, McDonald K, Byrne EJ, Burns A. (2011a). Disability and quality of life in Parkinson's disease is strongly associated with behavioural disorders in Parkinson's disease. *Age and Aging,* (in press).

Leroi I, Harbishettar V, Andrews M, McDonald K, Byrne EJ, Burns A. (2011b). Carer burden in apathy and impulse control disorders in Parkinson's Disease. *International Journal Geriatric Psychiatry,* (in press)

Marin RS, Biedrzycki RC, Firinciogullari S. (1991). Reliability and validity of the Apathy Evaluation Scale. *Psychiatry Research,* Vol. 38, pp. 143-162.

Marin RS, Firinciogullari S, Biedrzycki RC. (1993). The sources of convergence between measures of apathy and depression. *Journal of Affective Disorders*, Vol. 29, pp. 117-124.

Martínez-Martín P, Benito-León J, Fernando Alonso F. , José Catalán M et al. (2005).Quality of life of caregivers in Parkinson's disease. *Quality of Life Research.* Vol. 14(2), pp. 463-472

McPherson S, Fairbanks L, Tiken S et al. (2002). Apathy and executive function in Alzheimer's disease. *Journal of the International Neuropsychological Society*, Vol. 8, pp. 373-381

Mulin E, Leone E, Dujardin K, Delliaux et al. (2011). Diagnostic criteria for apathy in clinical practice. *International Journal of Geriatric Psychiatry*, Vol.26(2); , pp. 158-165

Peto V, Jenkinson C, Fitzpatrick R, Green hall R. (1995). The development and validation of a short measure of functioning and well being for individuals with Parkinson's disease. *Quality of Life Research*, Vol. 4(3), pp. 241-248

Pluck GC, Brown RG. Apathy in Parkinson's disease. (2002). *Journal of Neurology Neurosurgery and Psychiatry*, Vol. 73, pp. 636-643

Robert PH, Clairet S, Benoit M, Koutaich J, Bertogliati C et al. (2002). The Apathy Inventory: assessment of apathy and awareness in Alzheimer's disease, Parkinson's disease and mild cognitive impairment. *International Journal of Geriatric Psychiatry*, Vol. 17(12), pp. 1099-1105.

Robert PH, Berr C, Volteau M et al. (2006a). Apathy in patients with mild cognitive impairment and the risk of developing dementia of Alzheimer's disease: A one-year follow-up study. *Clinical Neurology and Neurosurgery*, Vol. 108, pp. 733-736

Robert PH, Berr C, Voleau M et al. (2006b). Neuropsychological performance in mild cognitive impairment with and without apathy. *Dementia and Geriatric Cognitive Disorders*, Vol. 21, pp. 192-197

Robert P, Onyike CU, Leentjens AFG, Dujardin K, Aalten P et al. (2009). Proposed diagnostic criteria for apathy in Alzheimer's disease and other neuropsychiatric disorders. *European Psychiatry*. Vol 24(2), pp.98-104 Senanarong V, Poungvarin N, Jamjumras P et al. (2005). Neuropsychiatric symptoms, functional impairment and executive ability in Thai patients with Alzheimer's disease. *International Psychogeriatrics*, Vol. 17, pp. 81-90

Schrag A, Jahanshahi M, Quinn N. (2000). What contributes to quality of life in patients with Parkinson's disease? *Journal of Neurology Neurosurgery and Psychiatry*, Vol. 69(3), pp. 308-312

Schrag A. Quality of life and depression in Parkinson's disease. (2006). *Journal of the Neurological Sciences*, Vol. 248, pp. 151-157.

Schulz, R.,& Beach, S. R. (1999). Caregiving as a risk factor for mortality: The Caregiver Health Effects Study. *Journal of the American Medical Association*, Vol. 282, pp. 2215-2219.

Schwab R, England A. Project technique for evaluating surgery in Parkinson's disease. (1969). In: Gillingham, J., Donaldson, I. (Eds.), *Third Symposium on Parkinson's Disease*. E&S Livingstone, Edinburgh, Scotland, pp. 152–157

Sockeel P, Dujardin K, Devos D, Deneve C, Deste´e A, Defebvre L.(2006). The Lille Apathy Rating Scale, a new instrument for detecting and quantifying apathy: validation in

Parkinson's disease. *Journal of Neurology Neurosurgery and Psychiatry*, Vol. 77, pp. 579 -584

Sperry SD, Strauss ME, Landes AM. (2001). Relation of apathy to depression, cognition, and daily function in dementia. *Journal of the International Neuropsychological Society*, Vol. 7, pp. 190

Starkstein SE, Mayberg HS, Preziosi TJ, Andrezejewski P, Leiguarda R, Robinson RG. (1992). Reliability, validity and clinical correlates of apathy in Parkinson's disease. *Journal of Neuropsychiatry*, Vol. 4(2), pp. 134-139

Starkstein SE, Petracca G, Chemerinski E, Kremer J. (2001). Syndromic validity of apathy in Alzheimer's disease. *American Journal of Psychiatry*, Vol. 158, pp. 872-877

Starkstein SE, Ingram L, Garau ML, Misrahi R. (2005). On the overlap between apathy and depression in dementia. *Journal of Neurology, Neurosurgery and Psychiatry*, Vol. 76, pp. 1070-1074

Starkstein SE, Jorge R, Mizrahi R, Robinson RG. (2006). A prospective longitudinal study of apathy in Alzheimer's disease. *Journal of Neurology Neurosurgery and Psychiatry*, Vol. 77(1), pp. 8-11

Weintraub D, Mobert PJ, Duda JE, Katz IR, Stern MB. (2004). Effect of Psychiatric and Other Nonmotor Symptoms on Disability in Parkinson's Disease. *Journal of the American Geriatrics Society*, Vol. 52(5), pp. 784–788

Williams-Gray CH, Foltynie T, Brayne CEG, Robbins TW, Barker RA. (2007). Evolution of cognitive dysfunction in an incident Parkinson's disease cohort, *Brain*, Vol. 130(7), pp. 1787-1798

Zarit, SH, Reever KE, Bach-Peterson J. (1980). Relatives of the impaired elderly: Correlates of feelings of burden, *The Gerontologist*, 20, Vol. 20, pp. 649-655.

10

Gastrointestinal Dysfunction in Parkinson's Disease

Klaus Krogh
Department of Hepatology and Gastroenterology V, Aarhus University Hospital Denmark

1. Introduction

Swallowing difficulties and constipation were included in the first description of Parkinsons´s syndrome from 1817 (Parkinson 1817). Since then, numerous studies have confirmed the magnitude of symptoms and addressed their pathophysiology. In spite of this, much remains to be determined and treatment of gastrointestinal dysfunction in Parkinson´s disease (PD) is often unsatisfactory.

Parkinson´s disease is now considered a multiorgan syndrome (Den Hartog 1960; Eadie 1963; Ohama and Ikuta 1976) and gastrointestinal dysfunction is one among a number of other complications. Gastrointestinal symptoms affect the quality of life of many patients with PD and altered gastric and small intestinal transit may cause unpredictable absorption of medication further aggravating the classical motor symptoms of PD. The severity of gastrointestinal dysfunction in PD is often closely associated with progression of the disease in general. This makes treatment even more difficult as the patient may be severely handicapped by motor and general autonomic symptoms. In spite of recent progress, the conclusion from the latest Cochrane review on treatment of bowel dysfunction in central neurological diseases still holds true: "Bowel management for these people must remain empirical until well-designed controlled trials with adequate numbers and clinically relevant outcome measures become available" (Coggrave 2006).

2. Normal gastrointestinal function

2.1 Gastrointestinal transit

Transit through the gastrointestinal tract depends on a number of factors of which contraction of muscle cells and coordinated function of sphincters are the most important. While most of the gastrointestinal tract consists of smooth muscle cells, the oral part of the oesophagus at one end and the external anal sphincter at another are striated muscles.

Contraction patterns of the stomach and the small intestine depend on time since last meal. The postprandial or feeding pattern consists of irregular contractions promoting mixing and absorption. The interdigestive or fasting pattern starts approximately three hours after a meal. It serves to empty the stomach and clear the intestine of mucus, bacteria and debris. The interdigistive phase consists of runs of strong propulsive contractions approximately every 90 minutes. Gastric emptying is faster for liquid than for solid content but it is usually less than four hours while the normal small intestinal passage is less than six hours. Transit through the colorectum is much slower than through the small intestine. Normal colorectal transit is usually less than three days. The colon is characterized by two types of contractions: localized (also termed haustral) contractions and high amplitude propagating contractions (also termed mass contractions). Haustral contractions occur all the time and serve to mix contents. Mass contractions occur a few times each day and propel stools over large distances in the colon. They often initiate defecation.

2.2 Normal defecation

Defecation depends on coordinated interaction between the colorectum, the puborectalis muscle and the anal sphincters. When mass contractions move stools to the rectum the rectal wall is stretched. This causes relaxation of the smooth muscle internal anal sphincter but contraction of the rectum itself, changing its properties from a reservoir to a conduit. Rectal contractions are further enhanced by the defecation reflex through the sacral segments of the spinal cord. The puborectalis muscle is relaxed thereby straightening the rectoanal angle and allowing passage from the rectum through the relaxed anal canal. If the striated external anal sphincter muscle is not contracted defecation takes place. The process is usually supported by a Valsalva manoeuvre. If any of the steps involved in defecation are impaired defecation becomes incomplete. This is felt by the subject as difficult defecation and an unpleasant feeling of residual stool in the rectum.

3. Gastrointestinal function in Parkinson´s disease

3.1 Parkinson´s disease and neuromuscular control of gastrointestinal transport

The basis for normal gastrointestinal transport is coordinated contraction of smooth muscle cells. Gastrointestinal smooth muscle cells contract when the membrane potential becomes more positive than -50 milli Volts. The frequency of contraction is determined by the interstitial Cells of Cajal, also termed gastrointestinal pacemaker cells. The smooth muscle cells are connected by gap-junctions making them function as a syncytium. Contractions and local reflexes are coordinated by the enteric nerve system located in the bowel wall. The enteric nervous system consists of approximately 10^8 neurons and a large number of neurotransmitters are found within it. One of these is dopamine. The direct effect of dopamine is inhibition of cholinergic transmission via D2 receptors (Walker 2000, Anlauf 2003). However, the *in vivo* result may be the opposite as there are indications that dopamine stimulates gastric and colonic contractions, possibly through other receptor types (Vaughan 2003).

Levi bodies are found in the enteric nervous system of patients with PD (Kupsky 1987, Wakabayashi 1990) and the concentration of dopamine in the colon is also reduced (Singaram 1995). This strongly indicates that enteric neurodegeneration as part of the multisystem involvement is a major factor in the pathogenesis of bowel dysfunction in PD. Also, there are indications that constipation in PD is associated with parasympathetic i.e. vagal dysfunction (Wang 1993).

3.2 Dysphagia in Parkinson´s disease

Abnormal swallowing is found in 50 to 95% of patients with PD (Bushmann 1989, Logemann 1975, Nowack 1977). In most patients this causes no or only minor symptoms, but when severe, dyshagia may cause pain and discomfort. In very severe cases dysphagia causes insufficient intake of food and medication. Dysphagia in PD is mainly due to insufficient cricopharyngeal relaxation and reduced oesophageal peristalsis (Eadie and Tyrer 1965 a, Nowack 1977). Insufficient chewing due to stiffness of the masticatory muscles may contribute to symptoms (Eadie and Tyrer 1965 b).

3.3 Gastric and small intestinal dysfunction in Parkinson´s disease

Gastric emptying of solids is prolonged in 88% of patients with PD and 38% have delayed emptying of liquids (Goetze 2006, Hardoff 2001). Accordingly, nausea and bloating are more frequently reported by patients with PD than by healthy controls (Edwards 1991). Delayed gastric emptying is associated with motor response fluctuations, probably due to unpredictable absorption of medication (Djaldetti 1996). Also, delayed gastric emptying is associated with use of levodopa (Hardoff 2001). Small intestinal transit in PD has only received little attention. In a single study using the hydrogen breath test patients with PD had longer than normal small intestinal transit time (Davies 1997). In the same study there was no sign of small intestinal bacterial overgrowth. As indicated, gastric emptying and small intestinal transit are important in PD not only because of gastrointestinal symptoms but also because they have profound effects on levodopa absorption.

3.4. Colorectal and anal sphincter dysfunction in Parkinson´s disease

Constipation is the most prominent bowel symptom in PD. It is a syndrome whose two main components are infrequent defecation and difficult rectal evacuation. The former mainly reflects slow colorectal transit and the later abnormal dynamics at defecation.
Infrequent defecation is commonly defined as two times or less per week. Following this definition between 35% and 81% of patients with PD have infrequent defecation (Edwards 1991, Sakakibara 2001, Siddiqui 2002, Singer1992, Ueki 2004). Comparing patients with PD to age adjusted control groups, PD patients have significantly less frequent defecation (Edwards 1991, Krogh 2008, Sakakibara 2001, Singer 1992) and more than one third regularly use oral laxatives (Eadie and Tyrer 1965, Krogh 2008, Singer 1992). It is likely that infrequent defecation is caused by enteric neurodegeneration in the colorectum. Accordingly, colorectal transit times, determined by the intake of radioopaque markers and subsequent abdominal x-rays, are prolonged in patients with primary PD (Jost and Schimrigk 1991, Edwards 1994, Sakakibara 2003) but not in those with non-idiopathic PD secondary to cerebral infarcts (Jost 1994).
Symptoms of difficult rectal evacuation are very common in PD (Edwards 1991, Krogh 2008). A subjective feeling of incomplete evacuation is reported by 23% and 17% need some sort of assisted defecation (digital evacuation, suppositories or mini enema) at least once per week (Krogh 2008). Studies with anorectal manometry have unambiguously shown that patients with PD and difficult defecation have dystonia of the external anal sphincter muscle (Ashraf 1995, Bassotti 2000, Edwards 1994, Mathers1988) and puborectalis muscle (Mathers1988). In contrast to normal external anal sphincter and puborectal muscle relaxation at defecation, patients with PD have paradoxical contraction. This obstructed defecation is the other main reason for constipation related symptoms in PD. In a comprehensive study of rectoanal physiology in PD rectal sensation to distension and rectal compliance were normal, but rectal contractions had significantly lower amplitude and there were significant post-defecation residuals (Mathers 1989, Sakakibara 2003). Reduced straining due to motor dysfunction may contribute to reduced colorectal transport at defecation (Sakakibara 2003). Some patients with PD have faecal incontinence, but compared to age matched control groups the prevalence is not increased (Krogh 2008, Singer 1992).

3.5 Gastrointestinal symptoms and severity of Parkinson´s disease

Infrequent defecation in otherwise healthy men is associated with increased risk of developing PD in later life. In a large American population based study mid aged men with bowel movement less than once per day had a 2.7 fold risk of developing PD within the next 24 years when compared to those with daily bowel movements (Abbott 2001). The information is of little clinical use, but underlines the multiorgan involvement in PD: in some the disease starts in the central nervous system in others it begins in the bowel. Several studies have confirmed that symptoms of constipation are strongly associated with the severity of PD assessed by the Hoen and Yahr staging (Eadie and Tyrer 1965, Edwards 1991, Krogh K 2008, Sakakibara 2001). It is also likely (Eadie and Tyrer 1965, Edwards 1991) but fully established (Bushmann 1989) that chewing difficulty and dysphagia are associated with increased severity of PD.

4. Evaluation of gastrointestinal symptoms in Parkinson´s disease

Evaluation and treatment of swallowing disorders in PD are beyond the scope of the present chapter.

4.1 Evaluation of gastric and small intestinal function in Parkinson´s disease

The gold standard for gastric emptying and small intestinal transit is scintigraphy with the liquid and the solid phase marked with each their isotope (Goetze 2006). The method is expensive and demands access to a gamma camera. It is therefore only used in a minority of patients. Absorption of paracetamol occurs in the duodenum and systemic absorption is therefore an indirect measure of gastric emptying of liquids. The method is of limited value in PD as most patients have delayed emptying of solid but not liquid contents. The wireless motility capsule (Kloetzer 2010) or the magnet based Motility Tracking System (Fynne 2011) may become clinically important alternatives. Endoscopy is indicated if structural changes or malignancy is suspected.

4.2 Evaluation of colorectal and anal sphincter function in Parkinson´s disease

No standardized instrument for assessment of colorectal symptoms in PD exists. The Cleveland Clinic constipation scoring system is often used (Agachan 1996), but it has not been formally evaluated in patients with neurological diseases. A neurogenic bowel dysfunction score has been developed for description of bowel symptoms in patients with spinal cord injury (Krogh 2006), but it is not valid in PD (Krogh 2008). A thorough anamnesis is therefore of paramount importance. Questions have to be specific and directly asked. Otherwise, symptoms will be underestimated. Important items are: Frequency of defecation, consistency of stools, number of unsuccessful attempts at defecation, time for each bowel movement, pain at defecation, need for digital evacuation of stools, a sense of incomplete defecation, abdominal pain, use of oral or rectal laxatives, bloating and blood in stools. Also, side effects to medication, including medication against PD, must be considered. Diet and fluid intake must be assessed. However, there is no evidence that the diet of constipated patients with PD differs significantly from that of asymptomatic controls (Edwards 1991).

In most patients treatment can be initiated just based on the anamnesis. Some bowel symptoms attributed to PD may be caused by colorectal cancer, especially if they have developed over a short period of time. Therefore, anorectal digital examination and endoscopy are relevant in a number of cases. In cases with severe symptoms not responding to first-line treatment determination of colorectal transit time and anorectal physiology tests may be performed. Colorectal transit time, or more correctly termed total gastrointestional transit time, can be assessed from the intake of radioopaque markers followed by one or more plain abdominal X-rays. A number of protocols exist. In general, the number of markers left after a specific number of days is counted. If only a single dose of markers (usually 24 small plastic rings) is taken and this is followed by a single x-ray the information is qualitative - transit time is either normal or prolonged. If markers (usually 10) are taken on a number of days (often six) before the x-ray is taken total transit time can be computed in days (Abrahamsson 1988). Also segmental transit times of the ascending colon, the transverse colon, the descending colon and the rectosigmoid can be computed. The advantages of radiographically determined colorectal transit time are that it is easy to perform, it provides an objective measure and it can be performed before and during treatment. The disadvantages are that intersubjective variation is very large and that the correlation between results and bowel symptoms in patients with PD is poor (Edwards 1994, Jost 1991). Examples of radioopaque marker studies are shown in figure 1.

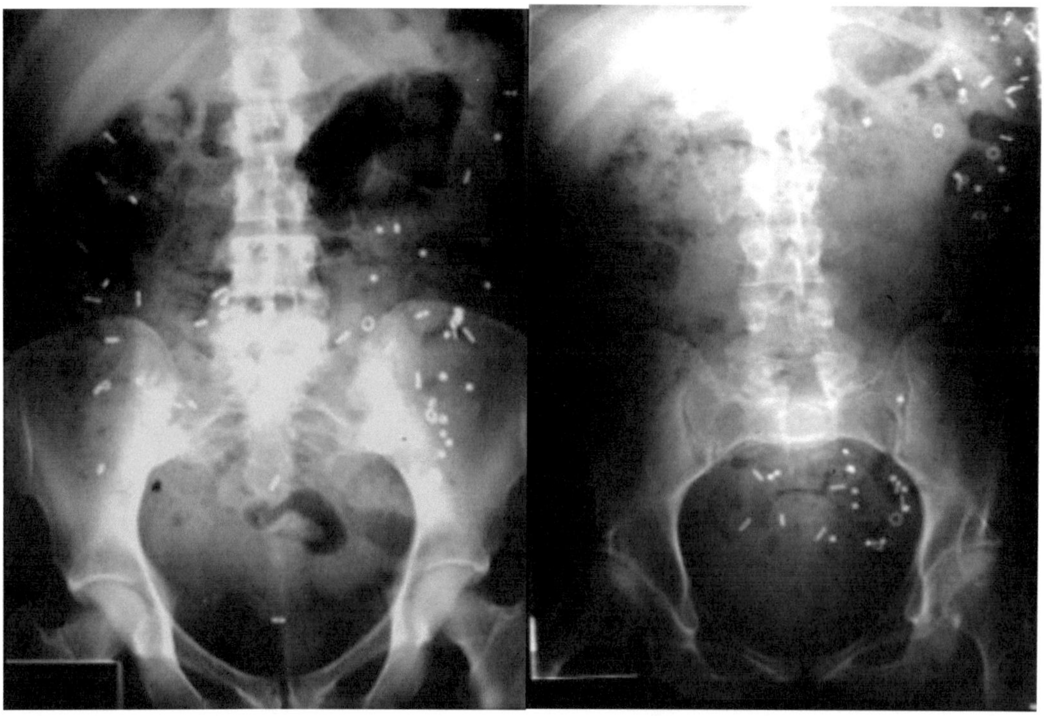

Fig. 1. Examples of radiographically determined colorectal transit times. Ten markes were taken each day on six consecutive days and an abdominal x-ray was taken on day seven. In healthy subjects there will be no more than 23 markers left. In the subject on the left the number of markers is increased and they are scattered throughout the colon. This indicaties generally slow colonic transit. In the subject on the right the number of markers is also increased but the are mostly located in the left colon and the rectum. This indicates difficult evacuation at defecation.

Anorectal physiology tests are only performed in a minority of patients with PD. The most common tests are manometry of the anal canal at rest and during squeeze, sensation during rectal balloon distension and anal manometry at attempted defecation of a balloon (Ashraf 1995, Edwards 1994, Mathers 1988). The later test is the most important in patients with PD as it may reveal abnormal contraction of the external anal sphincter during attempted defecation. Evacuation proctography is performed after installation of barium contrast in the rectum. The subject is seated on a commode in front of the camera and videoradiography is taken during attempted defecation. The method may show structural changes during defecation and it gives a semi-quantitative description of incomplete evacuation. It is, however, rarely performed in PD. New methods such as evacuation scintigraphy may have a future clinical role (Krogh 2003).

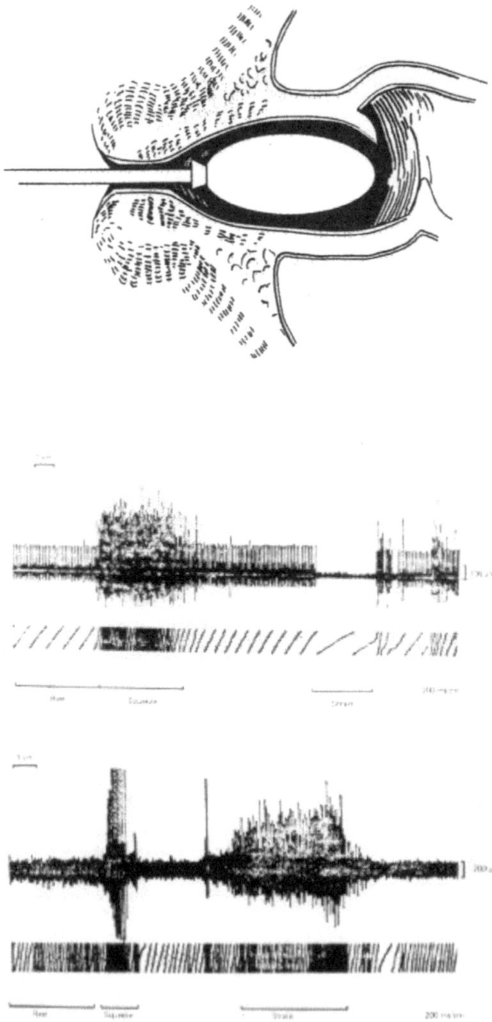

Fig. 2. Rectal balloon expulsion test. Pressure or EMG activity is registered in the anal canal while the subject tries to expel a balloon from the rectum (top). Under normal circumstances there is no increase in anal pressure or EMG activity (middle). In patients with Parkinson´s disease there is paradox contraction of the external anal sphincter (bottom).

5. Treatment of gastrointestinal complications in Parkinson´s disease

There are strong indications that levodopa may reduce dysphagia (Bushmann 1989, Logemann 1975) and constipation in PD (Krogh 2008). This is probably because levodopa reduces dystonia of the striated muscle muscle cells of the upper oesophagus and the external anal sphincter. Levodopa is absorbed in the duodenum and proximal ileum. Increased intake of insoluble dietary fibre not only alleviates constipation in PD patients (Astatloa 1993) but also increases the bioavailability of levodopa (Astarloa 1993, Garcia 2005 a+b). Use of levodopa is, however, associated with prolonged gastric emptying.

Symptoms of delayed gastric emptying can be treated with the dopamine antagonist domperidone which does not cross the blood-brain barrier (Shindler 1984, Soykan 1997). In contrast, dopamine antagonists that cross the blood-brain barrier, including metoclopramide and levosulpiride, should not be used in PD as they may worsen motor symptoms. Constipation can be alleviated with polyethylene glycol (Eichhorn 2001) or polycarbophil (Sakakibara 2007). Serotonin 5-HT4 receptor agonists including cisapride (Djaldetti 1995), tegaserod (Sullivan 2006) and mosapride (Liu 2005) may relieve constipation and reduced colonic transit time in patients with PD. Cisapride is now rarely used because of risk of cardiac arrhythmias and the clinical role of the other agents remains to be established. Many patients with PD use standard oral laxatives, suppositories and mini enema. Even though the use of such "older" agents is widespread their effects remain to be studies in clinical trials. Pilot data on Botolinum toxin A injections for relaxation of the puborectalis (Cadeddu 2005) or biofeedback for relaxation of the external anal sphincter muscle (Chiarioni 2006) in PD have been performed, but more data are needed to draw conclusions about future use.

Other methods commonly used for bowel dysfunction in other groups of patients with neurological disease include transanal irrigation through a catheter inserted in to the rectum (Shandling and Gilmour 1987), the Malone antegrade continence enema through a small stoma created from the appendix (Malone1990), sacral nerve stimulation (Kamm 2010), and colostomy. There is not enough evidence to recommend any of those methods for use in PD and they must until further be considered experimental.

6. Conclusions

Parkinson´s disease is a multi-system disorder including gastrointestinal dysfunction. Most gastrointestinal symptoms in PD can be attributed to dystonia of the striated muscle cells in the oesophagus and anal canal and to reduced stimulation of the smooth muscle forming the remaining part of the gastrointestinal canal. No guidelines to evaluation and treatment of gastrointestinal dysfunction in PD exist and evidence for treatment is generally poor. The majority of patients can be treated based on a thorough anamnesis. Initial treatment will often be increased fibre intake and oral laxatives. Advanced treatment of severe constipation in PD is still experimental.

7. References

Abbott, RD., Petrovitch, H., White, LR.,Masaki, KH., Tanner, CM., Curb, JD., Grandinetti, A., Blanchette, PL., Popper JS., & Ross GW. (2001) Frequency of bowel movements and the future risk of Parkinson´s disease. *Neurology*, Vol 57, No 3, 456-462.

Abrahamsson, H., Antov, S., & Bosaeus, I. (1998). Gastrointestinal and colonic segmental transit time evaluated by a single abdominal x-ray in healthy subjects and constipated patients. *Scand. J. Gastroenterol.*, Vol 152, Suppl, 72-80.

Agachan, F., Chen, T., Pfeiffer, J., Reisman, P., & Wexner, SD. (1996). A constipation scoring system to simplify evaluation and management of constipated patients. *Dis Colon Rectum, Vol* 39, No 6, 681–685.

Anlauf, M., Schafer, MK., Eiden, L., & Weihe, E. (2003). Chemical coding of the human gastrointestinal nervous system: cholinergic, VIPergic, and catecholaminergic phenotypes. *J. Comp. Neurol.*, Vol 459, No 1, 90-111.

Ashraf, W., Wszolek, ZK., Pfeiffer, RF., Nromand, M., Maurer, K., Srb. F., Edwards, LL., & Quigley, EM. (1995). Anorectal function in fluctuating (on-off) Parkinson´s disease: evaluation by combined anorectal manometry and electromyography. *Mov. Disord.*, Vol 10, No 5, 650-657.

Astarloa, R., Mena, MA., de la Vega, L., & de Yebenes, JG. (1992). Clinical and pharmacokinetic effects of a diet rich in insoluble fiber on Parkinson Disease. *Clinical Neuropharmacology*, Vol 15, No 5, 375-380.

Bassotti, G., Maggio, D., Battaglia, E., Giulietti, O., Spinozzi, F., Reboldi, G., Serra, AM., Emanuelli, G., & Chiarioni, G. (2000). Manometric investigation of anorectal function in early and late stage Parkinson's disease. *J. Neurol. Neurosurg. Psychiatry*, Vol 68, No 6, 768-770.

Bushmann, M., Dobmeyer, SM., Leeker, L. et al. (1989) Swing abnormalities and their response to treatment in Parkinson´s disease. *Neurology*, Vol 39, No 10, 1309-1314.

Coggrave, M., Wiesel, PH.,, & Norton, C. (2006). Management of faecal incontinence and constipation in adults with central neurological diseases. *Cochrane Database Syst. Rev.*, Vol 19, No 2, CD002115.

Davies, KN., King, D., Billington, D., & Barrett, JA. (1996). Intestinal permeability and orocaecal transit time in elderly patients with Parkinson's disease. *Postgrad. Med. J.*, Vol 72, No 845, 164-167.

Den Hartog Jager, WA., & Bethlem, J. (1960). The distribution of Lewi bodies in the central and autonomic nervous system in idiopathic paralysis agitans. *J. Neorol. Neurosurg. Psychiatry*, Vol 23, 283-290.

Djaldetti, R., Koren, M., Ziv, I., Achiron, A., & Melamed, E. (1995). Effect of cisapride on response fluctuations in Parkinson's disease. *Mov. Disord.*, Vol 10, No 1, 81-84.

Djaldetti, R., Baron, J., Ziv, I., & Melamed, E. (1996). Gastric emptying in Parkinson's disease: patients with and without response fluctuations. *Neurology*, Vol 46, No 4, 1051-1054.

Eadie, MJ. (1963). The pathology of certain medullary nuclei in parkinsonism. *Brain*, Vol86, 781-792.

Eadie, MJ., & Tyrer, JH. (1965 a). Radiological abnormalities of the upper part of the alimentary tract in parkinsonism. *Australas. Ann. Med.*, Vol 14, 23-27.

Eadie, MJ., & Tyrer, JH. (1965 b). Alimentary disorders in parkinsonism. *Australas. Ann. Med.*, Vol 14, 13-22.

Eichhorn, TE., & Oertel, WH. (2001). Macrogol 3350/electrolyte improves constipation in Parkinson's disease and multiple system atrophy. *Mov. Disord.*, Vol 16, No 6, 1176-1177.

Edwards, LL., Pfeiffer, RF., Quigley, EMM., Hofman, R., & Balluff, M. (1991). Gastrointestinal symptoms in Parkinson´s disease. *Mov. Disord.*, Vol 6, No 2, 151-156.

Edwards, LL., Quigley, EM., Harned, RK., Hofman, R., & Pfeiffer, RF. (1994). Characterization of swallowing and defecation in Parkinson´s disease. *Am. J. Gastroenterol.*, Vol 89, No 1, 15-25.

Fynne, L., Worsoe, J., Gregersen, T., Schlageter, V., Laurberg, S., & Krogh K. (2011). Gastric and small intestinal dysfunction in spinal cord injury patients. *Acta. Neurol. Scand.*, Epub ahead of print.

Garcia, JJ., Fernandez, N., Carriedo, D., Diez, MJ., Sahagun, A., Gonzalez, A., Calle, A., & Sierra, M. (2005). Hydrosoluble fiber (Plantago ovata husk) and levodopa I: experimental study of the pharmacokinetic interaction. *Eur. Neuropsychopharmacol.*, Vol 15, No 5, 497-503.

Fernandez, N., Carriedo, D., Sierra, M., Diez, MJ., Sahagun, A., Calle, A., Gonzalez, A., & Garcia, JJ. (2005). Hydrosoluble fiber (Plantago ovata husk) and levodopa II: experimental study of the pharmacokinetic interaction in the presence of carbidopa. *Eur. Neuropsychopharmacol.*, Vol 15, No 5, 505-509.

Goetze, O., Nikodem, AB., Wiezcorek, J., Banasch. M., Przuntek, H., Mueller, T., Schmidt, WE., & Woitalla D. (2006). Predictors of gastric emptying in Parkinson's disease. *Neurogastroenterol. Motil.*,Vol 18, No 5, 369-75.

Hardoff, R., Sula, M., Tamir, A., Soil, A., Front, A., Badarna, S., Honigman, S., & Giladi N. (2001). Gastric emptying time and gastric motility in patients with Parkinson's disease. *Mov. Disord.*, Vol 16, No 6, 1041-1047.

Jost, WH., & Schimrigk, K. (1991) Constipation in Parkinson´s disease. *Klin. Wochenschr.*, Vol 69, No 20, 906-909.

Jost, H., Jung, G., & Schimrigk K. (1994) Colonic transit time in nonidiopathic Parkinson´s syndrome. *Eur. Neurol.*, Vol 34, No 6, 329-331.

Kamm, MA., Dudding, TC., Melenhorst, J., Jarrett, M., Wang, Z., Buntzen, S., Johansson, C., Laurberg, S., Rosen, H., Vaizey, CJ., Matzel, K., & Baeten C. (2010). Sacral nerve stimulation for intractable constipation. *Gut*, Vol 59, No 3, 333-340.

Kloetzer, L., Chey, WD., McCallum, RW., Koch, KL., Wo, JM., Sitrin, M., Katz, LA., Lackner, JM., Parkman, HP., Wilding, GE., Semler, JR., Hasler, WL., & Kuo B. (2010). Motility of the antroduodenum in healthy and gastroparetics characterized by wireless motility capsule. *Neurogastroenterol. Motil.*, Vol 22. No 5, 527-533.

Krogh, K., Olsen, N., Christensen, P., Madsen, JL., & Laurberg S. (2003). Colorectal transport during defecation in patients with lesions of the sacral spinal cord. *Neurogastroenterol. Motil.*, Vol 15, No 1, 25-31.

Krogh, K., Christensen, P., Sabroe, S., & Laurberg S. (2006). Neurogenic bowel dysfunction score. *Spinal Cord*, Vol 44, No 10, 625-631.

Krogh, K., Ostergaard, K., Sabroe, S., & Laurberg, S. (2008). Clinical aspects of bowel symptoms in Parkinson's disease. *Acta. Neurol. Scand.*, Vol 117, No 1, 60-64.

Kupsky, WJ., Grimes, MM., Sweeting, J., Bertsch, R., & Cote, LJ. (1987). Parkinson´s disease and megacolon: concentric hyaline inclusions (Lewy bodies) in enteric ganglion cells. *Neurology*, Vol 37, No 7, 1253-1255.

Liu, Z., Sakakibara, R., Odaka, T., Uchiyama, T., Uchiyama, T., Yamamoto, T., Ito, T.,, Asahina, M., Yamaguchi, K., Yamaguchi, T., & Hattori, T. (2005). Mosapride citrate, a novel 5-HT4 agonist and partial 5-HT3 antagonist, ameliorates constipation in parkinsonian patients. *Mov Disord.*, Vol 20, No 6, 680-686.

Logemann, JA., Blonsky, ER., & Boshes, B. (1975). Dysphagia in Parkinsonim. *JAMA*, Vol 231, No 1, 69-70.

Malone PS, Ransley PG, & Kiely EM. (1990). Preliminary report: the antegrade continence enema. *Lancet*, Vol 336, No 8725, 1217-1218.

Mathers, SE., Kempster, PA., Law, PJ., Frankel, JP., Bartram, CI., Lees, AJ., Stern, GM., & Swash, M. (1989). Anal sphincter dysfunction in Parkinson´s disease. *Arch. Neurol*, Vol 46, No 10, 1061-1064.

Mathers, SE., Kempster, PA., Swash, M., & Lees, AJ. (1998). Constipation and paradoxical puborectalis contraction in anismus and Parkinson´s disease: a dystonic phenomenon? *J. Neurol. Neurosurg. Psychiatry,* Vol 51, No 12, 1503-1507.

Nowack, WJ., Hatelid, JM., & Sohn. RS. (1977). Dysphagia in Parkinsonims. *Arch. Neurol.,* Vol 34, No 5, 320.

Parkinson, J. (1817). An essay on the shaking palsy. Sherwood, Neely and Jones, London.

Sakakibara, R., Shinotoh, H., Uchiyama, T., Sakuma, M., Kashiwado, M., Yoshiyama, M., & Hattori, T. (2001). Questionnaire-based assessment of pelvic organ dysfunction in Parkinson´s disease. *Auton. Neurosci.,* Vol 92, No 1-2, 76-85.

Sakakibara, R., Odaka, T., Uchiyama, T., Asahina, M., Yamaguchi, K., Yamaguchi, T., Yamanishi, T., & Hattori, T. (2003). Colonic transit time and rectoanal videomanometry in Parkinson's disease. *J. Neurol. Neurosurg. Psychiatry,* Vol 74, No 2, 268-272.

Sakakibara R, Yamaguchi T, Uchiyama T, Yamamoto T, Ito T, Liu Z, Odaka T, Yamaguchi C, & Hattori T. (2007). Calcium polycarbophil improves constipation in primary autonomic failure and multiple system atrophy subjects. *Mov. Disord.,* Vol 22, No 11, 1672-1673.

Shandling, B., & Gilmour, RF. (1987). The enema continence catheter in spina bifida: successful bowel management. *J. Pediatr. Surg.,* Vol 22, No 3, 271-273.

Shindler, JS., Finnerty, GT., Towlson, K., Dolan, AL., Davies, CL., & Parkes, JD. (1984). Domperidone and levodopa in Parkinson's disease. *Br. J. Clin. Pharmacol.,* Vol 18, No 6, 959-962.

Siddiqui, MF., Rast, M., Lynn, MJ., Auchus, AP., & Pfeiffer, RF. (2002). Autonomic dysfunction in Parkinson´s disease: a comprehensive symptom survey. *Parkinsonism Relat. Disord.* Vol 8, No 4, 277-284.

Singaram, C., Ashraf, W., Gaumintz, EA., Torbey, C., Sengupta, A., Pfeiffer, R., & Quigley, EMM. (1995). Dopaminergic defect on enteric nervous system in Parkinson´s disease patients with chronic constipation. *Lancet,* Vol 346, No 8979, 861-864.

Singer, C., Weiner, WJ., & Sanchez-Ramos, JR. (1992). Autonomic dysfunction in men with Parkinson´s disease. *Eur. Neurol.,* Vol 32, No 3, 134-140.

Soykan, I., Sarosiek, I., Shifflett, J., Wooten, GF., & McCallum, RW. (1997). Effect of chronic oral domperidone therapy on gastrointestinal symptoms and gastric emptying in patients with Parkinson's disease. *Mov. Disord.,* Vol 12, No 6, 952-957.

Sullivan, KL., Staffetti, JF., Hauser, RA., Dunne, PB., & Zesiewicz, TA. (2006).Tegaserod (Zelnorm) for the treatment of constipation in Parkinson's disease. *Mov Disord.,* Vol 21, No 1, 115-116.

Ueki, A., & Otsuka, M. (2004). Life style risks of Parkinson´s disease: association between decreased water intake and constipation. *J. Neurol.* Vol 251, Suppl 7, 18-23.

Vaughan, CJ., Aherne, AM., Lane, E., Power, O., Carey, RM., & O'Connell, DP. (2000). Identification and regional distribution of the dopamine D(1A) receptor in the gastrointestinal tract. *Am. J. Physiol. Regul. Integr. Comp. Physiol.* Vol 279, No 2, R599-R609.

Wakabayashi, K., Takahashi, H., Ohama, E., & Ikuta F. (1990). Parkinson's disease: an immunohistochemical study of Lewy body-containing neurons in the enteric nervous system. *Acta. Neuropathol.,* Vol 79, No 6, 581-583.

Walker, JK., Gainetdinov, RR., Mangel, AW., Caron, MG., & Shetzline, MA,. (2000). Mice lacking the dopamine transporter display altered regulation of distal colonic motility. *Am. J. Physiol. Gastrointest. Liver Physiol.* Vol 279, No 2, G311-G318.

Wang, SJ., Fuh, JL., Shan, DE., et al. (1993). Sympathetic skin response and R-R interval variation in P